THE CARE

of the

OLDER PERSON

Fourth Edition

www.careoftheolderperson.com
www.rmcpublishingllc.com

The Care of the Older Person

ISBN: 978-1-7350093-4-6 (paperback)
        978-1-7350093-2-2 (epub)
Interior design by booknook.biz

CONTENTS

EDITORS/CONTRIBUTORS

Olivier Beauchet, MD, PhD, Professor of Geriatrics, Dr. Joseph Kaufmann Chair in Geriatric Medicine, Director of centre of excellence on aging and chronic diseases, McGill University

Howard Bergman, MD, FCFP, FRCP(C), Chair, Department of Family Medicine, Professor, Departments of Family Medicine, Medicine, and Oncology, McGill University

Ronald M. Caplan, MD, CM, FACS, FACOG, FRCS(C), Clinical Associate Professor Emeritus Obstetrics and Gynecology, Weill Medical College of Cornell University

Abraham Fuks, MD, CM, FRCP(C), Professor, Department of Medicine, McGill University

Serge Gauthier, CM, CQ, MD, FRCP(C), Director, Alzheimer Disease Research Unit, McGill Center for Studies in Aging, Professor, Departments of Neurology & Neurosurgery, Psychiatry, Medicine, McGill University

Phil Gold, CC, OQ, MD, PhD, FRSC, DSc (Hon), MACP, FRCP(C), Douglas G. Cameron Professor of Medicine, Professor of Physiology and Oncology, McGill University, Executive Director Clinical Research Center (MGH) McGill University Health Centre

Jose A. Morais, MD, FRCP(C), Professor, Faculty of Medicine, Director, Division of Geriatric Medicine, Lead, Dementia Education Program, McGill University, Co-Director, Quebec Network for Research on Aging

CONTRIBUTORS

Karen C. Altfest, PhD, CFP®, Executive Vice President and Principal Advisor, Altfest Personal Wealth Management, New York City

Paulina Bajsarowicz, MD, FRCPC, Geriatric Psychiatrist, Douglas Mental Health University Institute, Assistant Professor McGill University

Guy Hajj Boutros, MSc, Kinesiologist and Research Assistant, Research Institute of McGill University Health Centre

Lysanne Campeau, MDCM, PhD, FRCS(C), Assistant Professor of Surgery, Division of Urology, McGill University

Julia Chabot, MDCM, FRCPC, MSc, Assistant Professor, Faculty of Medicine, McGill University

A. Mark Clarfield, MD, FRCPC, Professor Emeritus of Geriatrics, Ben-Gurion University, Medical School for International Health, Faculty of Health Sciences, Ben-Gurion University of the Negev

Philippe Desmarais, MD, FRCPC, MHSc, Assistant Clinical Professor, Faculty of Medicine, University de Montreal

Liam Durcan, MD, FRCPC, Assistant Professor, Department of Neurology and Neurosurgery, McGill University, Consultant Neurologist, Stroke Service, McGill University Health Centre

Hao Feng, MD, MHS, Assistant Professor, Director of Laser Surgery and Cosmetic Dermatology, Department of Dermatology, University of Connecticut Health Centre

Catherine Ferrier, MD, Assistant Professor, Department of Family Medicine, Faculty of Medicine, McGill University

Jess Friedland, MD, FRCPC, Geriatric Psychiatrist, Douglas Mental Health University Institute, Program Director, Geriatric Psychiatry Sub-Specialty Residency Program, McGill University

Catalina Hernandez-Torres MD, FRCP(C), Geriatric Oncology, Ottawa Hospital Cancer Center

Tina Hsu, MD, FRCP(C), Assistant Professor, Division of Medical Oncology, University of Ottawa

Antony Karelis, PhD, Professor, Department of Exercise Science, Universite du Quebec a Montreal

Sathya Karunananthan, PhD, Postdoctoral Fellow, Ottawa Hospital Research Institute

Aziz Khan, MD, Assistant Professor, Department of Internal Medicine, University of Connecticut Health Center

Young-Sang Kim, MD, PhD, Associate Professor, Department of Family Medicine, CHA Bundang Medical Center, CHA University

Cyrille Launay, MD, PhD, department of medicine, division of geriatrics, University Hospital of Lausanne, Switzerland

Artin Mahdanian, MD, MSc, Department of Psychiatry, McGill University

Louise Mallet, B.Sc. Pharm., Pharm.D., BCGP, FESCP, FOPQ, Professor in Clinical Pharmacy, Faculty of Pharmacy, University of Montreal, Pharmacist in Geriatrics, McGill University Health Center

Silvia Monti De Flores, MD, FRCPC, DFAPA, Department of Psychiatry, McGill University

P. David Myerowitz, MD, FACS, FACC, Former Karl. P. Klassen Professor and Chairman Thoracic and Cardiovascular Surgery, The Ohio State University

Randy S. Perskin, Esq., JD, Elder Law Attorney, New York

Astrid F. Pilgrim, MD, MS, Fellow, Critical Care Medicine, University of Pittsburgh Medical School

Michael R. Pinsky, MD, CM, Dr hc, FCCP, MCCM, FAPS, Professor of Critical Care Medicine, Cardiovascular Disease, Anesthesiology, Clinical and Translational Sciences, Bioengineering, University of Pittsburgh Medical School

Samer Shamout, MD, MSc, Fellow, Division of Urology, McGill University

Michael Stiffel, MD, FRCPC, Assistant Clinical Professor, Faculty of Medicine, Universite de Sherbrooke

Norman Straker, MD, DLFAPA, Clinical Professor Weill Cornell Department of Psychiatry, Consultant, Sloan Kettering Cancer Center, Division of Behavioral Science

Dominique Tessier, MD, CCFP, FCFP, FISTM, Clinical Instructor, Family Medicine Department, University of Montreal, Medical Director, Travel Health Group, Montreal

Doreen Wan-Chow-Wah, MD, FRCPC, Assistant Professor, Faculty of Medicine, Division of Geriatric Medicine, McGill University Health Centre

Claire Webster, PAC, CPCA, Founder, McGill University Dementia Education Program

Mark J. Yaffe, MDCM, Professor of Family Medicine, Department of Family Medicine, St Mary's Hospital Centre and McGill University

Haibin Yin, MD, CCFP (COE) Assistant Professor, Director of Undergraduate Medical Education, Division of Geriatric Medicine, McGill University

INTRODUCTION

Jose A. Morais, MD, FRCP(C)

Professor, Faculty of Medicine, Director, Division of Geriatric Medicine,

Lead, Dementia Education Program, McGill University,

Co-Director, Quebec Network for Research on Aging

It is a well-recognized fact that our society is growing older. This aging of the population is observed in developed as well as in developing countries, albeit at a faster pace in the latter. From the days of the Roman Empire to the early XIX century, average life expectancy at birth remained stable at about 45 years. Since then, there has been a progressive increase in life expectancy with the introduction of improved hygiene and availability of food. The improvement in medical care also contributed to improved survival, especially in older individuals with chronic conditions. Nowadays, a cohort of newborns is expected to live an average of 80 years, with an excess of 3-4 years for baby girls compared with boys. The net effect of this increased longevity combined with the decline of birth rates is practically a doubling of the percentage of older adults, to reach about 25% of the population by 2030 in most developed countries. The prevalence of those above 85 years, the so-called "old-old" will in fact triple to attain 8% of the population. According to the World Health Organization, the aging of the population is an unprecedented phenomenon in human history. Although many anticipate this demographic revolution with apprehension, it is in fact a triumph of humankind over the adversities of the environment. Among many societal challenges posed by the aging of the population is a growing prevalence of multiple chronic diseases and functional impairments of older adults, giving rise to the geriatric syndromes, especially in those above 85 years of age. The shift in the prevalence from acute and communicable diseases to multiple chronic diseases calls for a realignment of the healthcare system that was previously organized to treat acute conditions. The solution resides in an integrated and coordinated system that is more expensive than one dealing with short term interventions, although many inefficiencies in care delivery and inappropriate interventions contribute to heighten the cost.

Why do we age?

Aging is a universal phenomenon defined as a progressive decline in the functional reserves of many body systems and organs once an individual has reached maturity, which in humans occurs between 20 and 30 years of age. These degenerative changes in organs are responsible for the loss of adaptive responses to stress and an increased risk for age-related illness and death. The theory of evolution proposes that the natural forces that shaped life allowed aging to occur because it would be better to perpetuate the species by investing in mechanisms promoting a high reproductive capacity in young individuals rather than in bodily mechanisms that would maintain individuals indefinitely but at greater risk of dying in a hostile environment. There are a number of theories of aging organized in several categories, but those gaining in popularity among scientists fall under the mechanistic theories of aging, grouped as the somatic mutation theory and the free radical theory. Both of these mechanisms are likely to be involved in aging as they implicate basic cellular processes and can explain other derangements at more complex levels of bodily organization such as dysfunction of neuro-endocrine and immune systems. The somatic mutation theory suggests that most somatic cells undergo replication and in this process, acquire damage by spontaneous mutations or by exposure to toxic products. The accumulation of damage will degrade cell function, leading to senescence. The telomere shortening theory can be considered as a special case of the mutation theory. The free radical theory explains that life is a dynamic process requiring metabolized energy that generates free radicals as by-products of normal redox reactions, e.g., reactive oxygen species. Such free radicals are the cause of oxidative damage to cell structures and impair their functions. The mitochondrial theory is considered a subcategory of the free radical theory. Although the body possesses many enzymes and surveillance systems to prevent cellular damage and mutations it is not a foolproof defense mechanism, which is in keeping with the theory of evolution.

What is Geriatrics?

The term "Geriatric" refers to old age that in most advanced societies has been set arbitrarily at 65 years. It is of interest that this age limit was proposed more than a century and a half ago by a German statesman, Baron Otto von Bismarck, based on the observations that at that time, life expectancy of civil servants aged 65 was on average only 2 years. He calculated that it would be more profitable for the state to offer them a retirement pension and to hire new, more productive young people. Since then however, life expectancy at age 65 has steadily increased in most developed countries to reach current levels of about 20 years for women and 15 years for men. Thus, even at age 65, there is opportunity to introduce preventive medicine and to educate people to adopt healthy and active lifestyles. At the same time, the prevalence of chronic diseases increases steadily with age, giving rise to co-morbidities and functional decline. Among older adults, 40-50 % have arthritis, hypertension and hearing deficiencies, 20-30% suffer from cardiovascular diseases, dementia, cancer, diabetes, chronic respiratory conditions, lack of teeth and impaired vision, and another 5-10% have strokes, Parkinson's disease and asthma. Hence, concomitant conditions, known as multimorbidity is highly prevalent as are impairments in activities of daily living. For the age group between 70-85 years of age, 25% have 5 or more diseases, another 25% will experience disabilities in basic activities of daily living, while 50% will be deficient in the instrumental activities of daily living. Geriatrics refers to the practice of medicine caring for older adults afflicted with many diseases and functional impairments. Geriatricians and family physicians with experience in the field know that a care plan needs to address not only a specific condition but also the interaction that results from all of them and their combined impact on the patient's autonomy. Fortunately, there is recent evidence from scientific literature that we are aging better compared with the previous generation with a decline in the incidence of dementia and disability. For many years, there was debate about the different rates at which the decrease in morbidity and mortality would progress. If lower morbidity would outpace mortality, then we would age better and into older years whereas the converse would have the opposite effect. These recent findings are optimistic, in that if further confirmed, persons can expect to live longer with less disability.

Active aging

Aging is a heterogeneous phenomenon that is the result of the interaction between the individual genetic background and environmental factors, not the least of which is the adoption of a healthy lifestyle. Certain families are more prone to develop specific diseases but the appearance of many of them can be delayed or even averted by the adoption of healthy habits. For example onset of type 2 diabetes can be delayed or prevented by regular physical activity and heathy eating habits. There are also several social and psychological determinants of health, including education, income, social status, social participation, perceived control over one's life, positive attitude, to name but a few. With so many factors at play, it is little wonder that each individual ages at his or her own pace. Gerontology has classified aging into three main categories: active aging (previously called heathy aging or successful aging), normal aging and frail aging. The distribution of these different types of aging varies according to different criteria but the majority falls within the active and normal aging categories with 15-25% considered to be frail. According to WHO (2002), active aging is the process of optimizing opportunities for health, participation and security in order to enhance quality of life as people age. The word "active" refers to continuing participation in social, economic, cultural, spiritual and civic affairs, not just the ability to be physically active or to participate in the labor force. Older people who retire from work, those who are ill or live with disabilities can still remain active contributors to their families, peers, communities and society.

Contribution of older adults to society

Contrary to common beliefs, many older adults are in good health, enjoying life and contributing to society. Such contributions extend to practically all domains of social life despite the challenge of ageism. At the familial level, older persons through their experience of life are of great support to their middle-age children, in counselling on many matters and in the upbringing of the grandchildren. In many instances, they provide financial support to them. At the community level, other than assisting a friend or a neighbor, they participate in organizing cultural and social events, thus to enriching their communities. Volunteering is definitely another non negligible contribution of unremunerated work of older people for the wider community. We all have had the experience of receiving information at the entrance of the hospital by an older person who is volunteering, but they also participate actively on boards of museums, art centers or charitable agencies, or in directly providing services to youth organizations and to more dependent older adults. By so doing, those engaged in volunteering also benefit from being socially active, since outreach and engagement enhance their own well-being and happiness. Finally, remaining part of the workforce is another way of contributing as well as of maintaining physical, cognitive and mental capacities. Society will need to continue its efforts to allow older adults to maintain their societal role as all derive benefits. The change in policies to make retirement age non-compulsory is a first step since we all age differently. Furthermore, facilitating different types of work and adjustments of schedules will permit older people to remain active and to contribute to society.

References

1. United population world Ageing 1950-2050, Population division, DESA, United nations, 2002, http://www.un.org/esa/population/publications/worldageing19502050

2. Brian T. Weinert and Poala S. Timiras. Invited Review: Theories of aging. J Appl Physiol 95: 1706–1716, 2003

3. Marti G. Parker, Mats Thorslund. Health Trends in the Elderly Population: Getting Better and Getting Worse. The Gerontologist 2007; 47:150–158.

4. World Report on Aging and Health http://www.who.int/ageing/publications/world-report-2015/en/

5. The Chief Public Health Officer's Report on the State of Public Health in Canada, 2010: Growing Older – Adding Life to Years. http://publichealth.gc.ca/CPHOreport

CARING FOR THE OLDER PERSON

Abraham Fuks MD, CM, FRCP(C),

Professor, Department of Medicine, McGill University

"…the secret of the care of the patient is in caring for the patient."

The epigraph is a phrase from a talk by Dr. Francis W. Peabody to medical students at Harvard and published in JAMA in 1927 under the title, *"The Care of The Patient."* It has been cited countless times over the past century by those describing a mode of medical practice that is desired, yet too often lacking. The idea has been repeated and promulgated by many speakers at medical school convocations and graduations and remarkably, Peabody's observations and admonitions remain vibrant and cogent today, and, I shall argue, are especially germane to the care of the elderly. The phrase served as an inspiration for the title of this book and certainly for this chapter whose objective is to examine the implications of the concept for contemporary practice and education.

We can better discern the intent of Peabody's comment by examining the words and syntax of his distinction. To be entrusted with the "care of the patient" is to receive a mandate to fulfill a duty. This is an obligation for a caregiver in any domain of medicine and is never taken lightly. Indeed, it is helpful to appreciate that clinical care is a duty of physicians, rather than a right that accrues to patients. That does not detract from a societal obligation to provide health care as a right that is owed to all persons rather than a transactional process. However, provision of care is the responsibility of the physician, though of course, the patient must provide consent. Peabody teaches us that care has additional dimensions and desiderata beyond the simple mandate or duty. "Caring for" a person refers to someone who is important or valued, often in a relationship, and for whose well-being one's concern may extend beyond the requirements and duty of care. The distinction can also be applied to objects, as care of a car indicates a need for maintenance and function while care for a new automobile suggests a deeper connection than with a simple mode of transport.

Peabody explains the relational aspect implicit in "caring for the patient" as follows: "The significance of the intimate personal relationship between physician and patient cannot be too strongly emphasized, for in an extraordinarily large number of cases both diagnosis and treatment are directly dependent on it, and the failure of the young physician to establish this relationship accounts for much of his ineffectiveness in the care of patients." This description is important in that Peabody's reason for stressing the imperative for a relationship is not one of warmth or friendship or even a moral obligation. Rather, the clinical relationship is valuable in leading to accurate diagnoses and effective treatments. He provides a helpful exposition, "What is spoken of as a 'clinical picture' is not just a photograph of a man sick in bed; it is an impressionistic painting of the patient surrounded by his home, his work, his relations, his friends, his joys, sorrows, hopes and fears." This is a simple but wonderful description of the clinical method that chooses to understand the patient as a person embedded in a family, community and possessing an emotional inner life. It also notes that clinical observations are shaped by the observer who gathers meaningful impressions of an ill person and not simple black and white photos of a diseased patient. I should hasten to add two glosses: Peabody today might have referred to both male and female patients rather than "a man sick in bed." Second, when he speaks of the "ineffectiveness" of young trainees, Peabody does not attribute this to ignorance or apathy but simply to the need for clinical experience accrued over time with strong role models.

Peabody tells us that clinical work is painstaking and demands time and effort. Yet, the human relationships so constructed are rewards in themselves. Finally, he concludes that an appreciation and regards for persons in their full humanity is both necessary for good clinical work and is also the source of its deep satisfaction: "The good physician knows his patients through and through, and his knowledge is bought dearly. Time, sympathy and understanding must be lavishly dispensed, but the reward is to be found in that personal bond which forms the greatest satisfaction of the practice of medicine. One of the essential qualities of the clinician is interest in humanity, for the secret of the care of the patient is in caring for the patient."

Older Persons

The use of the word older, rather than old, indicates that there is no clear line of division between those who are old and those who are not. We live on a functional continuum and each person's trajectory depends on the individual's sense of self, functional capacity, physical capability, and ability to accomplish those aspects of life that bring satisfaction and a lived sense of well-being and purpose. The use of the word person, rather than patient, notes that care for the elderly is not primarily an activity that takes place in a hospital or even a clinic, but enfolds the older person in all aspects of daily life. Clearly, the caregiver must be concerned not simply with the intercurrent episodes of acute illness that readily come to medical attention but the demands of daily living and the impositions on the person by chronic maladies that may not be cured but whose burdens may be lessened.

The misplaced emphasis of care on acute illnesses and the hegemony of diagnosis that afflicts most systems of health care are articulately described by Dr. Jason Mutter in an article entitled, "Neglected in the House of Medicine" that appeared in the Hedgehog Review in a special issue whose theme was "The Evening of Life." These entrenched elements of the US health care system have an especially deleterious effect on care for the elderly. The author states that the "American health care system that, despite its remarkable technological capacities, achieves poor outcomes for older adults." He attributes this failure to several factors including an emphasis on acute care, urgent care, trauma, and high-tech interventions. While these are certainly necessary, such spheres of medical care have displaced attention to chronic illnesses and the needs of the older person whose ailments need a more deliberate, longer-term horizon with different goals and aspirations. Dr. Mutter goes on to note that a person "becomes visible to the health care system when diagnosed with an acute ailment but then returns to invisibility once that episode has been managed." This stems from a model of care that is focused on diseases, the ICD classification and supported by payments based on DRGs, complex diagnostic tests and expensive atomized interventions. Lastly, he draws a sharp contrast between two rather different visions of care: "If diagnosis asks, 'What does this person have?' then prognosis asks something quite different: 'In view of the whole person—health, illness, vulnerabilities, and social supports—how is this person doing, what is their probable course, and how can we alter that course for the better?'"

This proactive and expansive vision of health care is appropriate for all but especially germane to care for older persons. Individuals are complex systems with a biopsychosocial nexus within which multiple functions are interconnected and socially embedded. Many components may each function at the limit of capacity yet the whole works in a set of precarious balances. Intervention in one may disrupt the efficacy of another, seemingly unrelated organ system and upset the fragile functional web. In that sense, 'care of' may permit an adjustment of a single anti-hypertensive medication in response to blood pressure readings whereas 'care for' insists on a concern with a broader assessment of risks and benefits to daily function. Thus, Peabody's call to care for the patient entails an integrative, holistic perspective of clinical practice.

The Current State of Care

Both basic research on aging and clinical research to improve the management and support for the frail elderly have advanced significantly over the past three decades. Peabody's plea has been echoed over the past hundred years and calls for holistic models of care are heard regularly at conferences and in articles and editorials. Why then is the state of care for the elderly still a poor relation and a neglected domain in health care systems throughout the Western world? Part of the explanation lies in the stigmas associated with aging that are evident in our culture and reflected in our language and behaviors. We have become accustomed to phrases such as silver tsunami, grey plague, and impending demographic disaster that consider the aging of the population in the same urgent terms used to address climate change. The descriptions of dementia and memory loss in apocalyptic terms evokes fear and dread amongst those who wish to grow old, namely, virtually all of us. We now launch wars against amyloid as a newfound enemy and bemoan the failures of such heroic interventions as intrathecal monoclonal antibodies. In brief, the barriers to improving care for the elderly may lie not in a lack of innovative concepts for support, care and the amelioration of the quality of life, but rather in our entrenched attitudes to those who grow old. This bias, often referred to as ageism, is reminiscent of ancient stigmas associated with mental illness and creates perceptions of aging as a period of decline and dependence and the elderly as the corresponding book end to infancy and its need for constant support. Other societies and cultures appreciate the later years of life as a period of continuing growth with new opportunities but that is hardly the case in Western society. It is little wonder then that health policies favor the young and those with acute conditions—these reflect superficial considerations but stem from deeply embedded biases. This was sadly evident in the enormous rates of mortality in residences for the elderly and related health care facilities during the COVID pandemic and in the results of subsequent investigations that uncovered the poor care and inappropriate living conditions in many such institutions. A society's interests and concerns can be assessed in part on how it rewards various occupations: perhaps it is not by accident that we underpay teachers and caregivers while concurrently trumpeting our commitment to growing children and aging adults. In reality, we may have simply decided that the tough challenges of both public education and health care are too complex and difficult to repair; we now simply ignore them, hoping they will somehow disappear while placing our societal investments in other domains, for example, space travel and military technology. Nonetheless, we continue to pay the enormous costs for our biases and consequent neglect. Becca Levy and colleagues examined the economic consequences of ageism that they described as "discrimination aimed at older persons, negative age stereotypes, and negative self-perceptions of aging." They found that "the 1-year cost of ageism was $63 billion…and ageism resulted in 17.04 million cases" of eight expensive health conditions in those aged 60 or above. They conclude that reducing bias would result in major economic gains and concurrently improve the lives of the elderly by decreasing the risk of major illnesses. A win-win for all!

Care for the older person cannot be provided in models used to look after younger patients who often need management for acute illnesses or those in middle-age who may require intensive high-tech but short-term interventions. While such transactional systems are not ideal, they work to provide care in well-developed societies and for patients with significant personal resources and independence. However, staccato care from referral networks of specialists cannot be expected to offer the requisite quality of care for the elderly. Older persons require and respond well to relational models of caregiving, in which attention is continual and anticipatory rather than stroboscopic and reactive. Support and trust are the results of a personal bond with a clinician who is willing and able to listen and who is able to enjoy the anecdotes and reminiscences of older patients and consider these as benefits, not burdens, of caring for those with a wealth of instructive experiences of long and rich lives. Thus, it helps to genuinely care for such individuals since that will motivate clinicians to provide the attention required to nurture and maintain the sense of well-being that enriches daily life—for both parties.

Language and Rhetoric

As noted above, the words we use may reveal our biases and perceptions of aging. Moreover, and perhaps more powerfully, language may shape our thinking and our consequent behaviors. A very instructive example was presented in an experimental study of the effects of 'elderspeak' in a facility caring for patients with dementia. Elderspeak describes a mode of infantilizing speech sometimes used by caregivers working with elderly persons that uses syntax and words more commonly heard in addressing the very young. For example, "how are we doing today, my dearie?" couched in a singsong prosody, or, "are we ready for some treats?" The research compared the behaviors of elderly subjects addressed in one of three registers, elderspeak, normal adult speech, or silence. The highest incidence of aggressive behaviors, such as resisting care by kicking or biting was displayed by persons addressed in elderspeak and the lowest in those spoken to in a normal voice. Silence led to an intermediate level of resistance. It is quite remarkable that in patients with dementia for whom the words themselves may have lost clear meaning, the sensitivity to the disrespect and perhaps degradation of infantilizing speech is retained and is robust.

A counterexample of the benefit of careful linguistic choices was provided by Daniel Busso and colleagues who examined the effect of different framing interventions on implicit age bias in a large sample of American adults. They found that messages that describe aging as "building momentum" and "The energy that we build up as we get older is what powers us to take up new ideas, advance toward new goals, and continue to move our communities forward," reduce bias against aging. A similar effect was noted after messages that speak of intergenerational communities, "By providing opportunities for older people to participate in and contribute to their communities, intergenerational community centers provide benefits for older people and strengthen the whole community." Thus, just as language can reflect and elicit inappropriate behaviors, thoughtful framings and an attention to different tropes may help ameliorate the problem. Judy Segal, a scholar of rhetoric, noted that simply convincing the elderly that aging can be "successful" and "healthy" runs the risk of blaming the older persons when growing old proves difficult. Rather, she recommends that understanding aging as a normal phase of life, and an identity that we all will share, shifts the discourse from a rhetoric of classification and hierarchy to a rhetoric of identification. As Segal notes, "Becoming old is not simply a matter of waning health or waxing decline; becoming old is growing into a person as complex as, arguably more complex than, that person when they were young." This is an optimism worth understanding and sharing as we continue to learn how to care for the older persons in our midst, and for our future selves.

1. Busso, Daniel, Volmert, Andrew, and Kendall-Taylor, Nathaniel (2019). Reframing Aging: Effect of a Short-Term Framing Intervention on Implicit Measures of Age Bias. *J Gerontol B Psychol Sci Soc Sci.* 74:4:559.
2. Levy, Becca, Slade, Martin, Chang, E-Shien et al. (2020) Ageism Amplifies Cost and Prevalence of Health Conditions. *Gerontologist,* 2020, 60:1:174.
3. Mutter, Jason. (2018) Neglected in the House of Medicine. *The Hedgehog Review* 20:3.
4. Peabody, Francis. (1927). The Care of the Patient. *JAMA* 88:12:877.
5. Segal, Judy Z. (2020). Ageism and Rhetoric. In *Routledge Handbook of the Medical Humanities*, ed. Bleakley, Alan. Routledge, Oxford. UK.
6. Williams, Kristine, Herman, Ruth, Gajewski, Byron, and Wilson, Kristel. (2009) Elderspeak Communication: Impact on Dementia Care. *American Journal of Alzheimer's Disease & Other Dementias* 24:1:11.

FRAILTY

Sathya Karunananthan PhD
Postdoctoral Fellow
Ottawa Hospital Research Institute

Howard Bergman MD, FCFP, FRCPC
Chair, Department of Family Medicine
Professor of Family Medicine, Medicine and Oncology, McGill University

Mrs. Black is a seventy-one year-old widow with four adult children. Her medical history includes mild osteoarthritis and diabetes, for which she takes acetaminophen as required. She lives alone, tends to be socially isolated, and has mild depressive symptoms. She walks without aids but seems to have slowed down lately. Her cognition is normal, and she is completely independent for all instrumental (IADLs) and basic activities of daily living (ADLs).

Is she frail? What is frailty, and can it be identified in the clinical setting? Are there interventions that effectively delay the onset of frailty or prevent adverse outcomes?

Most geriatricians affirm that they can identify frailty in patients when they see it[1,2]. Experts generally agree that frailty in older persons refers to a state of vulnerability to adverse health outcomes. It is considered different from aging per se, since some individuals live to an old age without becoming frail. Furthermore, individuals of the same age can be quite different in terms of how frail they are. Frailty would be the opposite of what many consider successful aging[3].

However, after three decades of research, there remains considerable uncertainty around the concept of frailty and its clinical usefulness. Conflicting ideas abound on the definition of frailty, what criteria should be used for its recognition, and its relationships with aging, disability, and chronic disease[3-6] .

Definitions and conceptualizations of frailty

Most experts agree that frailty is the manifestation of impairments in multiple organ systems that results in increased susceptibility to poor health outcomes[2]. The specific characteristics of frailty, however, remain an important point of contention.

Some have proposed that frailty fits the model of a medical syndrome, whereby all of its symptoms are linked through a single underlying biological mechanism. The most widely used definition of frailty fitting that approach includes five criteria:

1. shrinking (i.e., weight loss)
2. weakness (i.e., loss of muscle strength)
3. exhaustion
4. slowness (i.e., decreased walking speed)
5. low levels of physical activity.

An individual with any three or more of these five criteria is classified as frail[2].

Another widely applied approach is to define frailty as an indicator of global health status, whereby an individual's level of frailty is ascertained through a wide range of factors that may contribute to their well-being. A definition fitting this approach may pull together up to a hundred different characteristics ranging from visual impairment to poor social conditions, chronic diseases, and disability, into a single index of frailty[7]. For each characteristic, an individual is rated as either having a deficit or not. The frailty index is calculated as a proportion representing the number of deficits over the total number of characteristics assessed. By this approach, the more individuals have wrong with them, the more likely they are to be frail.

These approaches represent very different notions of what it is to be frail. The choice of approach has important implications for clinical applicability as well as the potential interventions and prevention of frailty. The number of frailty scores related to these and other approaches is constantly growing. A recent study identified

67 frailty scores with important heterogeneity across scores in the identification of individuals as frail[5].

What can be done about frailty?

Interventions to prevent or reduce frailty have included physical activity, nutrition, memory training, and individually tailored geriatric care models[8,9]. Effectiveness of these interventions has been mixed and the body of evidence is limited, given that the definition of frailty is not consistent across studies. Furthermore, these interventions largely overlap with those recommended for prevention or management of chronic diseases related to aging. Researchers have yet to establish whether targeting these interventions to frail individuals has added value.

Thus far, research has provided substantial evidence that frailty, however it may be defined, is a risk factor for various poor health outcomes. Individuals identified as frail are more likely to experience medical complications, disability, institutionalization or even death, compared to their non-frail counterparts, especially when exposed to stressors such as surgery, chemotherapy or falls. Based on this, many experts are advocating screening for frailty in all older patients. It has been shown, however, that risk factors that demonstrate high statistical significance may not be good predictors at the patient-level. In fact, very little is known about the contribution of frailty in improving patient-level prediction[10]. This needs to be investigated much further in order to justify the adoption of frailty as a clinical tool.

What frailty means to older persons

Older persons themselves may have their own perspectives of what it means to be frail. For example, factors such as mood, have been cited as important to patients and their families; often these are overlooked by clinicians and researchers[3,11]. Psychological health plays an important role in older persons' beliefs about aging successfully. In a study of older persons where only 15% experienced absence of physical illness, 92% reported feeling like they were aging successfully[12].

The research evidence has demonstrated that stereotypes of aging, both positive and negative, are internalized by older persons. This can have both short- and long-term effects on their health[13]. For example, when older adults are exposed to negative aging stereotypes, performance on memory tasks, handwriting and walking speed, as well as physiological measures such as blood pressure, pulse rate, and skin conductance become worse. In fact, in one study, the research showed that an increase in walking speed for those exposed to positive aging stereotypes was comparable to that seen with several weeks of rigorous exercise. Negative stereotypes act as cardiovascular stressors while positive stereotypes reduce evidence of cardiovascular stress. Positive perceptions about aging have impressive long-term effects as well. Individuals with positive self-perceptions of aging have been found to have better functional abilities over a period of eighteen years. These findings should serve as a caution about a potential self-fulfilling prophecy when labelling older persons as "frail".

Conclusion

Frailty is believed to be an early sign of declining health. As such, it may serve as a "red flag" prior to the occurrence of more severe or irreversible conditions, such as disability. In the example of Mrs. Black, the family and doctors would want to identify any factors that are contributing to her declining health and then attempt to address these. The goal is to prevent or at least slow down her decline.

However, after decades of research and discussion among experts, we are still far from a unified definition or diagnostic criteria for frailty. At this time, there is still very limited evidence on the added clinical value of frailty, and currently no evidence-based guidance on how to manage, treat of reverse frailty[9].

For Mrs. Black, better management of her chronic diseases and interventions to improve her social isolation can contribute to slowing down her decline. A diagnosis of frailty, however it is defined, is not likely to have an impact on the clinical care she receives and may only cause harm related to labeling.

References

1. Kaethler Y et al. Defining the concept of frailty: a survey of multi-disciplinary health professionals. Geriatric Today: J Can Geriatr Soc. 6: 26-31 (2003).
2. Fried, L. P. et al. Frailty in older adults: evidence for a phenotype. J. Gerontol. A. Biol. Sci. Med. Sci. 56, M146–156 (2001).
3. Bergman, H. et al. Frailty: an emerging research and clinical paradigm--issues and controversies. J. Gerontol. A. Biol. Sci. Med. Sci. 62, 731–737 (2007).
4. Hogan DB, MacKnight C, Bergman H. Models, definitions, and criteria of frailty. Aging Clin Exp Res. 15(Suppl 3):1–29 (2003).

5. Aguayo GA et al. Agreement Between 35 Published Frailty Scores in the General Population. Am J Epidemiol. 186(4):420-434 (2017).

6. Sternberg SA, Wershof Schwartz A, Karunananthan S, Bergman H & Clarfield AM. The identification of frailty: a systematic literature review. J. Am. Geriatr. Soc. 59: 2129–2138 (2011).

7. Rockwood, K. & Mitnitski A. Frailty in relation to the accumulation of deficits. J. Gerontol. A Biol. Sci. Med. Sci. 62: 722-7 (2007).

8. Puts MT et al. Interventions to prevent or reduce the level of frailty in community-dwelling older adults: a scoping review of the literature and international policies. *Age and Ageing*. 46(3): 383–392.

9. Walston J, Buta B, Xue QL. Frailty Screening and Interventions: Considerations for Clinical Practice. Clin Geriatr Med. 34(1):25-38 (2018).

10. Sourial, N. et al. Implementing frailty into clinical practice: a cautionary tale. J. Gerontol. A Biol. Sci. Med. Sci. 68: 1505-11 (2013).

11. Grenier, A. & Hanley, J. Older Women and 'Frailty' Aged, Gendered and Embodied Resistance. Curr. Sociol. 55: 211–228 (2007).

12. Montross, L. P. et al. Correlates of self-rated successful aging among community-dwelling older adults. Am. J. Geriatr. Psychiatry Off. J. Am. Assoc. Geriatr. Psychiatry 14: 43–51 (2006).

13. Richardson, S., Karunananthan, S. & Bergman, H. I May Be Frail But I Ain't No Failure. Can. Geriatr. J. CGJ 14: 24–28 (2011).

PHYSICAL ACTIVITY AS A COUNTERMEASURE TO FRAILTY

Guy Hajj Boutros, MSc
Kinesiologist and Research Assistant.
Research Institute of McGill University Health Centre.

Antony D. Karelis, PhD
Professor, Department of Exercise Science,
Université du Québec à Montréal.

Clinical vignette

A 78-year-old Caucasian man has difficulty standing up. His body mass index (BMI) is 20 kg/m² and he has lost more than 7 pounds in the last three months. He has been diagnosed with type 2 diabetes and suffers from hypertension. He fell a few years ago and uses a walker for indoor mobility. Since then, his mobility has been reduced, and he walks less than 1000 steps per day and fears walking outside. He started to suffer from low back pain and needs assistance to accomplish instrumental activities of daily living such as going to the grocery store and visiting friends and family. He spends most of his time alone watching television and waiting for someone to visit him.

The reduction of physical capacity in performing activities of daily living affects many older adults and should be taken seriously. There is a need to establish the presence of frailty, determine its risk factors, and propose a plan for assessment and management in which exercise has an essential role.

Why is being sedentary an important clinical problem?

Sedentary behavior may be defined as adopting a sitting or lying posture where little energy is being expended. In older individuals, there is evidence to suggest that most of their time is spent in a sedentary state (e.g. sitting) during the day. Almost 60% of older adults reported sitting for more than 4h per day. Accordingly, 65% of older adults sit in front of a screen for more than 3h daily and over 55% report watching more than 2h of TV. However, when energy expenditure was measured objectively in a small study, it was found that 67% of the older population was sedentary for more than 8.5h daily. Several studies have shown that long periods of sedentary behavior, such as sitting, may be associated with negative clinical outcomes including metabolic complications (i.e.insulin resistance, dyslipidemia), hypertension, cognitive impairments, functional incapacities, and a decrease in muscle mass and strength as well as an increase in fat mass. Interestingly, there is evidence to suggest that obese individuals sit 2 hours longer than lean subjects.

One could argue that sedentary behavior decreases cumulative energy expenditure due to the loss of a large amount of muscle contractions that could occur throughout the waking day. This quantity of energy expenditure has been coined as non-exercise activity. Evidence has shown that the energy expenditure from non-exercise activity is higher than structured exercise such as walking for 30 min a day 5 times per week or running 35 miles a week, a confirmation of sedentary time. Health professionals should not neglect this type of energy expenditure. It should be noted that sedentary behavior for prolonged periods in physically active individuals has been explored. For example, there is evidence to suggest that high sedentary time may be associated with chronic diseases independent from overall physical activity. Thus, sedentary behavior appears to be an important predictor of health outcomes that goes beyond the level of physical activity of an individual.

What are the risks related to a sedentary state?

Prolonged sedentary behavior seems to be associated with an increased risk of all-cause mortality, cardiovascular diseases, type 2 diabetes, Alzheimer's, depression and cancer. In addition, high sitting time has been reported to increase cardiovascular disease mortality 2.7-fold compared to those in the elderly population who spend less time sitting. Moreover, higher amounts of sedentary behavior, such as sitting, have been shown to be associated with a 73% increase in the risk of metabolic complications. As mentioned earlier, older individuals are associated with a decrease in muscle mass and strength, which has been termed sarcopenia. The loss of muscle mass could lead to an increased risk of falls, fractures and being hospitalized for prolonged periods.

Frailty is another common complication that appears in this population. Interestingly, a stressful event in the older individual's life seems to precede frailty. This condition is the consequence of a cumulative decline in many systems (physiological, neurological and musculoskeletal) over one's lifespan. Often a minor infection or a fall results in a dramatic and disproportionate change in health state and the patient goes from being independent to being dependent on another person. Frailty can commonly precede death (27.9%), and be associated with organ failure (21.4%), cancer (19.3%), dementia (13.8%) and other conditions (14.9%). Frailty is more prevalent in women (9.9%) than men (5.1%) and increases with age: 65-69 years: 4%; 70-74 years: 7%; 75-79 years: 9%; 80-84 years: 16%; >85 years: 26%. Frailty is not entirely caused by physical inactivity and sedentary behavior. Other factors that are associated with frailty are:

- Lower educational level
- Current smoker
- Current use of postmenopausal hormone therapy
- Depression or use of antidepressants
- Intellectual disability

The figure below explains how a certain stress can lead to a higher risk of frailty.

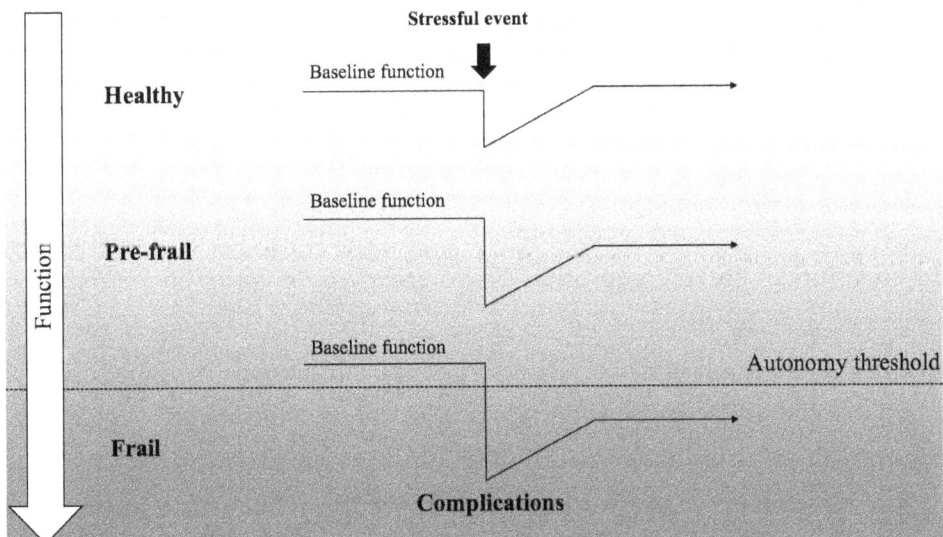

Kinesiophobia (the fear of walking) is another problem that usually appears in the older population, often following a previous fall. Kinesiophobia may decrease mobility, which could lead to isolation, dementia, sarcopenia, cardiovascular disease and mortality.

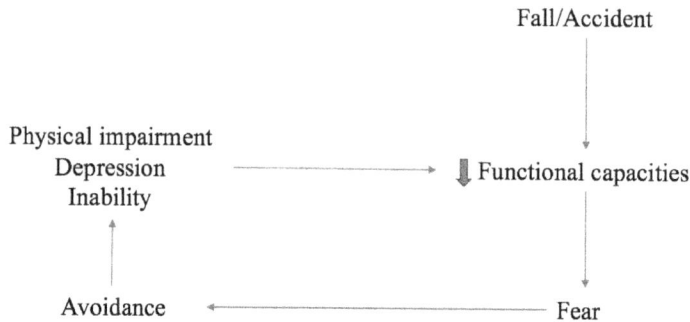

Fall/Accident

Physical impairment
Depression ⟶ ⬇ Functional capacities
Inability

Avoidance ⟵ Fear

How is frailty diagnosed?

The prevalence of frailty varies depending on the tool used to define frailty. The studies performed in the United States found that the percentage of frail individuals ranges from 4 to 16% in men and women aged 65 years and older. Injuries and diseases, such as cancer, increases the prevalence of frailty to 43 percent. Patients with pre-frailty also exist. Pre-frail patients fulfill some but not all the criteria and represent 28 to 44 percent in several studies. A variety of frailty measures have been performed in many epidemiologic studies. However, the most common cited frailty tool is the Physical Frailty Phenotype, also known as the Fried's criteria as discussed in the chapter dedicated specifically to frailty. This evaluation was developed based on progressive weakness and declines in the quality of life of older adults that usually follow an accident or diseases that decrease muscle mass and increase cardiovascular risk.

Frailty is not only based on the physical ability of the patient. The accumulation of illnesses, functional and cognitive declines and social situations must be taken into consideration by the clinician. A questionnaire with 10 or more medical and functional related questions could be used by the clinician during the screening as in the Frailty Index (see chapter on frailty). The higher the number of deficits, the greater the patient is considered as frail. Today, finding a fast and quick tool to examine frailty is important because clinicians have limited time with their patients. A tool that takes only few minutes to perform and can be incorporated into history-taking is the FRAIL scale. The component questions listed below define if the patient is frail or pre-frail.

- **Fatigue** ("Are you fatigued?")
- **Resistance** ("Can you climb one flight of stairs?")
- **Ambulation** ("Can you walk one block?")
- **Illnesses** (greater than five)
- **Loss of weight** (greater than 5 percent)

If patients answer 'Yes' to three or more of the questions, this indicates that they are frail. If patients answer 'Yes' to one or two of the questions, this indicates that they are pre-frail.

Another simple questionnaire that is used in many clinical settings is 'The Study of Osteoporotic Fractures' (SOF) frailty tool. A positive answer to the first question, and negative answers to the next two indicate frailty. The patient is considered frail if two of the three questions are responded to in this way.

- Did you lose more than 5 percent of your weight during the last year?
- Are you able to rise from a chair five times without the use of your arms?
- Do you feel full of energy?

The clinical frailty scale is a rapid screening questionnaire based on self-reported comorbidities and the need of assistance in activities of self-care and daily living. It is scored between 1 (very fit) and 7 (severely frail).

Many studies used several tools to identify frailty. The most commonly utilized screening tools were comparable in predicting health risks leading to mortality. Unfortunately, the presence of cognitive impairment increases the risk of frailty and deteriorates general health even further. Patients who meet criteria for physical frailty combined with cognitive problems must be considered more at risk than patients without cognitive impairment. Some clinicians use scales that define cognitive status to further refine their judgment and to prescribe assistance in case the patient is in need.

What are the interventions that can potentially reverse frailty?

Prevention is a better intervention than waiting until the patient is frail. For this reason, it is very important to explain and clarify at a young age the importance of a healthy lifestyle. Fortunately, the beneficial effects of physical activity can be observed at any age. Current recommendations of physical activity by the American College of Sports Medicine in older adults are a minimum of 30 minutes of moderate intensity endurance physical activity 5 days per week or 20 minutes of vigorous intensity 3 times per week during non-consecutive days. In addition, the guidelines recommend performing muscle-strengthening activities at least twice a week during non-consecutive days. A single set of 8-10 exercises with 10-15 repetitions should be performed for each exercise at a moderate to high level of effort using the major muscles of the body to maintain or increase muscle strength and endurance. Unfortunately, only 12 percent of the elderly population in Canada follow these recommendations. It is important to note that somewhat active older adults that do not achieve these numbers still have better health benefits when compared to inactive older adults. Health professionals could encourage different options/activities to older adults that may limit sitting time such as stand up desks for computers, interactive video games, standing when using public transportation, devices that vibrate when one is sitting too long and the use of stairs. Specifically decreasing the amount of sitting time in future physical activity guidelines, especially in frail and pre-fail patients, should be considered.

An important question that remains unsolved is whether standing for long periods throughout the day is enough to minimize the risk of disease and decrease the risk of falls. A potential method that could counteract the negative health effects of prolonged sedentary behavior is increasing the number of break up times. Accordingly, breaking up sedentary time (3-5 min walks every 30 min) appears to have positive effects on multiple metabolic risk factors. In addition, for the pre-frail and frail populations, it is important to practice resistance training to increase muscle strength and bone mineral density. Resistance training is a form of exercise that has been recommended as a safe, feasible, effective and preferred strategy in preventing the loss of muscle strength and increasing muscle mass in older adults. This type of exercise performed two to three time per weeks appears to have a positive impact on muscle mass, gait speed and strength.

Exercises for very frail patients

Unfortunately, many frail and pre-frail persons can not achieve these recommendations for resistance training due to muscle weakness and movement limitation. Some patient can not even walk a distance of 10m without a pause, stand up from a chair without help or even perform their everyday self-care. For this type of population, it is recommended to start with seated exercises such as knee extension, arm raise, hip flexion and standing up from the seated position with or without the assistance of their arms. Before starting the exercises, it is crucial to provide a steady base, so the patient will be safe and secure while she/he moves the body during the workout. Once the patient is able to perform 10 to 12 repetitions of these exercises, it is recommended to add a level of difficulty by asking the patient to stand up and to perform the same exercises while holding on to a counter or other stable surface. In addition, it is possible to add more exercises such as hip abduction, hip extension and calf raises. These movements could help to strengthen their lower limb muscles and eventually lead to improved balance. It takes balance to have a safe gait and to prevent falls. To ameliorate balance, a few specific exercises (see figure below) such as semi tandem position (one foot ahead of the other as if taking a step) and full tandem (heel of one foot directly in front of the toes of the other foot) are required. Once these exercises are well performed by maintaining the position for 20 to 30 seconds, it is possible to try the one-foot balance but always within reach of a stable support. Frail patients must be supervised by a kinesiologist or a physiotherapist during the first few sessions, and the evolution of the exercises (number of repetition and intensity) must be slower than in healthy aging patients.

Aerobic training

Aerobic training is another alternative to improve health outcomes in the elderly. Using equipment that has a lower impact on joints is important, especially in frail patients. Elliptical machines and seated ergocycles are preferred over treadmills because they increase stability and reduce the risk of falls. Some participants must start with exercises in the pool (aqua gym) to prevent negative impacts on joints.

Lately, high intensity interval training (HIIT) has been used to counteract physical, cognitive and metabolic declines. HIIT consists of repeated alternating short bouts of high intensity exercise with recovery periods of low intensity exercise. Different types of exercise equipment can be used to perform this kind of training such as the treadmill, ergocycle and elliptical. Several studies have shown that this kind of exercise decreases cardiovascular risk and improves muscle mass and gait speed more than continuous moderate intensity aerobic exercise. HIIT training sessions are shorter than aerobic continuous moderate intensity exercise sessions. Thus, interval training has become an interesting and a more time efficient option for exercise training protocols since it can help to break the barrier to engaging in physical activity due to a lack of time. Furthermore, some studies reported that this type of training is not only time efficient, but even more enjoyable than other forms of exercise.

Nutrition, as mentioned in another chapter of this book, is another alternative to counteract frailty in the elderly population. The combination of a proper amount of protein intake (1.0 to 1.2g/kg of weight) with physical activity has been found to improve muscle mass, functional capacities and the metabolic profile, which in turn improves frailty.

Resolution of the clinical vignette

The patient in our case study has several medical issues. Unfortunately, many older adults of the same age suffer from several conditions as described in the present case. First, a weight loss of more than 7lbs in the last three months, the low number of steps taken daily, and the reduced mobility all establish that he is frail. Second, the metabolic complication of type 2 diabetes with hypertension worsens the situation since diabetes is associated with a lower gait speed. Further, social isolation by spending days alone increases the risk of dementia and depression. The fear of going outdoors is making the patient even more sedentary. The assistance of a physiotherapist or a kinesiologist is vital to counteract the fears and to improve self-confidence. The therapist must start the interventions at a place familiar to the patient, usually his or her home. This decreases the risk of falls.

The intervention must start with a warmup seated on a chair with neck rotations followed by ankle rotations 10 times each. To improve lower muscle strength and balance, participant is asked to go from a seated position to standing tall (with or without help) for 10 repetitions. This exercise is functional and used in daily life. Once the patient is standing still and holding to a stable counter, he is asked to raise his heels and his toes 10 times each. To improve balance, semi tandem and tandem exercises are performed for 20 to 30 seconds and for standing on each foot. This workout could be performed 3 to 4 times a week with a day off between the sessions. After a few weeks, the therapist can take the patient outside or to an exercise facility for training. Moreover, since the goal of a training program is to improve the quality of life of the patient, the therapist must provide the patient with some exercises to do by themselves, which allows them to become more autonomous. Once the patient is comfortable in performing the exercises cited above. such as a stand up from a chair, calf raises and tandem, 8 to 12 repetitions, the addition of an external force will help the patient to have greater improvement in muscle mass. Exercises for upper limb muscle strength are important too. Seated shoulder press and seated biceps curls using lightweight dumbbells, bottles of water or a resistance elastic band, could help the patient in performing activities of daily living such as opening doors and storing personal effects in cabinets. To raise the degree of difficulty, all exercises mentioned above could be done when the patient is standing. It is very important to ensure that the patient is 100% able to perform these exercises by himself especially when the level of difficulty is increased. Aerobic exercise is essential to improve cardiovascular health. Starting the exercises using an ergocycle or an elliptical machine could help to reduce the impact on joints, especially because this population has a high prevalence of arthritis. Depending on the capacity of the patient to perform exercises, aerobic workout could last 5 to 10 minutes with a very low intensity. Combined exercises (resistance and endurance) could have a better impact on the general health of the patient since our goal is to increase muscle mass and strength and cardiovascular fitness levels. After several weeks, this exercise program at a frequency of 2 to 3 times a week should overcome the sedentary habit and allow the patient to feel the difference and look for other kinds of workout. Overall, being more active will help the patient to reduce many impairments and prevent health-related complications related to being sedentary, especially in older adults.

Example of an exercise session

Warm up:

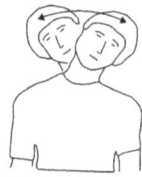 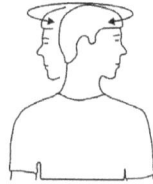 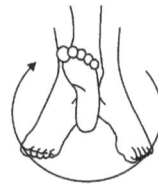

Neck Flexion   Neck Rotation   Ankle rotation

Strength and balance:

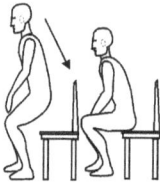 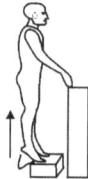 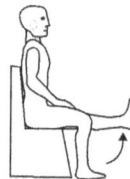 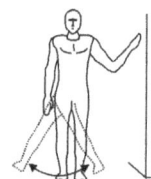

Sit and stand   Heels raise   Knee flexion   Hip abduction

Balance:

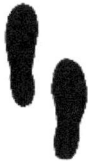 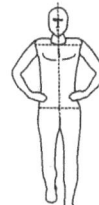

Feet together   Semi tandem   Tandem   1leg balance

Upper limb: Aerobic:

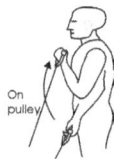 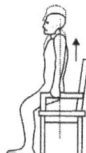 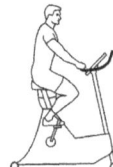

Elbow flexion   Elbow extension   Ergocycle

References:

1. Fried LP, Ferrucci L, Darer J, Williamson JD, Anderson G. Untangling the concepts of disability, frailty, and comorbidity: implications for improved targeting and care. J Gerontol A Biol Sci Med Sci 2004; 59 3:255–263.

2. Rockwood K, Mitnitski A. Frailty in relation to the accumulation of deficits. J Gerontol A Biol Sci Med Sci 2007; 62 7:722–727.

3. Lin F, Roiland R, Chen DG, Qiu C. Linking cognition and frailty in middle and old age: metabolic syndrome matters. Research

4. Bonnefoy M, Boutitie F, Mercier C, Gueyffier F, Carre C, Guetemme G, et al. Efficacy of a home-based intervention programme on the physical activity level and functional ability of older people using domestic services: a randomised study. J Nutr Health Aging 2012; 16 4:370–377.

5. Cesari M, Vellas B, Hsu F-C, Newman AB, Doss H, King AC, et al. A physical activity intervention to treat the frailty syndrome in older persons—results from the LIFE-P study. J Gerontol A Biol Sci Med Sci 2015; 70 2:216–222.

6. Romero-Ortuno R, Walsh C, Lawlor BA, Kenny RA. A frailty instrument for primary care: findings from the survey of health, ageing and retirement in Europe (SHARE). BMC Geriatr 2010; 10:57.

DOCTOR, MY WIFE IS GETTING FORGETFUL

Serge Gauthier, C.M., C.Q., MD, FRCPC
Director, AD Research Unit, MCSA
Professor, Departments of Neurology & Neurosurgery, Psychiatry, Medicine, McGill University
McGill Center for Studies in Aging

Exemplary case

A 78 year old lady is accompanied by her husband and daughter. The family is concerned about a memory decline over the past two years, worse the past six months. For example she forgets conversations, is losing interest in going out, and was twice late paying some household bills. She does not appear concerned about any of this. The family wants to know if this is early dementia and what can be done about it.

On further questioning she has forgotten some of the grandchildren's birthdays in the past year, is looking for things in the house and gets upset about it. She cooks only simple meals and gets flustered when her daughter's family is visiting. She drives in familiar areas, mostly to visit her daughter. The husband has taken over most of the household finances through their common bank account. There is no advance power of attorney for medical and financial decisions. She is independent for self-care. Her medical history is of mild labile arterial hypertension, controlled by a diuretic. She takes vitamin D supplements on a weekly basis. Her mother died of Alzheimer's at age 85.

The physical examination showed a pleasant and healthy looking elderly woman. Her Mini Mental State Examination (MMSE) is 21/30, with wrong day, date, month, year, name of the clinic, forgetting 3 words after distraction, unable to copy the drawing. She is unable to complete the short version of Trail B found in the Montreal Cognitive Assessment (MoCA), and to set the time at 11:10 on her clock.

The initial clinical impression is of a dementia due to Alzheimer's disease (AD). A head un-infused ("plain") head computer tomography showed generalized atrophy compatible with the age of the patient.

At the follow-up visit the MMSE score was 20, and the diagnosis of AD was disclosed to the patient and the family. A road test by an occupational therapist and an advance power of attorney to be drawn by a legal professional were recommended. A cholinesterase inhibitor (CI) was prescribed.

General work-up and diagnostic recommendations

Screening for cognitive decline in older persons without symptoms using tools such as the MMSE and the MoCA is not recommended in routine clinical practice. When symptoms suggestive of a progressive cognitive decline are spontaneously brought forward by reliable family members, there has to be a systematic assessment. First a semi-structured questionnaire about the types of cognitive symptoms (memory, language, orientation, judgment), how they affect daily life, and if they are accompanied by mood, personality or behavioral changes, is utilized. Then a general physical examination and a basic neurologic examination are done, looking for evidence of factors that may suggest a vascular etiology to the cognitive decline. For instance systolic hypertension associated by an asymmetry of deep tendon reflexes and of plantar responses would suggest a silent stroke.

The latest (4th) Canadian Consensus Conference on the Diagnosis and Treatment of Dementia published in 2012 an update of its recommendations reiterating that structural imaging using computer tomography (CT) or magnetic resonance imaging (MRI) is needed in a specific set of circumstances (Table 1).

The most common finding on CT or MRI in persons with mild dementia is generalized atrophy, which may be asymmetric, and is compatible with AD. Small (lacunar) infarcts may be found, and are not considered clinically significant towards the cognitive decline unless they are in a strategic area of the brain such as the thalamus or the head of the caudate, in which case a mixed etiology (AD and stroke) dementia is diagnosed.

TABLE 1: Recommendations from the CCCDTD about structural imaging needed if cognitive decline and:
• age less than 65
• rapid (1 or 2 months) unexplained decline in cognition and function
• short duration of symptoms (less than two years)
• recent and significant head trauma
• unexplained neurological symptoms such as headaches or seizures
• history of cancer
• use of anticoagulation or history of bleeding disorder
• early urinary incontinence and gait disorder
• lateralizing signs (hemiparesis, unilateral grasp or Babinski)
• prominent gait disturbance

The other relatively common type of late-onset dementia is Lewy Body (DLB), a mixture of AD and Parkinsonian features, which translates into visual hallucinations early in the course of the cognitive decline, fluctuations of symptoms from hour to hour, and motor changes such as rigidity with cogwheeling (the racket-like feeling when manipulating the neck or arms of a patient).

General treatment considerations

An accurate diagnosis of dementia can be made by all clinicians if there is reliable historical information, some basic cognitive tests and structural brain imaging when appropriate. The etiology of the dementia over age 75 is essentially, AD, AD with stroke, AD with some Parkinson features, or DLB.

What is not as easy is the disclosure of the diagnosis which should be as transparent as for someone with cancer. Most patients with dementia have relative indifference (anosognosia) to their symptoms and to their cause, but clinicians should be on the look out for someone with depressive symptoms. Practically speaking, the accompanying family member should be made aware of the diagnosis and potential consequences on driving and managing finances. If the patient asks he can be told about being in "early stages of a common brain aging condition", and if he specifically asks about AD tell the truth about the likelihood of this specific diagnosis (80% accuracy using clinical diagnosis) unless there is concern for a catastrophic reaction, which is very uncommon.

The loss of autonomy for instrumental and basic activities of daily living is progressive over many years, best handled by gradual adjustments of the family, and is facilitated by support groups. There is no need to make a list of all the changes to occur over five years at the time of diagnosis, but is it wise to anticipate losses though the annual or bi-annual follow-ups: driving, banking, cooking, traveling on foot, day programs, long term care, end-of-life care will be handled over time.

The mood and behavioral symptoms of dementia are often worse that the cognitive decline and the gradual loss of autonomy. Apathy, irritability and suspiciousness are common in the early stages of AD, and may be helped by antidepressants acting on serotoninergic pathways. Hallucinations in DLB improve with CIs. Aggressive behavior not manageable by environmental non-pharmacological approaches may require an atypical neuroleptic such as risperidone (attention to the black box warning about increased risk of stroke and death). Sometimes aggressive behavior is improved by antidepressants and/or the NMDA receptor antagonist memantine, reducing the need or the dose of a neuroleptic.

References

1. Gauthier S, Patterson C, Chertkow H et al. 4th Canadian Consensus Conference on the Diagnosis and Treatment of Dementia. Can J Neurol Sci 2012; 39: Suppl 5:

UPDATE ON ALZHEIMER'S DISEASE DIAGNOSIS AND MANAGEMENT

Serge Gauthier. C.M., C.Q., MD, FRCPC
Director, Alzheimer's Disease Research Unit,
McGill Center for Studies in Aging
Montreal, Canada

Introduction

Although there are important changes in the research definition of Alzheimer's disease (AD) using biomarkers for amyloid (A), tau (T) and neurodegeneration (N) (REF), the clinical definition of AD in day to day medical practice is still based on a history of cognitive decline affecting daily life, often accompanied by changes in mood and behavior. This chapter will illustrate the various modes of presentation of AD that many clinicians will come across.

In terms of treatment of AD, there will be no magic pill in the near future, so we must treat symptoms as they emerge over time and help both the person with dementia and the caregivers. A stage by stage management approach is discussed.

Diagnosis of AD – Initial assessment

Most persons with AD have memory complaints for one to three years before the memory lapses start interfering with their daily life. There are some gender and cultural differences in how significant these lapses are: a grand-mother forgetting her grand-children's birthday is more significant than a grand-father. A man who used to drive around without a problem and now needs help for navigation on a regular basis is significantly changed. Less commonly the person has progressive difficulties getting the words out, not just names of people but names of common objects. The handyman is now looking for his tools and taking much more time than before to fix things in the house. The mother who used to regularly invite the family for dinner now finds it too much of a burden because of the need to plan the meal and cook it properly. These are examples of common complaints in early stages of AD, but there can be variations, such as not recognizing people's faces, or being very suspicious about family members or neighbors stealing things, or having visual hallucinations of persons coming to the house.

When meeting a person with cognitive complaints for the first time, the health professional will ask about various symptoms as illustrated above, and will try to estimate their impact on daily life such as reliability in paying bills, taking medications, planning an outing. If the person is seen alone there is a need to get complementary information by talking with family or friends. It is sometimes necessary to talk to the accompanying person separately from the person with cognitive complaints, since there may be embarrassment about disclosing functional and behavioral changes. Some families will send the clinician a short email ahead of, or right after the first visit.

The history needs to be expanded to general health issues including past or current medical diagnosis such as sleep apnea, depression, alcohol abuse, etc. Medications in use are examined carefully since some of them may interfere with attention and memory, such as anticholinergic drugs prescribed for bladder urgency, or amitriptyline prescribed for headaches.

Screening memory tests are done, including the Mini Mental State Examination (MMSE) and the Montreal Cognitive Assessment (MoCA). They can be supplemented by other cognitive tests if required, such as the Short Version (15 pictures) of the Boston Naming or the Frontal Assessment Battery.

The physical examination is focused on blood pressure and circulation, including listening to the carotid arteries looking for a murmur, evidence of a general medical problem such as an enlarged thyroid, and asymmetry of the motor examination which can suggest a stroke or space occupying lesion.

The blood work is generally the same done on a yearly basis for a general preventive assessment, including AST/ALT, B12, BUN/creatinine, electrolytes, glycemia, TSH levels. A head computerized scan (CT) is often done but rarely influences the diagnosis when the history of a gradual cognitive decline over at least one year is associated with a normal general physical examination.

When the person is younger than 65, if there are atypical symptoms such as primarily language or visual complaints, asymmetry on the neurologic examination, a history of cancer or taking anticoagulants, a CT scan is indicated, and may be supplemented by other tests such as magnetic resonance imaging (MRI) of the head, or a position emission tomography (PET) of the brain using various radioisotopes, the most common being fluorodeoxyglucose (FDG), or a lumbar puncture (LP). These are usually ordered by a specialist in a "memory clinic" setting.

Diagnosis of AD – Differential diagnosis

Two visits usually six months apart allow to compare the performance on sequential MMSE's (it is preferable not to use the MoCA more often than once a year because of practice effects), and determine if there is improvement or worsening of symptoms. A diagnosis of mild cognitive impairment (MCI) is made if there is evidence of a cognitive decline not interfering with daily life compared to other persons in the same age, education and cultural group. A diagnosis of dementia is made if the cognitive decline is causing a loss of autonomy for some activities of daily living. AD is the most common cause of MCI with memory complaints (amnestic MCI) and of dementia over age 65, but other factors may be at play such as stroke, leading to a diagnosis of "mixed dementia". Less commonly there is a mix of Parkinson and Alzheimer symptoms (dementia with Lewy bodies -DLB) and fronto-temporal dementia (FTD).

The diagnosis of the cause of dementia may change over time. For instance a person with a normal motor examination at the initial assessment suggesting AD may show after two years one sided Parkinson-like changes, suggesting cortico-basal degeneration (CBD) or start falling backwards with rigidity in the neck muscles, suggesting progressive supra-nuclear palsy (PSP).

Natural history

Knowledge of the natural progression of AD and related disorders will help plan the management over time.

Many but not all persons with MCI will progress to dementia within five years. The general figure is 15% per year for such a progression, which may be delayed by careful attention to risk factors and enhancing protective factors. Some genetic factors such as the apolipoprotein E 4 (ApoE4) genotype are known to accelerate the rate of progression to dementia

Mild dementia (needs assistance for directions while driving, needs advice for financial decisions) may be already present at the time of diagnosis, and will progress over an average of eight years to moderate stage (needs supervision for grocery shopping, accompaniment to the bank, turn the oven off and use microwave) to moderate-severe stage (needs assistance for personal care), severe stage (cannot walk safely, incontinence) and terminal stage (difficulty swallowing leading to aspiration pneumonias). A classification from 1 to 7 is often used as a reference for staging the disease.

This pattern of progression is relatively predictable in AD but less so with other types of dementia. Mixed AD-vascular dementia usually shows a slower decline until a heart attack or stroke intervenes, leading to a shorter survival time. Dementias with an early motor component (DLB, CBD, PSP) are associated with falls that can lead to complications such as hip fractures and head injuries.

Some persons with AD have a slow rate of progression, with little functional decline for five years (they are usually older than 85 and in good general health). Other persons have a more rapid decline (they are often younger with higher education). The variability in speed of progression is partly determined by the brain reserve (more highly educated persons start symptoms of AD later than uneducated persons, but show a more rapid decline), co-existing diseases such as heart failure, social isolation and poor nutrition.

Depressive symptoms are common in the MCI and mild dementia stages of AD, since the person is still aware of the cognitive and functional decline. These symptoms tend to improve over time as the person loses awareness of the disease (anosognosia).

Agitation and aggressivity are usually more common in moderate stage dementia, and they often are worse at the end of the day (sundowning). Sleep disturbances with being up at night are more common in moderate to severe stages of dementia.

Physical impairment such as shuffling gait and falls occur usually in the severe stage. Difficulties in swallowing causing aspiration pneumonia usually follow.

Management of AD

Disclosure of the diagnosis of dementia due to AD or other cause is more easily done with the accompanying person, particularly if that person is also the legally designated representative. The person with dementia rarely asks, and there is a risk of catastrophic reaction in some individuals with anxiety about the future or with depression. In doubt, the clinician may state something like "you were right to come for an assessment of your memory; there is indeed a problem and we will work on it together".

Persons with MCI or with mild dementia are advised to indicate in writing who they trust in case of future needs: "Who can we ask permission if you have a car accident, you are unable to give an answer about your treatment, and bills need to be paid?". The document used is an Advance Directive called a Specific Power of Attorney. It takes effect immediately and allows a representative chosen by the affected person to act on behalf of that person for personal health care and financial issues. In case of incapacity, the document can be filled in at home with two witnesses, or executed at a notary or lawyer's office (which is preferable). It is recommended to designate a principal and a backup legal representative, or to designate one person for personal care issues and one for financial decisions. A General Power of Attorney allows for broader powers to the representative appointed and is a useful complement to the Advance Directive. Advance Directives can only be put in place when the person has capacity to do so.

Incapacity Homologation is the process by which a judge signs off on the documents in cases of incapacity. (see Chapter: How Do I Protect My Patient? Randy S. Perskin Esq., J.D.)

Improvement of cognitive abilities can be achieved by optimal care of other medical conditions such as sleep apnea, deafness, vitamin or nutritional deficiencies. Participation in social activities and being physically active may help in prevention of cognitive decline but does help people with MCI or dementia.

Current medications for dementia due to AD, mixed Alzheimer and vascular dementia, Parkinson's disease-associated dementia and DLB are of two classes: one class increases acetylcholine levels in the brain by inhibiting enzymes that break it down (acetylcholinesterase inhibitors: donepezil, rivastigmine, galantamine), the other class decreases the activity of the neurotransmitter glutamate (NMDA receptor blocker: memantine). These medications have been in use for more than a decade and may improve or stabilize symptoms for six to twenty-four months. Other medications used in managing dementia include antidepressants and low doses of antipsychotics.

Non-pharmacologic interventions include a quiet environment, more lights in the evening, and education of the caregivers about dementia-associated behaviors.

Persons with dementia are usually diagnosed and taken care of by their family doctor and his/her nurse and other community resources. A referral to a neurologist, psychiatrist or geriatrician may be required if there are issues that the local team has difficulty with. There are also persons with MCI or dementia that wish to participate in research, and they can be referred to memory clinics.

References using a case-based approach

1. Feldman HH, Jacova C, Robillard A et al. Diagnosis and treatment of dementia. 2. Diagnosis CMAJ 2008; 178(7):825-36.
2. Cherkow H, Massoud F, Nasreddine Z et al. Diagnosis and treatment of dementia. 3. Mild cognitive impairment and cognitive impairment without dementia. CMAJ 2008; 178(10):1273-85.
3. Hogan DB, Bailey P, Black S et al. Diagnosis and treatment of dementia. 4. Approach to management of mild to moderate dementia. CMAJ 2008; 179(8):787-93.
4. Hogan DB, Bailey P, Black S et al. Diagnosis and treatment of dementia. 5. Nonpharmacologic and pharmacologic therapy for mild to moderate dementia. CMAJ 2008; 179(10):1019-26.
5. Herrmann N, Gauthier S. et al. Diagnosis and treatment of dementia. 6. Management of severe Alzheimer disease. CMAJ 2008; 178(12):1279-87.

References on diagnosis and management using a consensus approach

Australia

Laver K, Cumming RG, Dyer SM et al. Clinical practice guidelines for dementia in Australia. Med J Australia 2016;204:1-3. Full guidelines: http://sydney.edu.au/medicine/cdpc/documents/resources/LAVER_Dementia_Guidleines_recommendations_PRVW%20%284%29.pdf

Canada

Gauthier S, Patterson C, Chertkow H et al. 4th Canadian Consensus Conference on the Diagnosis and Treatment of Dementia. Can J Neurol Sci 2012;39: Suppl 5: S1-S8. Being updated October 2019.

France

Haute Autorité de Santé. Guide parcours de soins des patients présentant un trouble neurocognitif associé à la maladie d'Alzheimer ou à une maladie apparentée. Les Parcours de Soins, Mai 2018.

Germany

Deuschl G, Maier W et al. S3-Leitlinie Demenzen. 2016. In: Deutsche Gesellschaft für Neurologie, Hrsg. Leitlinien für Diagnostik und Therapie in der Neurologie. Online: www.dgn.org/leitlinien

Singapore

Nagaendran K, Chen C, Chong MS et al. Ministry of health clinical practice guidelines: dementia. Singapore Med J 2013: 54: 293-299.

UK

https://www.guidelines.co.uk/mental-health/nice-dementia-guideline/454244.article

USA

Petersen RC, Lopez O, Armstrong MJ et al. Practice guideline update summary: Mild cognitive impairment
Report of the Guideline Development, Dissemination, and Implementation
Subcommittee of the American Academy of Neurology. Neurology® 2018;90:1-10. doi:10.1212/WNL.0000000000004826. Being updated Dec 2019.

NAVIGATING THE JOURNEY OF
DEMENTIA AS A CAREGIVER

By Claire Webster
Certified Alzheimer Care Consultant (PAC)
Certified Professional Consultant on Aging (CPCA)
Founder, McGill University Dementia Education Program

Patient Scenario

Mrs. L is a 74-year-old woman whose daughter brought her to the Neurologist after consulting with their family physician about her mother's unusual behaviour and significant change in personality following the recent death of her husband. Mrs. L had been a physically active, independent and outgoing woman, but over the past 18 months had become socially withdrawn and impatient, suffering from severe mood swings ranging from bouts of anger to depression. She had increasing difficulty managing her finances or preparing meals for herself. She developed a fear of stairs and zero tolerance for loud noise, often putting her hands over her ears while rocking back and forth in distress. She was often confused, had difficulty finding her words and started to use odd and inappropriate language. A few symptoms began appearing a year prior to her husband's passing. Mrs. L had become obsessed with the next-door neighbor, who she believed was operating a cocaine lab. Her car had numerous dents and marks indicative of accidents.

When the symptoms began to increase after her father's death, her daughter, who had been the primary caregiver for over thirty years, thought her mother was suffering from post-traumatic caregiver stress and grief, as she had been the primary caregiver for over 30 years. Mrs. L began donating money to the same charity multiple times a year and incurring random expenses. Her daughter noticed that she had been hoarding hundreds of empty plastic fruit containers in her kitchen cabinets and keeping expired food in the refrigerator.

Mrs. L's medical history included high cholesterol, and she had suffered a minor transient ischemic attack (TIA) at the age of 68. There was a history of cardiac issues in her family.

Against her mother's will and in full denial of anything being wrong, her daughter made an appointment with a Neurologist. The doctor asked the daughter a series of questions about her mother's cognitive and physical well-being while the mother sat beside her, in great frustration, refusing to accept or admit to any of the information that was being shared. The Neurologist performed the MOCA (Montreal Cognitive Assessment Test) wherein Mrs. L scored 17/30. The Neurologist informed Mrs. L that she had Alzheimer's Disease, and upon learning that she was still driving, immediately called the license bureau, and without any warning, cancelled her driver's license.

In shock and completely unfamiliar with dementia, Mrs. L's daughter asked the doctor if he could explain what Alzheimer's Disease is, how to manage the disease, what to expect and whether her mother could still live on her own. The doctor answered, "No, she cannot live on her own. There is information about the disease on the Internet, and GOOD LUCK." Mrs. L and her daughter left the doctor's office without being provided any information on the symptoms of the disease or guidance on how to plan for the future. They were not counseled on the importance of accessing support services or told what the next steps should be.

Mrs. L's 38-year-old daughter was her only child, and she was raising a family of three young children while holding a full-time job managing a company with her husband. Over the next few years, she would get caught up in a cyclone of caregiving that resulted in severe burnout and post-traumatic stress disorder. The Neurologist's inability to provide information and guidance would have a significant impact on the quality of care and safety of Mrs. L in the coming years, as well as a ripple effect on the mental and physical health of her daughter.

Who are Caregivers?

It is important for the physician to know who the primary caregiver is to the Person Living With Dementia (PLWD) as the disease progresses. By asking this question, the physician can help the newly-diagnosed patient and their caregiver recognize that their relationship will change as the disease progresses. This is particularly important since many informal caregivers do not recognize themselves as "caregivers", which may also contribute to stress. A caregiver may be the person's spouse or partner, friend, adult child or other family member, and may not realize that their role in their loved one's life will ultimately change. The caregiver may also have health issues of their own that will impact the level of care they are able to provide.

In their report, *Improving the Quality of Life and Care of Persons Living with Dementia and their Caregivers*, the Canadian Academy of Health Sciences (CAHS, 2019) notes that assessing the needs of caregivers is key to identifying the support that each caregiver is likely to require.

The health and well-being of the caregiver directly affects the care they are able to provide to their loved one. Upon receiving a diagnosis of dementia (or soon thereafter), a needs assessment should be performed for the caregiver using a validated instrument designed to complete a comprehensive psychosocial assessment that identifies caregiver needs and key areas of concern such as the Caregivers' Aspiration, Realities, and Expectations Tool (CARE Tool). This type of assessment has been found to increase the health practitioner's awareness of the caregiver's needs and can help them refer timely supports and improve access to appropriate services (Keefe, J. et.al., 2014). The fact of having participated in such an assessment recognizes and validates the caregiver's role in addition to providing information about services, an opportunity to tell their story and permission to express their feelings (Keefe, J. et. al., 2014).

The Ripple Effect of Dementia on the Caregiver

Understanding and caring for someone with Alzheimer's Disease or other dementia-related illnesses is a long, stressful and intensely emotional journey. PLWD progress along an unpredictable path to complete loss of self and autonomy. The diagnosing physician needs to consider that the person who accompanies the patient is receiving devastating news about their loved one, and it is imperative to provide them with as much information as possible on that first visit and offer the necessary resources to ensure the best quality of care and safety for both the patient as well as the caregiver's physical, mental and financial health and well-being.

A diagnosis of Alzheimer's Disease affects all intimate family and friends of the PLWD. Caregivers need support to care for themselves in order to avoid becoming overwhelmed. They are at an increased risk of developing significant health problems as their loved one's cognitive, physical, and functional abilities diminish.

The Risks of Not Providing Education and Support about Dementia to Caregivers

A lack of education about dementia will have a significant impact on the quality of care and safety of the individual who has been diagnosed as well as on the caregiver. Unlike other diseases, the patient who is diagnosed with dementia and their caregiver are rarely provided with information on how to navigate the challenges associated with managing and living with this disease. The medical community does not automatically educate individuals about the disease and/or refer them to the available support services or inform them how to access support from the public health care system.

Caring for someone known previously as a vital and independent individual is incredibly stressful. The caregiver is grieving their loss at the same time as they are looking after their loved one, who often may resist and resent their efforts to help and protect them as the disease progresses. As dementia is a disease that is continuously evolving, robbing the PLWD of their cognitive and physical skills throughout the process, it is important to recognize that the care partner is constantly in a state of anticipatory grief as they witness and mourn the evolving loss of independence and skills of their loved one with dementia. There is also an overwhelming sense of responsibility when it comes to making important daily life and end-of-life decisions on behalf of the person they are caring for.

Caregivers depend on the physician's guidance, support and intervention, but that rarely occurs without a direct request for help from the caregiver. In over 40% of all cases of dementia, there will be at least one member of the informal care team whose own emotional and/or physical health deteriorates to a degree that they are unable to continue looking after their loved one and in most cases, only reach out for support when they have reached a crisis point. Inevitably, this results in feelings of helplessness, grief, anger, guilt and terrible sadness which can lead to coping mechanisms involving excessive amounts of alcohol, cigarettes, drugs, food, gambling and/or shopping, turning into addictive behaviours.

Providing care to PLWD is known to take more time and cause more distress to caregivers than caring for seniors with other issues. On average, caring for a PLWD requires up 26 hours per week of informal versus 17 hours of care for other seniors, and 45 % of caregivers of PLWD exhibit signs of distress compared to 23 % of those caring for seniors without dementia (CIHI, 2018). Logic tells us that a caregiver who is informed about what to expect as the disease progresses and the services available to aid them is more likely to understand what is going on with their loved one and be prepared to access those services. Similarly, a caregiver who is aware of the various safety issues around the home is going to be able to avoid emergencies by making the environment safer for their loved one. Finally, being recognized as a caregiver, and having the difficulties of that role acknowledged, will open the door to asking for and receiving assistance before emotional and/or physical breakdown occur.

What Caregivers Need to Know

Physicians have a role to play in assisting caregivers navigate the dementia journey of a loved one. From the moment that an individual is diagnosed with dementia, their care journey will require the assistance of a multidisciplinary team of health care and legal professionals. All physicians who are in a position to be giving a diagnosis of Mild Cognitive Impairment, Alzheimer's Disease or other dementia-related disease should have on hand material about the disease and resources to help their patients and caregivers understand what they are facing.

Information helps caregivers and the PLWD ensure the best and most appropriate care possible. This could include: knowing the different types of dementia and how they are likely to progress; understanding and responding to challenging behaviours; various treatments that exist for some of the symptoms; how to plan for the future in terms of financial matters; how to provide assistance and support with activities of daily living (dressing, bathing, grooming, eating, etc); the types of care available; and end-of-life choices. Caregivers need to understand at the outset that the disease is constantly evolving, that they will need to constantly adapt to a changing situation, and that they will need help along the way if they wish to remain resilient throughout the journey.

Physicians should be prepared for questions such as: how to communicate with a PLWD throughout the various stages of the disease; how to maintain a connection with a PLWD; what types of activities they can do throughout the various stages of the disease; what are the household safety hazards; when to stop driving; the use of medication or non-pharmacological treatments to manage challenging behaviour; what strategies can be employed to prevent falls and injury; when should transition to a residence/long term care facility be considered. It is also imperative that caregivers know how to access the various public health agencies and resources that are available in their community to assist with home care support, respite and eventual transition to long-term care.

Physicians should remind PLWD and their caregivers to discuss and make their preferred financial, care and living arrangements as soon as possible, unless this has already been determined prior to diagnosis.

Resolution of Clinical Vignette – A Prescription of Care for Informal Caregivers

When diagnosing patients like Mrs. L, it is recommended that the physician take the time to ensure that the primary caregiver is given the following "Prescription of Care":

1. Education about the disease and its progression

Dementia affects the individual both cognitively as well as physically over a 7- to 10-year period. Knowing as much as possible about the disease, how it will progress, and how to plan for the future prepares caregivers for the journey and provides them with the necessary information and tools to ensure the best care possible.

2. Accept the diagnosis and avoid denial

Accepting the diagnosis and learning how to adapt to the various cognitive and physical changes that the disease will place upon the person will allow for best care practices. It is important to recognize that the person with dementia is doing the best they can, and if something is not working, it's the responsibility of the care partner to change their approach and behavior towards the person.

3. Plan for the future

Planning for the future is an important part of the journey as it relates to making decisions concerning health and personal care, living arrangements, finances as well as legal and estate planning. As the disease progresses, it will become difficult to communicate needs and make choices without assistance. While the person with dementia is still able to, it is highly recommended to meet with family members and legal experts in order to arrange for a mandate/notarized power of attorney authorizing someone to legally make decisions on their behalf when they are no longer able.

4. Ensure a safe home environment

As the disease evolves, a person's vision, mobility and cognitive decline will all have a direct impact on their activities of daily living such as cooking, eating, bathing, grooming, dressing, sleeping as well as other facets of their day-to-day life. Keeping the person safe at home thus becomes a priority in order to prevent falls and injuries. Certain rooms in the home such as the kitchen and bathroom, and stairs, have higher risks. Meet with a physical or occupational therapist, recreation therapist or a specialist who can properly assess the home in order to ensure a safe home environment.

5. Identify and accept as much support as possible

Caring for someone with dementia can be one of the most stressful situations for a family member to be faced with and it is not possible to do it alone. In order to prevent caregiver burnout, it is extremely important to identify additional family members, friends, community and/or private resources that can provide assistance with household chores, caregiving tasks, transportation as well as psychological support and respite care. Seek out the necessary support services immediately upon diagnosis in order to understand the various available options in order to be properly prepared.

6. Understanding and responding to challenging behaviour

Dementia often leads to communication challenges and unexpected behaviors from the individual who has the illness. These behaviors can sometimes be attributed to changes in the brain, other health issues, the environment, relationships with others, how the person is spending his/her time as well as the individual's own personality prior to diagnosis. In order for the caregiver to be able to assess what may be causing the individual to respond in a certain way, it is important to understand their personal history prior to diagnosis. Information about previous occupations, personality traits, fears, likes/dislikes, music preferences, milestones, food preferences, body temperature, and activity level can be used to help a caregiver figure out why some behaviours are occurring and ways to address them.

7. The importance of self-care

Caregivers need to preserve as much energy as possible in order to be able to fulfill their daily tasks. It is recommended that they become more protective of personal time and commitments and ensure that they surround themselves as much as possible with people and projects that add positive energy into their lives. Learning to say no and becoming selective of where, how and with whom they invest their time is key. Establishing a regular exercise routine, healthy eating and quality time spent with friends, family and colleagues is important to maintaining a balanced life.

References

1. *Improving the Quality of Life and care of Persons Living with Dementia and their Caregivers*, the Canadian Academy of Health Sciences (CAHS, 2019)
2. *Caregiver Assessment: An Essential Component of Continuing Care Policy* (2014) Janice Keefe, Nancy Guberman, Pamela Fancey and Lucy Barylak.
3. *Alzheimer Society of Canada* - www.alzheimer.ca
4. *"Claire's Prescription of Care"* - Caregiver Crosswalk 2016 -www.carecrosswalk.com
5. *McGill University Dementia Education Program* - www.mcgill.ca/dementia

HOW TO DIAGNOSE AND MANAGE DELIRIUM

Haibin Yin, MD, CCFP(COE)
Assistant Professor, Director of Undergraduate Medical Education,
Division of Geriatric Medicine, McGill University

Clinical vignette

An 84-year-old female living at home with mild mixed dementia and Parkinson's disease was admitted for right intertrochanteric fracture after a fall. Functionally, she required assistance for most instrumental activities of daily living, and could perform most basic activities of daily living. She had 24-hour private help at home.

Her past medical history included congestive heart failure, Parkinson's disease and atrial fibrillation on Coumadin. On POD #2, she began to have visual hallucinations and became disoriented. She also had delusion of persecution. Her mental status fluctuated, from trying to get out of bed to sleepiness. She refused to eat and to take her medications.

She was in abdominal restraints. She was alert and calm, but hesitated for 15 seconds or more to answer questions. Her vital signs were normal. There were no additional heart sounds. Her JVP was slightly elevated. Her lung examination revealed decreased air entry bilaterally. Her abdomen was soft and bowel sounds were present. Her wound was clean with no surrounding edema. Both lower extremities were edematous (R>L) but non-tender. There were no neurovascular damages distally. She had bilateral upper extremity resting tremors and cogwheeling rigidity.

Her medications included Morphine 1.25mg SQ q 2 hours PRN (none taken in past 24 hours), Haldol 0.5mg IM tid PRN (received 2 doses in past 24 hours), Sinemet 100/25 1 PO tid, Coumadin 5mg PO qd with Lovenox (prophylactic dose) bridging and Lasix 20mg PO bid. What could be the potential causes of this patient's delirium and how should it be managed?

What is delirium? Why is it important to recognize it?

Delirium is also known as acute brain failure, toxic-metabolic encephalopathy or acute confusional state. DSM-V defines it as acute changes (with fluctuating course) in attention, awareness and cognition, that are caused by an underlying medical condition or medication. Different studies show that it affects one third of patients over 70 years old on general medical units, amongst which half are delirious on admission. Among geriatric patients in the Emergency Room, 15% are delirious. In the ICU, prevalence could reach 70%.

The most useful tool for diagnosing delirium is the Confusion Assessment method (Table 1). This systematic-review-validated tool reaches sensitivity and specificity of over 90%. It has also been adapted for patients in the ICU (CAM-ICU). Other tools (Delirium Symptom Index, The 4-AT Test etc.) could also be used.

The pathophysiology of delirium is poorly understood. Several hypotheses include primary or secondary neuroinflammation and cholinergic deficiency. The predisposing factors of delirium include old age, functional impairment, cognitive deficits, multiple medical comorbidities and sensory impairment. The precipitating factors can include many medical conditions, medications and interventions (restraints, indwelling devices etc.).

TABLE 1: Confusion Assessment Method (Positive if criteria 1,2,3 or 1,2,4 are present)
1. Acute change in mental status from baseline and fluctuation in behaviour during the day, AND
2. Attention impaired, easily distractible, difficulty keeping track of what is being said, AND
3. Disorganized/incoherent thinking or illogical conversation, OR
4. Altered mental status (hyperalert, lethargic, difficult to arouse)

One of the reasons why it is important to recognize and manage delirium is its poor outcome. A meta-analysis which follows 3000 patients for 2 years showed that delirium was associated with a 2-fold increase in death, 2.4-fold in institutionalization and 12.5-fold in new dementia. Despite traditional view that delirium was a transient and reversible condition, recent evidence has shown that persistence of delirium occurs in many patients, and is associated with poor long-term outcomes.

Unfortunately, despite this, delirium is often underrecognized by physicians. Several factors could explain this reality. Firstly, hyperactive delirium, which is the most noticeable subtype, represents only 25% of the cases. Hypoactively delirious patients attract less attention of the medical team, despite their poorer prognosis. Secondly, physicians often have a snapshot of their patient once per day, however, by definition, delirium is a fluctuating syndrome. Thirdly, diagnosing delirium could be time-consuming as it often involves detailed interview with collateral historians as well as chart reviews to identify the acute change and fluctuation. Finally, in some cases, delirium could be difficult to distinguish from other conditions, such as Lewy Body dementia, depression and mania. Therefore, clinicians should always have a high index of suspicion and be diligent in their assessments.

What are the causes (precipitating factors) of delirium? How to investigate?

The causes of delirium are vast. Any acute medical illness or medication can precipitate delirium. Infections are the most commonly diagnosed. Any infection has the potential of being the underlying cause. The presence of asymptomatic bacteruria, however, often leads to a misdiagnosis of UTI causing delirium. Recent studies show that antibiotic therapy in these patients does not change the course of delirium. Electrolyte imbalances, especially of sodium, calcium and glucose, could cause delirium. Cortisol excess or insufficiency could be manifested as hyperactive and hypoactive delirium, respectively. In patients with history of falls presenting with delirium, intracranial bleeding should be considered in the differential diagnosis. In patients with hypoactive delirium, particular attention should be paid to rule out hypoxia and CNS infections. In patients with cirrhosis, hepatic encephalopathy should be ruled out. Hypoxia or shock due to any cause could cause acute confusion due to brain hypoperfusion. In patients that develop delirium days after admission, alcohol or benzodiazepine withdrawal should be considered. Other precipitants include physical restraints, indwelling devices (Foley catheters, central venous catheters etc.), immobility, urinary retention, fecal impaction and uncontrolled pain.

Many medications can precipitate delirium. Common candidates are benzodiazepines, opioids, anticholinergics, antiparkinsonians, antipsychotics, antidepressants (especially TCAs and MAOIs) and NSAIDs.

In order to summarize the above precipitants, the following mnemonics provided by Wise, M.G. (1986) is helpful (Table 2):

Taking history of delirium (mostly taken with the collateral historian) should include a detailed timeline of the acute confusion as well as symptoms leading to or co-occuring with the onset of the acute confusion. A detailed review of systems could help diagnose the underlying causes of delirium. A thorough medication review is important not only for deciphering changes that can contribute to the acute confusion, but also for addressing polypharmacy which could potentially prolong and exacerbate delirium. Past medical history can also provide cues because acute exacerbation or decompensation of many chronic medical conditions could lead to delirium.

On physical examination, the general appearance can provide information such as hydration status, nutritional status, attention and sensorium. Special attention should be given to vital signs. For example, hypotension and tachycardia could indicate ischemia, sepsis or severe dehydration. Fever could indicate infection or pulmonary embolism. Desaturation could indicate cardiac and pulmonary causes. A thorough physical examination should be focused on the potential underlying acute medical conditions. A well-documented mental status examination could help clinicians track the evolution of delirium. If possible, a mini-mental status examination could be done to quantify the cognitive changes during delirium, which could serve the purpose of a point of comparison when delirium improves in the future.

TABLE 2: Causes of delirium – I WATCH DEATH
I – infectious: pneumonia, UTI, CNS infections, abscesses, osteomyelitis, endocarditis etc.
W – withdrawal: from benzodiazepines, alcohol
A – Acute metabolic changes: acidosis/alkalosis, hypo/hyperNa, hypo/hyper Ca, acute kidney and liver failure
T – Trauma: Intracranial bleeding, brain injury
C – CNS pathology : Intracranial tumor, post-ictal state
H – Hypoxia : Anemia, pulmonary embolism, CHF, myocardial infarctions
D – Deficiencies: Vitamin B1, B12
E – Endocrine: hypo/hypercortisol, hypoglycemia
A – Acute vascular : hypertensive emergency, stroke
T – Toxins and drugs : benzodiazepines, opioids, anticholinergics
H – Heavy metals

What initial investigations should be requested for delirium?

Investigations should include basic laboratory tests, including complete blood count, biochemistry profile (including urea, creatinine, calcium and magnesium), glucose, coagulation profile, TSH, Vitamin B12, and liver function tests. An EKG could be ordered, not only to identify potential cardiac causes if indicated by history, but also to document baseline QTc, as many medications (including antipsychotics and antibiotics) have potential to cause QTc prolongation.

Other investigations may be required depending on the history and examination. If the patient is febrile, septic work-up (blood cultures, urine analysis and culture, CxR etc.) should be ordered before starting antibiotics. If there is suspicion of meningitis or encephalitis, a lumber puncture should be done. Urine or serum toxicology should be ordered if there is suspicion of medication, alcohol and drug toxicity. For patients with suspicion of hypoxemia, hypercapnia or shock, arterial blood gas and lactate could be ordered. If cardiac ischemia is suspected, serial troponins should be ordered. For patients with history of falls, CT-head should be considered. For patients with suspicion of urinary retention, a post-void residual should be obtained.

Table 3 summarizes initial work-up for patients with delirium.

TABLE 3: Investigations for delirium	
Essential	CBC, SMA-10, glucose; INR, PTT; TSH; Vitamin B12, LFTs, ECG
May be required	Blood cultures x 2, Urinalysis and culture, Urine toxicology Lactate, Venous Blood Gas, Serial Troponins, EtOH level
	Post-void residual, Tot & conj Bilirubin, Albumin, Amylase CT-head, Chest X-ray

How to manage delirium

Most patients with delirium require hospitalization, not only for investigation and medical therapy purposes, but also for behavioral management, to manage acute functional deficits, to manage complications and for rehabilitation. For the management of neuropsychiatric symptoms of delirium, a non-pharmacological approach is favoured. For aggressive patients, distraction and de-escalation strategies should be adopted. For patients with day-night reversal, it is important to promote good sleep hygiene by ensuring adequate light during the day and darkness at night. For all patients with delirium, physical restraints should be avoided, as they not only prolong delirium and cause immobilization syndrome, but also increase risk of strangulation. Ensuring proper hydration and nutrition could prevent delirium from worsening. It is also important to monitor and prevent the development of pressure ulcers. It is important to compensate for patients' sensorial deficits, by encouraging uses of glasses and hearing aids. Orientation cues such as photos of family members and calendar, should be used if possible. Early mobilization could be helpful to prevent deconditioning and immobilization syndrome. Occupational therapy assessments are helpful for discharge planning purposes when delirium improves.

When and how to use medications for behavioral disturbances?

Non-pharmacological approaches should almost always be attempted first to curb agitation. One of the only circumstances where pharmacological approaches should be used first is if the patient's agitation poses a risk of self-harm or a threat to others.

Antipsychotics such as Haloperidol, Quetiapine, Risperidone, Olanzapine and Ziprasidone are first-line pharmacological treatments for agitation in delirium. Haloperidol is the most efficient against aggression, however, high doses of haloperidol (>4.5mg per day) are associated with an increase in extrapyramidal side effects. Based on limited evidence, it is recommended that low-dose haloperidol (0.5mg to 1.0mg PO or IM) should be used for the control of agitation and psychotic symptoms, up to a maximum of 3mg per day. Its onset is 30 to 60 minutes after parenteral administration, longer if PO. Please note that IV haloperidol should be avoided due to QTc prolongation. Seroquel is the most sedating antipsychotic, and causes less extrapyramidal signs and symptoms. Its main limitation is that it can only be given per os. Its starting dose is 12.5mg to 25mg with a maximum dose of 50mg per day.

It is worth mentioning that a recent meta-analysis of randomized trials showed that antipsychotics do not alter the duration or severity of delirium, and do not reduce ICU admissions or mortality. Therefore, clinicians should be cautious when prescribing antipsychotics, by weighing apparent benefits with the risks of antipsychotic side-effects and complications (i.e. falls, stroke, increased mortality).

Benzodiazepines are second-line agents, due to respiratory depression, paradoxical excitation, fall risk and oversedation. However, benzodiazepines such as Ativan could be used first-line in specific situations where antipsychotic use should be avoided. These include patients with seizures, in those in alcohol or benzodiazepine withdrawal, and in those with a history of neuroleptic malignant syndrome or Lewy Body Dementia (who are very sensitive to antipsychotics).

Benadryl, Gravol and other medications with significant anticholinergic effects should be avoided, as they may exacerbate and prolong delirium.

All medications for agitation should be discontinued as soon as possible and should usually not be continued beyond the hospitalization for delirium. In the minority of patients who require antipsychotics on discharge, caution needs to be exerted so that the prescription has a finite duration and should be reassessed frequently with appropriate follow-up.

Table 4 summarizes the above choices of initial pharmacological regimen.

TABLE 4: Pharmacological management of hyperactive delirium – Standard order
• Risperidone 0.25-0.5 mg PO bid PRN
• Haloperidol 0.5-1mg PO/IM q1h PRN severe agitation. Reassess after 3 doses.
• If patient has history of Parkinson's disease or Lewy Body Dementia:
• Seroquel 12.5mg PO bid PRN agitation. Lorazepam 0.5-1mg IM q1h PRN severe agitation. Reassess after 3 doses.

Conclusion

As the population ages, clinicians will encounter delirium more frequently as more patients have dementia and have multiple comorbidities. Prompt and efficient management of delirium is essential to preserve a patient's cognition and function, and of course, to decrease mortality.

Among non-delirious hospitalized patients who are at risk, prevention techniques such as the HELP (Hospital Elder Life Program) could reduce the incidence of delirium. One area of research also focuses on finding a delirium risk-prediction score. Hospital resources could then be used to provide prevention techniques targeting those patients who are at high risk of developing delirium, with the potential to decrease its sometimes-catastrophic consequences.

The clinical vignette revisited

Pre-operatively, this patient was already at high risk for delirium, due to her age, dementia, functional impairment and multiple comorbidities. Initial investigations mentioned above should be performed. The potential causes and management plan are summarized in the following table:

The non-pharmacological management of this patient includes removal of restraints, early mobilization, nutrition and speech-language pathology consult and promotion of night-time sleep.

Possible causes of patient's delirium	Management plan
Opioids (morphine)	Change to Dilaudid, and consider regular Dilaudid for 6-12 hours as delirious patients might not ask for pain medications
CHF exacerbation due to overhydration	Chest X-ray; increase Lasix if needed
Anemia due to blood loss	Follow Hb, transfuse if needed
Right lower extremity DVT	Venous Duplex
Worsening of Parkinson's disease due to Haldol and refusal to take Sinemet	Change Sinemet to equivalent dose per rectum
	Use Seroquel PO or Ativan IM for agitation if non-pharmacological approaches fail

Uncontrolled pain	Monitor and manage pain
Constipation	Mobilization, laxatives, DRE to R/O impaction
Urinary retention	PVR, in/out if needed
Stroke despite Coumadin bridging	Thorough neurological examination, CT/CTA head if high suspicion
Aspiration pneumonia due to Parkinsonism	Chest X-ray

FURTHER READING

1. Wise, M. G. (1986). Delirium. In R. E. Hales & S. C. Yudofsky (Eds.), American Psychiatric Press Textbook of Neuropsychiatry (pp. 89–103). Washington, DC: American Psychiatric Press Inc.
2. Marcantonio, E. R. Delirium in Hospitalized Older Adults. N Engl J Med 2017; 377:1456-1466. DOI: 10.1056/NEJMcp1605501
3. Chew, M.L. Anticholinergic activity of 107 medications commonly used by older adults. J Amer Geri Soc 2008; 56,7:1333-1341. DOI: 10.1111/j.1532-5415.2008.01737.

WHY DOES MY PATIENT HAVE GAIT & BALANCE DISORDERS?

Olivier Beauchet, MD, PhD

Professor of Geriatrics, Dr. Joseph Kaufmann Chair in Geriatric Medicine, Director of centre of excellence on aging and chronic diseases,
McGill University

Patient Scenario

An 87-year-old woman walks into your office unaided, without any noticeable gait abnormality. She reports that she has balance difficulties with fear of falling but denied any fall. The patient's medication list includes amlodipine 5 mg QD, metformin 500 mg BI, aspirin 80 md QD, atorvastatin 10 mg, donepezil 5 mg QD and temazepam as needed for sleep. Her body mass index is 18 kg/m². The daughter hands you an X-ray report indicating that the patient has severe osteoporosis, moderate spinal (cervical and lumbar) osteoarthritis associated with dorsal kyphosis.

Since your patient has a high risk of falls, you would like to determine the reason of balance complaints to decide whether she needs specific interventions.

Why is this question important?

Gait - the medical term used to describe the human locomotion - and balance disorders are prevalent in older individuals. It is difficult to ascertain prevalence as no accepted definition exists. However, it is estimated that at least 35 percent of individuals 65 and older report difficulty walking three city blocks or climbing one flight of stairs, and approximately 20 percent require the use of a mobility aid to ambulate. The prevalence of gait and balance disorders can reach 80 percent in the oldest-old (i.e., ≥ 85 years) individuals who live in residence.

Gait and balance characteristics change over the individual's lifetime with a decline of performance. Gait and balance disorders are usually defined as a decrease of performance (for instance, a slow gait speed) causing instability and falls. Gait and balance disorders are the most common cause of falls in individuals 65 and older. They are associated with an increased morbidity and mortality, disability, loss of independence, institutionalization and limited quality of life. Early identification and appropriate interventions may prevent gait and balance disorders and their related adverse consequences.

Which are the causes of gait and balance disorders?

Gait and balance disorders are usually multifactorial in origin and require a comprehensive assessment to determine contributing factors and targeted interventions. Most changes in gait and balance that occur in older individuals are related to physiological aging of the sensorimotor system combined with adverse consequences of chronic and acute medical conditions. The causes of gait and balance disorders fall under three categories of factors:

- The predisposing factors which are individually related and result from adverse consequences of physiological aging of the sensorimotor system combined with chronic medical conditions leading to chronic gait and balance instability.
- The precipitating factors which may be separated in two subtypes: those related to individual acute medical conditions and those related to physical activity inducing gait and balance instability.
- The environment combined with the physical activity while falling.

There is a complex synergic interaction between factors provoking gait and balance instability, explaining why gait and balance instability may fluctuate with time.

The main chronic medical conditions which affect gait and balance stability are:
- Visual impairment with abnormal distance vision including low visual acuity and low contrast sensitivity.
- Lower limb proprioception impairment.
- Lower limb poor muscle mass and strength.

- Lower limb joint deformity, podiatric abnormalities and back deformity (e.g.; kyphosis, scoliosis) related to osteoarthritis and osteoporosis.
- Obesity.
- Myelopathy.
- Normal-pressure hydrocephalus.
- Parkinson disease.
- Cerebellar dysfunction or degeneration.
- Vascular brain disease.
- Vestibular disorders.
- Cognitive impairment: from mild cognitive impairment to severe dementia.
- Depression.
- Fear of falling.

Any acute medical condition may increase gait and balance instability within hours and cause a motor deconditioning (i.e.; loss of body postural reflexes and inability to stand up and/or walk without assistance) in older individuals with predisposing factors to gait and balance disorders.

Who should be screened for gait and balance disorders?

- Adults aged 65 and over should be asked about or examined for gait and balance disorders at least once per year.
- Adults aged 65 and over who report a fall or have an acute medical condition should be asked about difficulties with gait and balance, and should be examined for gait and balance disorders.

What is the clinical assessment?

Clinical assessment should be separated into two main parts: global and analytic clinical assessment. The global assessment detecting gait and balance difficulties begins with watching individuals as they rise from a chair or as they walk into the examination room. The use of a walking aide and its nature (i.e.; cane, walker, personal assistance and supervision) should be noticed and the individual should be asked about his/her subjective perception of gait and balance difficulties using a single question: "Do you have any difficulty walking?" with a graduated answer (i.e., never, almost never, sometimes, often, and very often).

This visual observation should be completed with three standardized motor tests providing an objective measure of gait and balance performance: The Timed up & Go (TUG) test, the five time to sit to stand test and the gait speed (distance divided by ambulation time) when walking a distance of 4 meters at a steady-state pace. The TUG measures in seconds the time it takes an individual to rise from a chair, walk a distance of 3 meters, turn, walk back to the chair and sit down. This test has been used extensively in geriatric medicine to examine balance, gait speed, and functional ability that would be required for the performance of basic activities of daily living in older people. A score ≥ 20 second should be considered as an abnormal performance. The Five-Times-Sit-to-Stand test (FTSS) measures in seconds the time it takes an individual to stand up from a chair five times as quickly as possible. This clinical test explores postural control and lower limb muscular strength. A score ≥ 15 seconds should be considered as an abnormal performance. Walking speed is a simple, objective, performance-based measure of lower limb neuromuscular function which not only allows detection of subtle impairments and preclinical diseases, but also is a sensitive marker of functional capacity in older adults. A gait speed at usual pace under 1 m/s should also be considered as abnormal.

The analytic clinical assessment includes collection of:

- Demographic (i.e., age in years and sex) and anthropometric items (height in meters [m], weight in kilograms [kg], body mass index (BMI) in kg/m^2), should be systematically assessed because each may influence gait and balance stability. In addition, the place of living should be considered as a binary variable home versus institution, and an institutionalized individual should be considered to have a higher risk of gait and balance disorders.

- Given that the burden of disease can influence gait and balance performance, it is important to assess this information as well. Different scales have been developed to score morbidity burden, but they remain difficult to use in clinical routine among older adults, especially because of possible recall bias in individuals with cognitive disorders, and lack of feasibility in daily practice. Medication data, including the number of drugs taken daily provides a global measure of morbidity status, and has been associated with physician-rated disease severity as well as with individual-rated health status. Hence, recording the use of drugs in the clinical assessment is required. Polypharmacy is defined as use of more than four different medications per day. The use of psychoactive drugs (i.e., benzodiazepines, antidepressants, neuroleptics), needs to be specially recorded.

- Information about falls, with a fall being defined as an event resulting in a person coming to rest unintentionally on the ground or at another lower level, not as the result of a major intrinsic event or an overwhelming hazard, in the previous 12 months period before the assessment, should be recorded. Information on recurrence (i.e.; >2 falls) and severity (defined as fractures, cranial trauma, large and/or deep skin lesion, post-fall syndrome (including an association of fear of falling (FOF), postural instability with absence of postural reflexes), inability to get up alone from ground, time on the ground > one hour, and hospitalization) are proposed for the data collection.
- FOF using the single question: "Are you afraid of falling?" with a graded answer (i.e., never, almost never, sometimes, often, and very often) should be asked to the patient as FOF is associated with a greater gait and/or balance instability.
- Collecting information on disorders or diseases that directly influence gait performance is also recommended. First, information on neurological disease (limited to the existence or non-existence of dementia) and other diseases (coded as yes or no) should be collected. Information on memory complaints, MCI, nature of dementia (i.e., Alzheimer Disease (AD), non-AD neurodegenerative, non-AD vascular, mixed), Parkinson disease, idiopathic normal pressure hydrocephalus, cerebellar disease, stroke, myelopathy and peripheral neuropathy should be recorded. A quantification of global cognitive functioning is also recommended, using for example The Mini Mental State Examination (/30) and The Montreal Cognitive Assessment (MoCA) if MMSE score is above 19/30.
- In addition, among the neuropsychiatric disorders, it is important to collect information about depression symptoms because they can lead to gait instability and falls. The 4-item geriatric depression scale should be used as a screening test. A measure of anxiety is also proposed using the 5-item Geriatric Anxiety Inventory.
- Information on major orthopaedic diagnoses (e.g., osteoarthritis) involving the lumbar vertebrae, pelvis or lower extremities, coded yes versus no, as well as the use of a walking aids, should also be recorded.

- Information on sensory and motor subsystems such as muscle strength, lower-limb proprioception and vision are required because the age-related impairment in the performance of these subsystems may affect gait performance. First, the maximum isometric voluntary contraction (MVC) of hand grip strength must be measured with a hydraulic dynamometer. The test should be performed three times with the dominant hand. The mean value of MVC over the three trials should be used as the outcome measure. Second, distance binocular vision should be measured at a fixed distance with a standard scale. Vision needs to be assessed with corrective lenses if used regularly. Third, lower-limb proprioception should be evaluated with a graduated tuning fork placed on the tibial tuberosity measuring vibration threshold.

Is there a need for complementary investigations?

The role of laboratory testing and diagnostic evaluation for gait and balance disorders has not been well studied.

There is no systematic investigation recommended to perform. The following complementary investigations are recommended:

- Bone radiography in the event of acute pain, joint deformation and/or functional disability.
- Standard 12-lead ECG in case of dizziness.
- Blood glucose level in patients with diabetes.
- Serum 25OHD concentration if there is no vitamin D supplementation.

Cerebral imaging in the absence of specific indication based upon the clinical examination may not be necessary.

Which are the possible interventions?

It is recommended to suggest to the patient with gait and balance disorders, irrespective of the place of living, an intervention combining several of the following domains:

- When possible, a revision of the medications to ascertain if the patient takes fall-related drugs (please see above) and/or the number of drugs is >5.
- The correction or the treatment of predisposing or modifiable precipitating factors (including environmental risk factors of falls);

- The wearing of shoes with broad, low heels (2 to 3 cm), and firm, thin soles with a high upper;
- The regular practice of walking and/or any other physical activity (the duration of exercise for prevention of recurrent falls remains unclear);
- A dietary calcium intake ranging from 1 to 1,5 gram per day;
- The use of an adapted walking aid;
- The correction of a potential vitamin D deficiency by a daily dose of at least 800IU.

It is recommended to prescribe physiotherapy, including:
- Working on static and dynamic postural balance;
- Increasing of the strength and muscular power of the lower limbs.
- Other techniques, including stimulation of sensory afferents or learning to stand up from the ground, may also be proposed.

Such interventions may involve rehabilitation professionals, such as occupational therapists. A regular physical activity should be performed at low to moderate intensity exercise. It is recommended to perform rehabilitation exercises with a professional, as well as between therapy sessions and after each session, in order to extend rehabilitation benefits to the daily life.

Scenario resolution

Your patient requires a specific gait and balance assessment as she is an oldest-old (i.e.; > 85 years) lady who reports balance difficulties.

Based on the information provided by the list of medications and the daughter, you can conclude that she has an objective gait and balance disorder caused by an accumulation of chronic medical conditions, which are:
- A polypharmacy: Six different medications are taken daily.
- A lower limb diabetic polyneuropathy causing proprioceptive impairment.
- An abnormal static posture due to spinal osteoarthritis and osteoporosis deformaties
- A poor muscle mass and strength because of a malnutrition status (body mass index score 18 kg/m^2).
- A cognitive impairment due to a dementia because of the prescription of donepezil.

You can confirm you first analysis by performing a TUG test.

You can propose:

- To discontinue the temazepam,
- To continue anti-osteoporotic treatment and vitamin D supplementation.
- To a regular practice of walking and/or any other physical activity.

You can prescribe physiotherapy including:

- Working on static and dynamic postural balance.
- Increasing of the strength and muscular power of the lower limbs.

References

1. Nutt JG. Classification of gait and balance disorders. Adv Neurol 2001;87:135-141.
2. Seidler RD, Bernard JA, Burutolu TB, Fling BW, Gordon MT, Gwin JT, Kwak Y, Lipps DB. Motor control and aging: links to age-related brain structural, functional, and biochemical effects. Neurosci Biobehav Rev 2010;34:721-733.
3. Beauchet O, Dubost V, Revel Delhom C, Berrut G, Belmin J, French Society of Geriatrics and Gerontology. How to manage recurrent falls in clinical practice: guidelines of the French Society of Geriatrics and Gerontology. J Nutr Health Aging 2011; 15:79-84
4. Panel on Prevention of Falls in Older Persons, American Geriatrics Society and British Geriatrics Society. Summary of the Updated American Geriatrics Society/British Geriatrics Society clinical practice guideline for prevention of falls in older persons. J Am Geriatr Soc 2011; 59:148-157.
5. Salzman B. Gait and balance disorders in older adults. Am Fam Physician. 2010;82:61-68.

COULD MY PATIENT BE MALNOURISHED?

Jose A. Morais, MD, FRCP(C)

Professor, Faculty of Medicine, Director, Division of Geriatric Medicine, Lead,
Dementia Education Program, McGill University, Co-Director, Quebec Network for Research on Aging

Clinical vignette

An 82 year old widow has a 4.5 kg weight loss over the last 6 months following the death of her beloved husband. Her present BMI is 21 kg/m^2 and her triceps skinfold thickness is in the 10th percentile for age. She is known to have diabetes and osteoarthritis of both knees for which she uses a walker for indoor mobility. She denies being depressed, but her family physician prescribed a tricyclic antidepressant medication, soon after the death of her spouse. Since then, she complains of dry mouth with difficulty swallowing food and is constipated. Her other medications are metformin 850 mg BID and naprosyn 250 mg BID. The pertinent blood tests available disclosed an albumin of 38 g/L, CRP 2 mg/L, A1C 6%, creatinine 98 umol/L.

Since involuntary weight loss in older adults should always be taken seriously, there is a need to ascertain the presence of malnutrition, determine its risk factors, and propose a plan for assessment and management.

Why is malnutrition an important clinical problem?

Malnutrition is common in older people and in those who are frail and ill. In the healthy community-dwelling older person, its prevalence is about 2-5%, whereas in the frail, dependent elderly, it can reach 20-30%. In those living in nursing homes or in hospital, levels as high as 50-70% have been reported.

Malnutrition or more precisely, undernutrition, is a state of reduced food intake below recommended daily allowances that leads to loss of body mass (weight) and functional impairment. The functional deficiencies comprise physical performance such as grip strength and gait speed, immunocompetence and tissue repair capacity. As a consequence, malnourished older persons have higher risks of falls and fractures, delirium, depression, cognitive deficits, infections, hospitalisations with prolonged stay, decubitus ulcers and death.

Other terminologies are often used in conjunction with malnutrition. These are protein-energy malnutrition (PEM), anorexia, wasting, cachexia and sarcopenia. PEM refers to a global decrease in food intake with its health consequences and is equivalent to undernutrition/malnutrition; anorexia is a lack of appetite and wasting that is synonymous with loss of body mass. Wasting follows a lack of appetite without inflammation, and therefore, a preferential loss of adipose tissue over muscle mass is a predominant feature. Cachexia on the other hand is a catabolic condition often involving a high degree of inflammation from a disease such as cancer or congestive heart failure. Its prominent feature is suppression of appetite with proportionally more muscle loss than adipose tissue and with fatigue. Sarcopenia refers to a selective loss of muscle mass and strength associated with aging that has a large number of factors contributing to its development.

What are the risk factors for malnutrition?

Older adults are predisposed to anorexia due to intrinsic as well as exogenous causes. At the intrinsic physiological level, one needs to consider the adjustment of energy balance that occurs with aging. Aging is associated with loss of lean body mass, especially muscle mass, a metabolically active tissue, and therefore its loss leads to a decrease in the basal metabolic rate (energy spent at rest to maintain bodily functions). Furthermore, since there is also a progressive decline in physical activity, the total amount of energy ingested needs to be reduced, otherwise the elderly would gain considerable weight over time.

A theoretical model of anorexia of aging proposes a dysregulation of the appetite control center in the hypothalamus. This dysregulation is in part related to changes in brain neurotransmitters, such as NPY and dynorphin, the latter decreasing the pleasure associated with meals. It is also recognized that there is a higher circulating gastrointestinal peptide cholecystokinin (CCK) upon food ingestion, which is a potent central anorexigen. At the fundus of the stomach, there is reduced nitric oxide production with meals which contributes to a lesser relaxation of the stomach, therefore contributing to a precocious sensation of fullness. Older persons have also alterations in their taste perception from changes in the odor and taste capacities. Thirst perception is equally affected with age, which predisposes to dehydration.

Although the above factors are present with aging, they are not by themselves responsible for the decrease in food intake of older persons. Multiple other causes contribute as well. These include:

- Uncontrolled medical conditions that predispose to anorexia through the effect of inflammatory mediators (TNF-α and cytokines), pain, distress, lethargy, delirium, etc.
- Social-economic factors including isolation, poverty and institutionalization
- Masticatory and swallowing difficulties: e.g., poor fitting dentures and dysphagia
- Decrease in functional capacity caused by mobility problems, poor endurance and multiple co-morbidities, which affect the capability to purchase food and prepare meals
- Mental and cognitive disorders e.g., depression and dementia
- Peculiar habits such as aversion to certain foods and alcoholism
- Medications, in particular: digoxin, SSRIs, NSAIDs, metformin, antibiotics and psychoactive drugs

It is often difficult to distinguish a single factor as responsible in the vast majority of the cases, as more often several factors interact. The above pathological/physiological/environmental changes can be summarised in a mnemonic MEALS-ON-WHEELS, proposed by Morley EJ and Silver AJ Ann Intern Med 1995;123:850-9.

Below is an algorithm to assist in evaluating causes of PEM. In general it is helpful to determine if the patient is eating well despite losing weight. If it is the case, the patient is either suffering from malabsorption (a relatively easy diagnosis to make because of GI symptoms) or having increased needs for energy in conditions such as hyperthyroidism, diabetes, cancer, chronic infections or advanced COPD or CHF.

Factors Contributing to Malnutrition

MEALS ON WHEELS acronym helps to remember the common risk factors and causes of undernutrition in older adults

Medications (polypharmacy, herbal preparations)

Emotional causes (dysphoria, depression, psychosis)

Appetite disorders (anorexia tardive, abnormal eating attitudes)

Late-life paranoia (social isolation)

Swallowing disorders

Oral factors (tooth loss, periodontal infections, gingivitis, poorly fitting dentures)

No money (poverty)

Wandering (dementia)

Hyperactivity/hypermetabolism (tremors, movement disorders, thyrotoxicosis)

Enteral problems (chronic diarrhea, malabsorption syndromes)

Eating problems (altered food preferences, decreased taste and flavor perception)

Low-nutrient diets (low-salt, low-cholesterol, antidiabetic, fad diets)

Shopping and food-preparation problems (impaired mobility, unsafe environment, inadequate transportation)

On the other hand, if the patient is not eating well, then a first step is to verify accessibility to food (poverty, mobility issues and meal preparation). If these are not factors, then consider masticatory and swallowing difficulties. If these are not an issue, it is likely that we are facing a case of anorexia from medications, depression, dementia or multi-morbidity.

Diagnostic evaluation of PEM

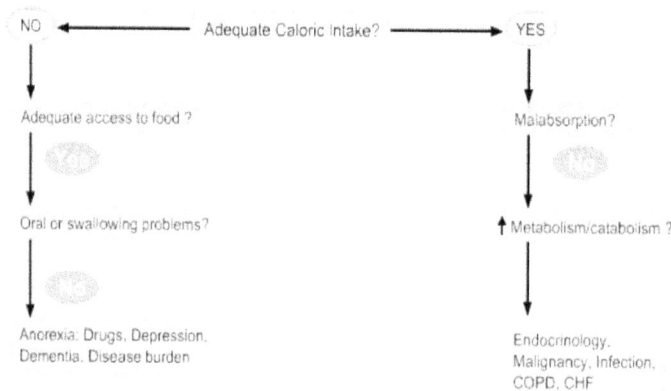

NO ←——————— Adequate Caloric Intake? ———————→ YES

Adequate access to food ?   Malabsorption?

Oral or swallowing problems?   ↑ Metabolism/catabolism ?

Anorexia, Drugs, Depression,   Endocrinology,
Dementia, Disease burden   Malignancy, Infection,
                                                   COPD, CHF

How is the diagnosis of malnutrition made?

On history taking, one reliable but often-ignored parameter of malnutrition is weight loss. A history of 5-10 % weight loss over 6 months (> 3 kg) or 2-3% in 1-2 months, is a significant amount that threatens the general health. Changes in food habits for any reason (difficulty swallowing, poverty) and GI symptoms (nausea, abdominal cramps, and diarrhea) are other important items of information. Any new drugs being prescribed? Typically, one eats three meals a day and eating less frequently puts one at risk. Food assessment is done by a registered dietician through different of dietary intake assessment methods, each with its own limitations.

On physical examination, in addition to a low weight for height or a low body mass index (BMI) < 22 kg/m^2, signs of ascites/edema or decreased skin turgor are suggestive of malnutrition. Loss of typical roundness of the face, shoulder and buttocks is often encountered as well as muscle loss at the temporal areas, biceps, thigh and calf. Specific vitamin deficiencies leading to angular stomatitis of the mouth and glossitis are late signs. All of these signs become more difficult to assess in the elderly due to lack of specificity and sensitivity. For example, a decrease in skin elasticity with aging and other causes such as venous stasis contribute to peripheral edema. Typically, it is the dietitian who carries out the relevant anthropometric measurements (body and limb circumferences and skinfold thickness). Values below the 15th percentile for sex and age are very suggestive of malnutrition. Physical performance tests such as handgrip strength using a dynamometer may corroborate the diagnosis.

At the laboratory level, the serum albumin level is the most useful parameter. This protein is produced by the hepatocytes when adequate amino acids and energy are available. The total body albumin pool is about 300 g with 1/3 lying in the interstitial space and its half-life is 20 days. The albumin value doesn't need to be at 35 g/L to be considered low. Any value below 40 g/L puts the patient at risk, although typically values < 38 g/L are used as cut-off for malnutrition. If coupled with a low cholesterol value of < 4 mmol/L, the likelihood of malnutrition is greatly augmented. Despite adequate dietary intake of both energy and protein, albumin and pre-albumin are decreased in 1) the presence of inflammation (cancer, immunological disorders, trauma, and infections), 2) patients who have received large amounts of intravenous fluids (dilutional), 3) protein losing enteropathies (losses through the gut) or 4) nephropathies (losses through the kidney). On the other hand, albumin in the interstitial space can be recruited to the circulation during periods of poor intake without inflammation, which is the case in simple anorexia (wasting).

Measurement of pre-albumin values is rarely required, since it is under the same regulatory control as albumin. It may however be useful in monitoring the response to a nutritional intervention due to its half-life of 2 days. Cut-off values for undernutrition are below 180 mg/L.

Low hemoglobin and lymphocyte counts are less specific and are a late manifestation of malnutrition. In the absence of any other cause, a lymphocyte count below 800 cells/mL is however a sign of severe malnutrition. Anergy testing is rarely performed but would likely demonstrate a reduced immune response.

Useful tools for the diagnosis of malnutrition

There is no single parameter with the requisite sensitivity and specificity; thus, it is recommended that a combination of 3 or 4 indices from different domains (history, physical examination and investigation) be assessed. In this regard, several screening and diagnostic tools are available. Among these, two have received significant attention, the Mini Nutritional Assessment (MNA) and the Subjective Global Assessment (SGA).

The MNA has been validated in many settings, including long term care and acute care hospital sites and can be used to screen and diagnose early undernutrition in frail persons. It comprises items that are related to cognition, mental and physical function as well as dietary intake and anthropometric measurements. The total possible score is 30--values below 17 are diagnostic of malnutrition, between 17-24 suggest a risk of malnutrition and above 24, signify good nutritional status. A shorter version based on the first 14 points of the MNA exists that is almost as reliable as the full version for screening and has the merit of precluding a full assessment if values are 12 or higher. If score of the shorter version is < 11, one should perform the full MNA. The MNA formula can be downloaded at no cost: http://www.mna-elderly.com/mna_forms.html

The SGA is a clinical assessment of nutrition status based on history and physical examination. In taking a history, one reviews changes in dietary intake, weight loss, GI symptoms and functional capacity and on physical examination, one should look for signs of undernutrition, including ascites and edema. It requires only minimal training. The rater then classifies patients subjectively as well-nourished, mildly/moderately malnourished or severely malnourished. This tool has been validated with respect to clinical outcomes and has a good inter-observer agreement. The form can be downloaded at no cost: http://nutritioncareincanada.ca/

What are the interventions to reverse malnutrition?

Before proposing an intervention, it is necessary to determine the factors contributing to undernutrition in the specific case instance (review the mnemonic MEALS-ON-WHEELS). Intervention can be as broad as helping with meal preparation, providing spoon feeding or diagnosing an underlying medical condition.

The first step in the management of undernutrition consists in identifying and treating the underlying causative factors. If the nutrition status does not show improvement in 1 week with this first-line approach, than nutritional support may be necessary. If not done previously, it is recommended at this stage to seek the advice of a dietician. Below is an algorithm with an approach to treatment of malnutrition.

The dietician will assess in detail the patient's food intake and preferences and will propose a meal plan with more frequent meals and snacks enriched with food additives to enhance energy intake to 30-40 kcal/kg/d and protein to 1.2 - 1.5 g/kg/d. If this doesn't suffice, an oral formula supplement can be offered together with food additives. It is best to provide such added formula feedings in the evening to avoid interference with meals resulting in meal replacement without higher total energy intakes. A high density formula supplement of 1.5 - 2 calories/mL can deliver up to 400 calories with as much as 15 g of protein per container.

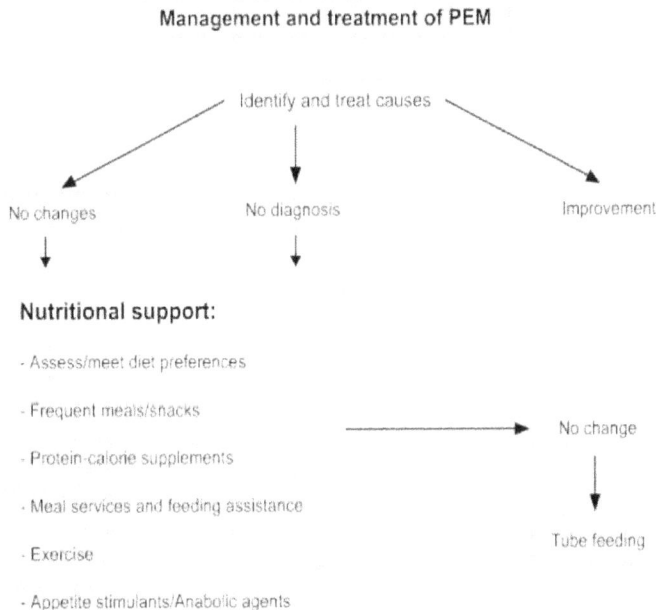

Management and treatment of PEM

Identify and treat causes

No changes   No diagnosis   Improvement

Nutritional support:

- Assess/meet diet preferences

- Frequent meals/snacks

- Protein-calorie supplements   No change

- Meal services and feeding assistance

- Exercise   Tube feeding

- Appetite stimulants/Anabolic agents

Whenever possible, combining some degree of physical activity such as frequent short walks with the dietary intervention can ameliorate appetite and food intake. The use of oral orexigenic medications is controversial in older adults, including the new synthetic tetrahydrocannabinol molecule, dronabinol. However, in case of depression, one should consider mirtazapine, a tetracyclic antidepressant with appetite stimulating properties. Hormones are useful only in those in whom a deficiency state has been diagnosed,

In cases in which malnutrition progresses rapidly, assessment in an acute care setting may be considered to provide access to the different specialists, investigational platforms and interdisciplinary teams. In certain cases, enteral feeding may be indicated and can be initiated.

Resolution of the clinical vignette

The higher the number of indices of malnutrition, the greater the certainty of its presence. In the case of the person described at the outset of this chapter, the weight loss of more than 3 kg in 6 months, a BMI of less than 22 kg/ m² and the low triceps skinfold percentile are very suggestive.

The risk factors comprise isolation (death of husband), recent bereavement, side effects from the medication (dry mouth, constipation), swallowing difficulties, chronic pains from arthritis and reduced mobility to purchase food. Consideration should include metformin due to its propensity to suppress appetite and naprosyn which can lead to peptic ulcer disease (nausea).

Serum albumin is often used as one of the criteria to diagnose malnutrition. In the present case, a value of 38 g/L can be misleading since there is mild dehydration (Cr 98 umol/L), that may be responsible for a factitious elevation. Since CRP is in the normal range, it rules out inflammation. The A1C level is also too low for this frail patient suggesting overly 'tight' control of capillary glucose putting the patient at risk of hypoglycemia.

The amount of weight loss indicates referral to a dietitian, but at this stage, one can emphasise the avoidance of food restriction or a severe diabetic diet, which is often the case in diabetic patients. The dietitian is likely to suggest high density food additives with regular meals and snacks as a first approach. If no change in weight is observed at follow-up in 2 weeks' time, an oral formula supplement should be provided for evening consumption, to avoid interference with regular meals, thus resulting in little gain in total daily calorie intake.

A medication review is mandatory. Metformin should be reduced to 250 mg po BID and Naprosyn discontinued. For pain management, one can offer acetaminophen. The tricyclic antidepressant should be stopped and clinical review after 2 weeks can ascertain if symptoms of dry mouth, swallowing difficulties and constipation have disappeared. If not, one would need to consider a GI assessment.

Finally, a functional evaluation should be undertaken and community support offered to this patient to compensate and support her life situation. Above all, we should help overcome her isolation and assess her meal preparation and food purchasing capacities.

References

1. Kucukerdonmez O, Navruz Varli S, Koksal E. Comparison of Nutritional Status in the Elderly According to Living Situations. J Nutr Health Aging. 2017;21(1):25-30.
2. Landi F Calvani R, Tosato M et al. Anorexia of Aging: Risk Factors, Consequences, and Potential Treatments. Nutrients 2016, 8, 69; doi:10.3390/nu8020069
3. Stajkovic S¹, Aitken EM, Holroyd-Leduc J. Unintentional weight loss in older adults. CMAJ. 2011 Mar 8;183(4):443-9. doi: 10.1503/cmaj.101471
4. Pirlich M, Lochs H. Nutrition in the elderly. Best Practice & Res Clin Gastroenterol. 2001; 15: 869-884
5. Gaddey H L., Holder K. Unintentional Weight Loss in Older Adults. Am Fam Physician. 2014;89:718-722

ARE THE IMMUNIZATIONS OF MY PATIENT UP TO DATE?

Dominique Tessier, MD, CCFP, FCFP, FISTM

Clinical Instructor, Family Medicine Department, University of Montreal, Medical Director, Travel Health Group, Montreal

Clinical vignette

Jeannette and Andrew are both 75 years old. Jeannette is healthy, but her strength has been put to a test in recent months as her husband was hospitalized on several occasions. Andrew was admitted 6 months ago with a diagnosis of myocarditis secondary to acute influenza. He was re-admitted to intensive care after contracting an invasive pneumococcal infection. After weeks of hospitalizations, 10 days after being back home, shingles appeared on his right chest. He still suffers from post-herpetic neuralgia. As he says, "he permanently lost something" and does not feel he will ever be the same. Jeannette would like to know if anything could be done to prevent her from going through what Andrew suffered. She is concerned with the fact she needs to remain healthy to care for her deteriorated husband.

Why are immunizations important?

Immunization programs are hailed as one of the greatest achievements in medicine. They saved more Canadian lives over the last 50 years, than any other health intervention. Still, every year, up to 50,000 people will die in North America alone due to vaccine preventable diseases. Influenza and invasive Streptococcus pneumoniae are responsible for most of the deaths.

The frequency and severity of infectious diseases increase with old age. Infections carry a substantial risk of illness, loss of independence, disability, and death in elderly persons. Unfortunately, immunization rates are relatively low, rarely above 50% in older adults, including in very high-risk groups. These infections are leading causes of catastrophic disability in older adults. In Canada, there is also significant differences in immunization rates between different ethnic and racial groups.

High risk groups

Many risk factors increase the rates and severity of complications and deaths in the older adult. With increasing age, even in people active and fit, the immune system undergoes characteristic changes, termed immunosenescence, which lead to increased incidence and severity of infectious diseases. Unfortunately, it is also responsible for insufficient protection following vaccination. Therefore, some vaccines are specifically designed for older adults and others are contraindicated. Without any other risk factor, this immunosenescence is responsible for hospitalisations with prolonged stay, and death.

Vaccination against SARS-CoV-2 virus that causes COVID-19 disease: see Chapter: COVID-19 in long-term care.

What are the risk factors that should alert you to recommend immunizations?

- Travel: influenza with a yearlong risk around the equator line, yellow fever, Japanese encephalitis, typhoid, enterotoxigenic Escherichia coli (ETEC)-cholera, …
- Cardio-vascular and ischemic diseases
- Diabetes
- Immunologic disturbances including HIV and cancer, use of medications affecting the immune system
- Mobility restrictions and activity limitations in daily life
- Chronic respiratory conditions
- Lifestyle: alcoholism, illicit drug use, smoking, inactivity, being homeless

The combination of chronic medical conditions can significantly affect the risk of complications and deaths related to vaccine preventable diseases.

Vaccine recommendations:

Influenza

Each year influenza is believed to infect 10-20% of the population. The highest risk of mortality occurs in patients > 65 years of age and those with underlying conditions. Annual vaccination is recommended in most provinces and states.

Direct and indirect potential complications of influenza include bronchitis and pneumonia, asthma and COPD exacerbations, ear and sinus complications, acute myocardial infarction, ischemic heart disease and cerebrovascular diseases, and exacerbation of renal disorder and diabetes.

At the individual level, the Centers for Disease Control and Prevention (CDC) and the National Advisory Committee on Immunization -Canada (NACI) recommends that high-dose trivalent influenza vaccine (HD-TIV) should be offered over standard-dose TIV to persons 65 years of age and older. NACI concludes that, given the burden of disease associated with influenza A(H3N2) and the good evidence of better efficacy compared to standard-dose TIV in this age group, HD-TIV should be offered over SD-TIV to persons 65 years of age and older (Grade A). There is insufficient evidence to make comparative recommendations on the use of MF59-adjuvanted TIV and QIV over standard-dose TIV (Grade I). HD-TIV is covered by Public Health programs in some provinces.

Diphtheria-Tetanus-Pertussis

In most provinces and Territories in Canada as well as in USA, a Tetanus and diphtheria (reduced toxoid) vaccine (TD) is recommended every ten years. Pertussis in adults is not common but complications include sleep disturbance, rib fractures, subconjunctival hemorrhages, rectal prolapse, and urinary incontinence, all from intense and persistent coughing. One booster dose per adult lifetime (and one at each pregnancy) of acellular pertussis-containing vaccines is recommended. In USA and Canada, pertussis vaccine for adult use is only available as an acellular preparation in a combination vaccine (Adacel®, Boostrix®).

Pneumococcal infections

Polysaccharides vaccine programs in Canada and USA (PP-23) are targeted at reducing the risk of invasive pneumococcal diseases, not pneumonia. The immune response is very different with the conjugated vaccine (PC-13), which induces a stronger and longer lasting secondary immune response. PC-13 have been demonstrated to prevent community acquired pneumonia et invasive pneumococcal infection. To allow for the best immune response, PC-13 should be administered 8 weeks prior to PP-23. If PP-23 was administered first, wait one year before administering PC-13.

Shingles

Any person who has had varicella is at risk of developing Herpes Zoster (HZ). However, HZ occurs most frequently among older adults and immunocompromised persons. Age is the most important risk factor with two-thirds of the cases occurring in individuals over 50 years of age. The severity of illness associated with HZ and its complications also increases markedly with age. Up to 10% of persons over 65 years of age will be admitted to hospital with an episode of HZ.

HZ infection is characterized by pain and a unilateral vesicular eruption, usually in a single dermatome. The most frequent complication of acute HZ is post-herpetic neuralgia (PHN) which is characterized by prolonged and often debilitating neurogenic pain that lasts for more than 90 days from the onset of rash. Because treatment options for PHN are of limited effectiveness, PHN often has major adverse impacts on quality of life. Older adults, people living with chronic conditions such as diabetes or autoimmune diseases, and persons who are immunocompromised may be at greater risk of developing PHN. They are also at risk of experiencing longer lasting HZ rash than the general population. Other potential complications of HZ include ophthalmic sequelae (herpes zoster ophthalmicus), central nervous system infection, nerve palsies including the Ramsay-Hunt Syndrome, neuromuscular disease including Guillain-Barré Syndrome, pneumonia, hepatitis and secondary bacterial infections.

Two different HZ vaccines are currently used in Canada: Zostavax II® (Live Zoster Vaccine, **LZV**), and Shingrix® (Recombinant Zoster Vaccine, **RZV** or sub-unit adjuvanted Zoster vaccine, **SU-Z**). All individuals ≥50 years of age without contraindications should receive HZ vaccine, preferably RZV. LZV is contraindicated in those with immunosuppression. In the USA, the CDC recommends that healthy adults 50 years and older get two doses of Shingrix®, 2 to 6 months apart.

What are the resources for immunizations ?

Most guidelines propose tables and immunization calendars for adults that will generally cover vaccines offered in Public Health programs. It is important to refer to your provincial or state Health Authority for vaccine coverage. The primary objective of provincial immunization programs for adults is to reduce hospitalizations and deaths associated with vaccine preventable diseases.

Health care providers goal should be to prevent morbidity and mortality at an individual level.

For vaccines not covered by a public health program, a prescription will be required to insure re-imbursement for those with insurance coverage or to receive a proper receipt for an income tax deduction related to medical care costs.

Here's a table including all the vaccines recommended, including those at the expense of the patient.

Table 1: Vaccines for older adults

Disease	Vaccines /Administration	Comments
Hepatitis A	Havrix® Vaqta® Avaxim® Combined with Hepatitis B : Twinrix Combined with typhoid : Vivaxim Two intramuscular doses: 0 and six months	Vaccinate: MSM ; users of illicit drugs orally, by inhalation or by injection under unhygienic conditions ; inmates in correctional facilities under provincial jurisdiction ; People in communities with outbreaks of hepatitis A (eg, the Hasidic community) or where hepatitis A is endemic. ; residential contacts of an adopted child who has arrived for less than three months and comes from a country where hepatitis A is endemic ; chronic liver disease ; planned travel and stay in endemic areas ; some workers
Hepatitis B:	Engerix®-B (20 µg/ml HBsAg) Recombivax HB® (40 µg/ml HBsAg) Combined with Hepatitis A: Twinrix Three intramuscular doses: 0, one and six months	Administer 40 µg per dose for vaccination of immunosuppressed persons. The dosage of anti-HBs is recommended between one and two months after the last dose to check the immune response. The combined vaccine for Hepatitis A and Twinrix® Hepatitis B (GSK) is not recommended (b) for vaccination of immunosuppressed patients. Use monovalent vaccines
Human Papilloma Virus	HPV2 : Cervarix® HPV4 : Gardasil® HPV9 : Gardasil® 9 Three intramuscular doses: 0, two and six months	HPV vaccines may be administered to women over 45 years of age and men 27 years of age and older who are at ongoing risk of exposure to HPV. MSM have a disproportionately high burden of HPV infection. The vaccine can be given even if the person has already had an HPV infection or an HPV infection-related lesion (eg, condyloma or abnormal screening test) since the acquired immunity is specific (type-specific) .
Influenza	Standard dose (SD) trivalent and quadrivalent High-dose trivalent influenza vaccine (HD-TIV) Annually	The quadrivalent live attenuated influenza vaccine (Flumist Quadrivalent) is a live attenuated, reassortant vaccine and is contraindicated in immonosupprimed persons NACI recommends that high-dose trivalent influenza vaccine (HD-TIV) should be offered over standard-dose TIV to persons 65 years of age and older.

Disease	Vaccines /Administration	Comments
Pneumococcal	PC13 : Prevnar 13® (conjuguated) PP23 : Pneumovax® 23 (polysaccharide) One dose PC13 followed 8 weeks later or more by 1 dose PP23 1 booster dose of PP23 at ≥ 65 (minimum 5 years interval)	Wherever possible, the conjugate vaccine (PC13) should be administered first with a minimum of 8 weeks of polysaccharide vaccine. If the PP23 was administered first, wait 1 year before administering the PC13.
Shingles	Recombinant Zoster Vaccine, RZV or sub-unit vaccine : Shingrix® Live Zoster Vaccine, LZV: Zostavax II® RZV : 2 doses at a recommended interval of 2 months Minimum 4 weeks LZV: One dose	RZV: Vaccinate all people aged 50 or over Preferential use of the RZV over LZV A person can be vaccinated against shingles regardless of their history of chicken pox, shingles or varicella vaccination. People with a history of ophthalmic zoster with ocular involvement may be vaccinated 12 months or more after the start of the shingles episode if at least 6 months have elapsed since the end of their active treatment. LZV should be used only if RZV is not available or contraindicated.
Tetanus-diphteria-Pertussis	Adacel® (dcaT) Boostrix® (dcaT) dT (dT) Booster : One dose (dT) every ten years. Administer at least one dose of vaccine containing the pertussis component in adult life	People who need a primary vaccination should receive one dose of the Tdap (or Tdap-Polio) vaccine and two doses of the Td (or dT-Polio) vaccine. In exceptional circumstances (for example, a long stay in a region where access to health care is limited), another reminder may be given if more than five years have elapsed since the last dose. Adults should be given a dose of Tdap without adhering to the usual interval since administering a dose of Td vaccine.

Table 2: vaccines for travellers

Disease	Vaccines /Administration	Comments
Cholera-ETEC	Dukoral 2 doses orally, 1-6 weeks apart Booster : 1 dose every 3 months (ETEC) or 1 dose every 2 years (cholera)	May be considered for prevention of travellers' diarrhea in persons with chronic illnesses such as, chronic renal failure, congestive heart failure, insulin-dependent diabetes mellitus, and inflammatory bowel disease, for whom there is an increased risk of serious consequences from travellers' diarrhea. If more than 5 years have passed since primary immunization or last booster dose, repeat primary series.
Japanese encephalitis	Ixiaro 2 doses	If the risk of exposure persists, give 1 dose after 12 months after a primary vaccination with Ixiaro and a second dose after 10 years.
Meningococcal ACWY	Menactra® Menveo® Nimenrix	Vaccinate those at high risk (asplenia, contact, travel)
Meningococcal B	Bexsero (GSK); Trumenba (Pfizer)	Vaccinate those at high risk (asplenia, contact, travel)

Disease	Vaccines /Administration	Comments
Polio Rabies	Imovax-Polio® : one booster dose at 0, 1 month ——————— Imovax-Rabies : multiple calendars possible. Refer to guidelines	A single polio vaccine booster is indicated for at-risk adults. Routine vaccination of adults (18 years of age or older) is not necessary in Canada. ——————— Pre-exposure immunization with ID is not recommended in immunosuppressed persons.
Typhoid	Injectable, recombinant vaccines : Typhim Vi® ou Typherix® Combined, recombinant with Hepatitis A : Vivaxim Oral, live attenuated vaccine : Vivotif®	Booster : A vaccination started with a hepatitis A vaccine or a typhoid vaccine can be continued with the combined vaccine against hepatitis A and typhoid, and vice versa, depending on the schedule and dosage of the vaccine used. Oral, live attenuated vaccine contraindicated in immunosuppressed.
Yellow fever	YF-VAX® : live attenuated vaccine	Since the entry into force of the amendment to the International Health Regulations on 11 July 2016, all international yellow fever vaccination certificates are considered valid for life, including certificates issued more than 10 years ago. Use of a one-time booster dose is recommended for travellers who may have received a primary dose of yellow fever vaccine during a period of reduced immunocompetence. This includes those who were pregnant, taking immunosuppressive medication, received a previous dose which may be inadequate for long term protection, and individuals diagnosed with an illness associated with an immunocompromised state. Individuals who underwent a hematopoietic stem cell transplant after having received yellow fever vaccine are included in this category (see Recommendations for expanded discussion.) A booster dose of yellow fever vaccine every 10 years is recommended for HIV-positive individuals prior to travel to endemic regions.

Antibody levels

Rarely, it will be necessary to do a serology to verify if a patient is protected against vaccine preventable diseases. Hepatitis B seroprotection is defined as anti-HBs titer of ≥10 IU/L. In adults, the immune response can be affected negatively by immunosuppression, in chronic conditions such as chronic kidney disease, among individuals with diabetes. For immunocompromised individuals, initial annual monitoring of HB antibody levels following HB immunization may be considered.

For yellow fever, for those previously immunized who are at very high risk or for whom a booster dose is recommended, measured neutralizing antibody titre to yellow fever virus can confirm ongoing protection and prevent the need for a booster.

For rabies, in both pre-exposure prophylaxis and post-exposure prophylaxis, a post-vaccination serology two to four weeks after the last dose should be considered if the person vaccinated is considered immunocompromised.

Resolution of the clinical vignette

Immunization is one of the greatest success stories in medical history. It has improved the lives of every Canadian and American and has saved more lives than any other health intervention. We have seen many diseases such as diphtheria, mumps, measles and rubella drop by over 99% with the introduction and integration of a vaccine into the immunization program. In older adults, immunization is a powerful tool to protect a vulnerable person from severe infections and their complications.

- Vaccinations provide efficient protection from infectious diseases.
- Age-related changes in the immune system may hamper successful vaccination.
- Vaccines tailored to the needs of the aging immune system will have to be developed
- Vaccination schedules will have to be adapted to improve protection in elderly persons.

For this particular couple, each member should have annual influenza vaccination with HD-TIV, and once in their lifetime a pneumococcal vaccine with PC-13 administered 8 weeks prior to PP-23, a shingle vaccination with Shingrix® and a Boostrix® vaccine against diphteria-tetanus-pertussis infections.

Older adults are predisposed to complications from vaccine preventable diseases due to intrinsic as well as exogenous causes. Aging is associated with a decrease in the efficacity of the immune system to fight infections, called immunosenescence. Therefore it leads to an increase risk of invasive diseases with agents such as pneumococcal infection.

To insure that all your patients keep their immunization status up-to-date, provide them with an immunization booklet and ask them to bring it to every medical consultation.

References

1. Protocole d'immunisations du Québec. MSSS. Québec. Mises à jours trimestrielles.

2. http://www.msss.gouv.qc.ca/professionnels/vaccination/protocole-d-immunisation-du-quebec-piq/

3. Provincial and Territorial Routine Vaccination Programs for Healthy, Previously Immunized Adults. Public Health Agency of Canada. February 2019. https://www.canada.ca/en/public-health/services/provincial-territorial-immunization-information/routine-vaccination-healthy-previously-immunized-adult.html

4. Sellers SA, Hagan RS, Hayden FG, Fischer WA 2nd. The hidden burden of influenza: A review of the extra-pulmonary complications of influenza infection. *Influenza Other Respir Viruses*. 2017;11(5):372–393. doi:10.1111/irv.12470

5. Hospitalisations et complications attribuables à l'influenza : rapport de surveillance 2017-2018

6. INSPQ Fevrier 2019. https://www.inspq.qc.ca/publications/2486 . https://www.inspq.qc.ca/sites/default/files/publications/2486_hospitalisations_complications_inluenza_2017_2018.pdf

7. Dr. Janet McElhaney

8. Member, CIHR Institute Advisory Board (IAB) on Indigenous Peoples' Health

9. http://www.cihr-irsc.gc.ca/e/50234.html

10. Vaccination contre le tétanos : pertinence de doses de rappel chez l'adulte. INSPQ septembre 2018.

MANAGEMENT OF OLDER PATIENTS IN THE EMERGENCY DEPARTMENT: THIS MAN IS OLD, BUT IS IT AN EMERGENCY?

Cyrille Launay, MD, PhD

Department of medicine, division of geriatrics,

University Hospital of Lausanne, Switzerland

Clinical vignette

An 88 year old man is brought to the emergency department (ED) by his daughter because he can no longer perform his basic activities of daily living (bathing, dressing, transferring). She also reports that her father was having difficulty preparing his meals and has lost weight. The patient cannot provide details and does not understand why he is at hospital. He has no complaints and states that even if he is "a little bit tired", he wants to go back home. He is coherent but he is not able to say the month or the year. He has a mild cough but has no fever. The chest examination reveals wheezing but no audible crackles. Blood tests available disclose leukocytes $7x10^9$/L, CRP 15mg/L, creatinine 67 umol/L. The physician diagnoses acute bronchitis, proposes discharge home and treatment with an opioid cough suppressant.

Why are older patients in the Emergency Department at risk of misdiagnosis?

The health status of older patients (i.e; 75 years and older) is highly heterogeneous and is related to the various and cumulative effects of aging, life habits and chronic diseases that are highly prevalent in this age group. Thus, older patients are generally sicker than younger ones and 80% of those aged 75 years and older present with at least 2 chronic diseases that increase the risk of developing acute diseases. Indeed, older patients often experience complex interactions between acute and chronic diseases but also geriatric syndromes (e.g., cognitive impairment) that may induce atypical clinical presentations such as functional decline or increasing disabilities. Thus, they may be admitted to ED with non-specific complaints (feeling "tired" or "weak") that arise due to cognitive impairment and communications problems, functional decline and comorbidities. Geriatric syndromes may not be recognized (misdiagnosed) and not managed (mistreated).

Therefore, 25% of older patients leave ED with no definite diagnosis whereas most of them suffer from an acute disease. Underdiagnosis and underestimation of patients with atypical clinical presentations may lead to adverse outcomes such as higher risk of hospitalization and in-hospital mortality.

How to deal with older patients in the Emergency Department

The adapted care plan of older patients is based on a multidimensional, interdisciplinary diagnostic process to determine the medical, psychological and functional capabilities called the comprehensive geriatric assessment (CGA). CGA is the most validated intervention dedicated to elderly patients and aims at assessing and addressing their needs.

Benefits of CGA have been confirmed through several meta-analysis, which have reported a reduction of admissions and readmissions to hospital, more discharges to home, increased lifetime spent at home, prevention of functional decline and decrease in mortality and in healthcare expenditures.

Despite its benefits, a systematic CGA for every older ED inpatient in daily practice remains impossible to implement because it is a complex and time-consuming process. Furthermore, it requires a multidisciplinary geriatric team that cannot alone support the care of all frail older ED patients due to limited availability.

The usual Emergency Department's mission is to quickly prioritize patients whose life is in danger; therefore, their triage often fails to detect the complex reasons that lead to the ED visits of older patients.

Thus, a two-step approach seems the best strategy to provide the appropriate care to the right patient at the right time, in order to identify those who are in greatest need of a geriatric intervention.

To implement such an approach, a screening tool is required to identify frail patients or patients at risk of adverse outcomes during hospitalization.

Useful tools to identify vulnerable patients in ED

Several tools have been developed to identify early frail patients or patients at risk of a prolonged hospital stay, 30-day readmission or mortality. There is currently no consensus on a screening tool for use in ED. The ideal tool would need to be multidimensional. Thus, most of the screening tools in use assess physical function, cognition, malnutrition and disabilities that are the main geriatric conditions.

To date, there is a consensus for the need for a screening tool in ED, but this tool needs to be adapted to the specific conditions of the medical practice in ED. This tool needs to be multidimensional, capable of being quickly performed and easy to use without specific geriatric training. Among those tools, Identification of Senior At Risk (ISAR), Emergency Room Evaluation and Recommendations (ER2) or Prisma 7 are meant to guide the appropriate levels of treatment to provide to older patients. According to their risk stratification, patients considered frail or at risk of prolonged length of hospital stay may require a geriatric intervention (i.e; to be hospitalized in a geriatric unit, or the intervention of a mobile geriatric team).

Key components of a comprehensive geriatric assessment	
Medical assessment	Problem list Comorbidities Medications Nutritional assessment Gait and balance assessment
Functional assessment	Activities of daily living Instrumental activities of daily living
Psychological assessment	Cognition Assessment of mood
Social Assessment	Family support Home help services
environmental assessment	Financial

If no screening tool is available, an assessment based on the components of the CGA may be performed.

CGA allows a coordinated and integrated plan of treatment, and thus may prevent complicated medical pathways characterized, for instance, by prolonged length of hospital stay. This intervention can be performed in different ways depending on the medical resources and organization of the structure. Most of the time, CGA is delivered on a geriatric ward, or by a mobile geriatric team.

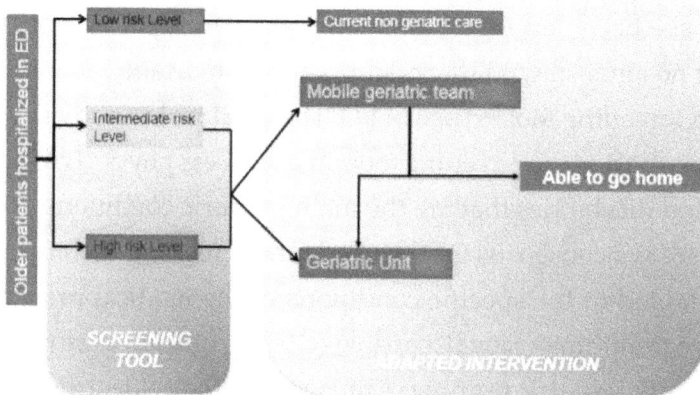

In EDs, mobile geriatric assessment provides an intervention with several objectives. The first one is to diagnose unrecognized geriatric syndromes such as delirium, frailty and gait impairment. Secondly, the mobile geriatric team may provide guidance on the level of care and recommendations on immediate care, prevention of functional decline or prevention of delirium. Finally, mobile geriatric teams may propose and coordinate a care plan that includes a discharge home or suggest the type of inpatient medical unit that may provide the most adapted care (e.g., a geriatric unit, an internal medicine unit) or institutionalization.

Continuation of the vignette

A mobile geriatric team is asked to assess the patient in order to help with the medical management and to coordinate the discharge.

Their geriatric assessment uncovers several geriatric syndromes. First, cognitive impairment is detected, using the Mini Mental State Examination (MMSE). Secondly, they gather information that the patient fell many times and always refused a walking aid. Finally, malnutrition is diagnosed considering a weight loss of 7kg in the last 6 months and a lower than expected weight of 61kg. The mobile geriatric team provided a plan for immediate care and proposed to transfer the patient to an acute geriatric unit.

How to deliver a geriatric assessment in ED?

Several areas must be considered to assess older patients. These areas have been grouped under the acronym of 5Ms as proposed by the American and Canadian Geriatrics Societies. These 5 Ms stand for:

- **Mind: refers to cognitive impairment and/or delirium and depression:**
  Delirium is highly prevalent in EDs (up to a quarter of patients) and should

not remain unrecognized considering related morbidity and adverse outcomes. The confusion assessment method (CAM) is a simple tool with high predictive performance that may be used to identify delirium. Patients with cognitive impairment are vulnerable and must be managed carefully because of the risk of delirium. Besides, assessing their cognitive status is mandatory to enable a safe return home from ED. For interventions to reduce or manage delirium, please refer to the chapter on delirium.

- **Mobility: refers to gait impairment and falls:** Half of those aged 80 years and over fall at least once a year. Thus the history of falls is a predictor of future falls and is also associated with greater disabilities and injuries. The intervention may assess the risk of falls and identify their risk factors, in order to implement multidisciplinary interventions to address them. For details on the management of mobility and falls in older adults, please refer to the dedicated chapter.

- **Multi-complexity: refers to the burden of chronic diseases and bio-psycho-social situations including functional status:** Functional decline and disabilities are relatively common reasons for visits to EDs by older patients and may be the clinical presentation of an underlying disease. That is why such non-specific complaints must trigger an exhaustive assessment of acute and chronic diseases and geriatric syndromes.

- **Medication: refers to optimization of prescriptions and adverse drug events**. Taking 5 different medications or more per day usually defines polypharmacy. Adverse drug effects increase with aging and number of drugs and may be a reason for ED visits in up to 14% of older persons. Furthermore, the number of drugs taken per day is associated with comorbidity burden and diseases' severity. For more information on polypharmacy, please refer to the appropriate chapter.

- **Matters most: refers to each individual's own meaningful health outcome goals and care preferences**. These important aspects can be discussed with the caregiver when the patient is unable to contribute. Emphasis should be placed on patient-centered care.

Resolution of the clinical vignette

Many geriatric syndromes may be evoked from the beginning of this vignette. The reason for admission is non-specific and the clinical presentation is mainly functional.

Such a visit could be considered inappropriate in ED whose aim is intended to treat acute diseases. However, nearly 60% of patients presenting with non-specific complaints to ED suffer from serious medical conditions. Acute functional decline may lead to disabilities. It is mandatory to provide specific interventions that improve the diagnostic process to manage patients adequately and prevent further decline. The main clinical elements suggest acute bronchitis without severity criteria. However an acute disease may expose a vulnerable patient with reduced physiological reserves to dependency.

The patient is described as not able to say the month or the year, suggestive of cognitive impairment. Indeed, temporal disorientation is related to acute and chronic cognitive impairment. Thus this item may help to identify delirium and/or dementia. Consequently, opioid treatment must be used with caution to avoid delirium and is not indicated to treat cough. A brief geriatric assessment that examines cognition is mandatory in this case. Confirmation of a diagnosis of dementia can be completed at a later stage along with a decision on treatment.

Finally, this clinical vignette shows the necessity to go beyond the assessment of acute diseases in ED and to consider geriatric syndromes and chronic diseases. A care plan to prevent functional decline, disabilities and delirium must be elaborated from ED to avoid inappropriate discharge home with its deleterious consequences.

References

1. Preston L et al. Southampton (UK): NIHR Journals Library; 2018
2. Ellis G, Whitehead MA, O'Neill D, Langhorne P, Robinson D. Comprehensive geriatric assessment for older adults admitted to hospital. Cochrane Database Syst Rev. 2011;doi: 10.1002/14651858.
3. Aminzadeh F, Dalziel WB. Older adults in the emergency department: a systematic review of patterns of use, adverse outcomes, and effectiveness of interventions. Ann Emerg Med. 2002;39:238-247.
4. Wachelder JJH, Stassen PM, Hubens LPAM et al. Elderly patients presenting with non -specific complaints: characteristics and outcomes. PlosOne.2017; 12(11): e0188954
5. Ellis G, Marshall T, Ritchie C. Comprehensive geriatric assessment in the emergency department. Clin Interv Aging. 2014; 9: 2033–2043.
6. Sternberg SA, Wershof Schwartz A, Karunananthan S, Bergman H, Mark Clarfield A. The identification of frailty: a systematic literature review.J Am Geriatr Soc. 2011 Nov;59(11):2129-38.

CRITICAL CARE OF THE OLDER PERSON

Astrid F. Pilgrim, MD, MS .Fellow, Critical Care Medicine, University of Pittsburgh Medical School
Michael R. Pinsky, MD, CM. Dr hc, FCCP, MCCM, FAPS, Professor of Critical Care Medicine, Cardiovascular Diseases, Anesthesiology,
Clinical and Translations Sciences, Bioengineering, University of Pittsburgh
Department of Critical Care Medicine, University of Pittsburgh Medical School

Clinical Vignette:

An 85-year-old non-smoking Caucasian male widower, previously self-sufficient and living alone, is brought into the Emergency Department by his daughter. She normally spoke to him daily, but the day before when she called him he sounded somewhat confused. On the day of admission she went to his home and found him confused and rambling, but in no acute distress. After calling his primary care physician she brought him into the local hospital Emergency Department. In the Emergency Department he was found to be sleepy but arousable, disoriented, but in no acute distress, with a good nutritional status and no evidence of trauma.

Temperature was 38.2 C, heart rate 85/min and regular, respiration rate 12/min and unlabored, blood pressure 135/60 mmHg. Neurological, cardiac and respiratory examinations were normal. The abdomen was slightly distended with tenderness but no rebound. There were no bowel sounds. Periphery had good pulses without edema. Capillary refill time was 1.5 seconds. Abnormal initial laboratory studies included a serum sodium of 125 mmol/dl, hemoglobin of 10.5 gm/dl, a white blood count of 10,000 with 3% bands and an arterial blood gas on room air of PO_2 55 mmHg, PCO_2 38 mmHg, pH 7.32. A chest radiography revealed some calcification of the aorta, thoracic vertebral fusion and free air under the diaphragm. An abdominal

95

CT scan revealed free air anteriorly, fluid in the abdominal cavity and thickened descending colon wall.

Based on these findings blood cultures were obtained and the patient placed on broad spectrum antibiotics and resuscitated with 500 ml of 0.9% NaCl. Surgical consultation was obtained and the patient was transferred to the intensive care unit where he was instrumented with a central venous and radial artery catheter. Over the next hour the patient received 1,500 ml of a balanced salt solution, but he progressively became unresponsive. He was electively intubated to protect his airway. Upon intubation, his blood pressure decreased to 95/40 mmHg and his heart rate increased to 95/min. His blood pressure did not respond to 1000 mL bolus infusion of 0.9% NaCl, so norepinephrine was initiated and titrated to achieve a mean arterial pressure greater than 65 mmHg while plans were made for an emergent exploratory laparotomy.

Upon opening the abdomen during laparotomy foul smelling feculent fluid was observed with fecal soiling; a ruptured descending colonic diverticulum was identified. A diverting colostomy and rectal mucus fistula was created, the abdomen was washed out three times, and then closed. A second look surgery the following day revealed no bowel leak or fluid collections. However, on post-operative day two his urine output decreased despite being 5,000 ml positive with a doubling of both BUN and creatinine. He was placed on continuous veno-venous hemofiltration for fluid management, which was weaned off after 5 days. His initial post-operative course was complicated by secondary fungal peritonitis treated with anti-fungal agents. However, his level of consciousness remained depressed despite holding all sedation. He remained ventilator and vasopressor dependent.

At 10 days post intubation, a discussion was had about tracheostomy. A spot cortisol level was drawn and came back 18 mg/dl. He was placed on hydrocortisone 100 mg intravenously every 8 hours. After 36 hours of hydrocortisone, his level of consciousness markedly improved and he was rapidly weaned off the ventilator and 12 hours later off norepinephrine. On his 14th hospital day he was transferred to a regular ward and by day 20 transferred to a skilled nursing facility.

Case Discussion:

This case highlights many of the features of critical illness in the older person. As people age their ability to cope with stress of any kind decreases. First, the typical clinical presentations of pneumonia, sepsis or myocardial infarction are often absent. The most common presentation of older patients with catastrophic illness is confusion and inactivity. This patient presented with confusion and minimal inflammatory changes, like fever and tachycardia, despite severe intra-abdominal sepsis. Some of this blunted response may be due to the immune senescence seen with aging. Also, his initial arterial blood gas revealed hypoxemia with an increased A-a gradient, but no pulmonary infiltrates. Aging causes alveolar dropout or senescent emphysema such that the normal PaO_2 of an 85-year-old person is 60 mmHg. With aging, all physiologic systems are impaired and homeostasis becomes "homeostenosis."

Second, when being treated with presumptively correct therapies, he did not rapidly improve. This is also frequent. Critically ill older people do nothing quickly except die. Thus, responses to dialysis, antibiotics and fluids need to be titrated much more closely than in the younger patient. The relative adrenal insufficiency documented on day 10 and treated appropriately would have resulted in a rapid improvement in level of consciousness in a younger patient. Our patient took 36 hours to respond.

Third, the older critically ill patient will recover and, surprisingly, if they had no pre-existing morbidities carry a similar mortality rate as younger patients. So do not allow age to be a primary factor in determining who to treat for critical illness.

Fourth and finally, the older patient will recover, but their recovery will be protracted so it needs to be viewed within a longer time frame. Our patient did not recover fully for 6 months.

Physiologic changes associated with aging: when Homeostasis becomes "Homeostenosis"

After about 25 years of age, further aging is associated with decrements in physiologic reserve of all organ systems although at different interindividual rates (1). These usually do not become noticeable except in elite athletes until the mid-40s and are not physiologically relevant until after age 60. The heart increases in size and weight, atherosclerosis progresses, and pacemaker cells are lost (2). Maximal heart rate and oxygen (O_2) delivery are reduced. The lung experiences loss of elastin fibers and collagen as alveoli drop out causing senescent emphysema, increased closing volumes and arterial to alveolar O_2 difference manifest as resting hypoxemia made worse by exercise and prolonged supine positioning (3). Thoracic cage deformity by kyphosis decreases chest wall compliance and increases residual volume in the lungs. The brain loses white matter which usually only manifests itself as confusion during stress. Renal concentrating capacity decreases such that measures of creatinine or BUN underestimate renal dysfunction. The gastrointestinal system displays decreased salivary production, dysphagia, delayed gastric emptying, development of diverticulae and hernias, and impaired vitamin absorption (4). A summary of the measured decrements in physiologic reserve seen with aging is listed in Table 1. The functional cumulative result of these decrements in physiologic reserve is fragility leading to the inability to maintain homeostasis in response to an otherwise minimal stressor.

Table 1: Systemic Changes with Aging (2,4)	
System	**Physiologic Changes**
Neurologic	Decreased number of neurons. Decreased action potential speed. Decreased axon/dendrite branches.
Cardiovascular	Heart increases in size and weight. Progression of atherosclerosis. Loss of pacemaker cells. Increased vascular intimal thickness and stiffness. Increased left ventricular (LV) wall thickness and left atrial (LA) size.
Pulmonary	Loss of elastin fibers and collagen, kyphosis with decreased compliance of chest wall, increased residual volume. Alveoli duct volume increases at the expense of the alveoli resulting in senile emphysema
Gastrointestinal	Decreased salivary production, dysphagia, diverticulae and hernias, delayed gastric emptying, impaired vitamin absorption
Genitourinary	Kidney size and weight decreases. The number of functional glomeruli and renal tubules decreases, GFR declines, concentrating ability of kidney declines. The bladder can develop trabeculation and diverticula. There is urethral mucosal atrophy.
Endocrinologic	Increased atrophy of certain glands (pituitary, thyroid, thymus) with resultant changes in hormone levels and function.
Hematologic	Loss of self-renewal capacity of hematopoietic stem cells
Immunologic	Gradual decline in the acquired immune system ("immunosenescence") including fewer naive and more memory T cells and decreased function of the B cell. Atrophy of the thymus. Increase in innate immune system activation leading to an elevated proinflammatory state marked by increased levels of cytokines and macrophage activation markers.
Musculoskeletal	Decreased bone density. Loss of cartilage thickness in synovial joints resulting in stiffness and less flexibility. Selective loss of type II muscle fibers. Lipofuscin and fat deposited in muscle tissue. Decrease in overall muscle mass.

These are important concepts to remember when treating the older patient with critical illness. They often appear well, living independent lives with good mentation and ambulation while handling their activities of daily living (Figure 1). Yet with some stressor, which could be as minor as moving to a new environment, they may become confused, belligerent or subdued. Regrettably, these are often the same presenting symptoms as a new infection or organ ischemia. They rarely have high fevers or tachycardia to the level seen in younger patients with the same illnesses. Similarly, they may not appreciate infarction or inflammation as pain. As in our case with fecal peritonitis, there was no rebound tenderness on abdominal examination.

The Impact of Aging on the Ability to Respond to Stress

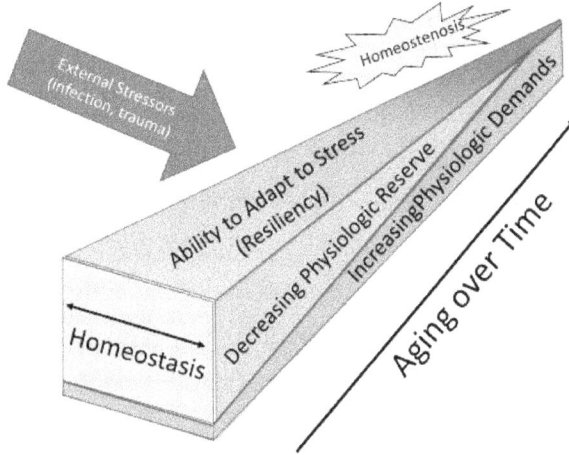

Figure 1: Schematic diagram of the effect of aging on the ability of the body to adapt to stress effectively.

Resuscitation of the critically ill older patient: Sick old people do nothing fast but die

Due to their markedly reduced physiological reserve, the older critically ill patient needs a more nuanced resuscitation approach that recognizes those differences. Regarding specific therapies for diseases, the same management principles apply to older patients, but with an understanding that too rapid fluid resuscitation, vasopressors and extubation from mechanical ventilation may be as dangerous as delayed resuscitation and prolonged mechanical ventilation.

The fundamental principles of resuscitation of the critically ill patient presenting with cardiorespiratory insufficiency remain unchanged. Regarding ventilation, maintain a pulse oximeter O_2 saturation >90% with supplemental oxygen as needed and defend the airway. If breathing is inadequate to sustain normal gas exchange artificial ventilation, an initially non-invasive trial could be done but if not successful, invasive ventilation via endotracheal intubation should be performed.

Regarding cardiovascular support, the priorities are pressure, flow, and function. Ensure that mean arterial pressure (MAP) is >65 mmHg or no more than 15 mmHg less than baseline in a previously hypertensive subject in order to sustain cerebral and coronary blood flow. This is usually done by rapid small bolus fluid resuscitation and vasopressor infusions. It is important to note that the recent Lamontagne et al. 65 TRIAL (5) which compared a MAP goal > 65mmHg to >60mmHg in patients older than 65 with vasodilatory hypotension demonstrated a non-significant trend towards higher mortality with higher MAP goal. While current practice dictates a MAP goal of 65, this may change in the future with more studies.

Once pressure has been corrected, and this should take less than an hour, the focus shifts to maintaining an adequate flow to meet the metabolic demands of the body as assessed by loss of skin mottling, short (<2 sec) capillary refill time, lactate levels falling to <2 mmol/dl, and resolution of metabolic acidosis if previously present.

Finally, once global blood flow appears adequate, resuscitating is fine-tuned by adjusting pressure and flow as needed to establish adequate renal blood flow as monitored by urine output, gut blood flow as monitored by bowel mobility, and sensorium as monitored by increased level of consciousness and lack of anxiety. Thus, there are no specific issues in management that are different in treatment of the older patients except that complications of those treatments will be more frequent.

A good example of that is the high incidence of confusion and acute psychosis in the elderly in response to sedative therapies. Older adults need time to adjust to treatments and once treated to recover. In a landmark study of ICU outcomes of critically ill older adults, Chelluri et al. in 1993 (6) found that in ICU patients aged 65 to 74 as compared to those aged 75 and older there was no significant difference in length of stay, mortality at 1 year, or quality of life at 1, 6, and 12 months. Thus, age alone cannot predict long term survival or quality of life in older adults admitted to the ICU. The study also suggests that older persons can eventually get back to their baseline function, but it takes more time and requires more involvement. In 2015 Ferrante et al. (7) performed a prospective cohort study on over 700 community dwelling older adults with three distinct pre and post ICU functional trajectories–minimal disability, mild to moderate disability, and severe disability. They found that while more than half the participants experienced functional decline after critical illness, pre-hospitalization functional status played a more important role than age with older adults having minimal disability often being able to return to their pre-hospitalization status.

There are certain drugs routinely used during critical care illness (e.g. for delirium, stress ulcer prophylaxis, arrhythmias, etc.) which show greater toxicity in the older patient. Every three years the American Geriatric Society (AGS) publishes the Beers criteria: a list of potentially inappropriate medications for older adults (8). Last updated in Jan 2019, the list includes 30 medications or medication classes to avoid in older adults. Most notable on this list with high quality of evidence and a strong strength of recommendation against use in older adults are tricyclic antidepressants, nifedipine, amiodarone, proton pump inhibitors, and non-selective NSAIDS. Lower on the list with moderate quality of evidence, but a strong strength of recommendation against use in older adults includes anticholinergics, second generation antipsychotics (except quetiapine, clozapine, and pimavanserin), benzodiazepines, non-dihydropyridine calcium channel blockers, and opioids. While the overall management strategies for diseases are the same for geriatric and non-geriatric patients, it's important to recognize the adverse effects that potentially inappropriate drugs can have in the geriatric patient population in case there is an equally efficacious but safer alternative therapy.

End of Life Care in the ICU

In an ideal world, end-of-life care is considered in the older person as part of the long-term healthcare discussion and would occur outside of the hospital in a setting where the patient is healthy enough to express their personal values. In reality, many older patients have never discussed end-of-life care and find their last days of life to be in the hospital where they are unable to share their own wishes and personal values and their family/caretakers are overwhelmed and unsure of the patient's personal values. When the place of care is the intensive care unit, this can make dying with dignity a challenge (9). Importantly, end of life care is just part of the palliative medicine spectrum of care. Palliative care is often provided within the intensive care environment, and can be done with all the appropriate trappings of dignity and respect for the patient, their wishes, and the family's sensitivities. The World Health Organization defined palliative care as "an approach that improves the quality of life of patients and their families facing the problem associated with life-threatening illness" (10). Thus, palliative medicine is complementary to critical care medicine and physicians in general, but intensivists in particular, should strive to enhance the patient's quality of life, provide treatment consistent with their personal values, and offer a support system to the patient and family/caretaker. For example, it is reasonable to initiate an aggressive treatment plan for organ failure scenarios in conjunction with palliative care goals. However, if the outcome appears bleak, it is important to re-align the treatment plan with the patient's values and if indicated, transition to end of life care. This often is associated with withdrawal of life supporting therapies, like mechanical ventilation and vasopressor therapy. Such a realignment of care goals is a process that will occur multiple times between the medical team and the patient/family over the course of a patient's admission. Overall, with end-of-life intensive care medicine, the prevention and relief of suffering becomes the primary goal.

The Unexpected Consequence of Aging – Cost of Care Decreases

The common belief is that with hospitalization and especially an ICU admission, older adults utilize more resources than their younger cohorts. Surprisingly, older age is actually associated with a lower total hospital cost. This was demonstrated in the 2003 Chelluri et al. (11) study which analyzed the hospital charges of 813 patients requiring mechanical ventilation; after adjusting for severity of illness (APS), ICU type, care insurance, and the Charlson comorbidity score, each decade of life was associated with a measurable decrease in costs. Further analysis showed decreased costs in the elderly occurs early on during the hospital stay and is not due to a limitation in care in the later days of the hospital stay.

Resolution of the clinical case

The patient remained in the skilled nursing facility for 2 months before being able to return home with daily home care nursing visits. By month 6 he resumed his normal level of activity and independence. His colostomy was taken down at that time without difficulty.

References

1. Brummel NE, Ferrante LE. Integrating geriatric principles into critical care medicine: the time is now. Ann ATS 15:518-522, 2017. doi.org/10.1513/AnnalsATS.201710-793IP

2. Strait, James B, and Edward G Lakatta. Aging-associated cardiovascular changes and their relationship to heart failure. Heart failure clinics 8:143-64, 2012. doi:10.1016/j.hfc.2011.08.011

3. Andrews P, Azoulay E, Antonelli M, Brochard L, Brun-Buisson C, De Backer D, Dobb G, Fagon JY, Gerlach H, Groeneveld J, Macrae D, Mancebo J, Metnitz P, Nava S, Pugin J, Pinsky MR, Radermacher P, Richard C. Year in review in Intensive Care Medicine 2006 II. Infections and sepsis,

haemodynamics, elderly, invasive and non-invasive mechanical ventilation, weaning, ARDS. Intensive Care Med 33: 214-228, 2007. doi:10.1007/s00134-006-0512-z

4. Medina-Walpole A, Pacala JT, Potter JF, eds. Geriatrics Review Syllabus: A Core Curriculum in Geriatric Medicine. 9th ed. New York, NY: American Geriatrics Society; 2016.

5. Lamontagne F, Richards-Belle AQ, Thomas K, Harrison DA, Sadique MZ, Grieve RD, Camsooksai J, Darnell R, Gordon AC, Henry D, Hudson N, Mason AJ, Saull M, Whitman C, Young JD, Rowan KM, Mouncey PR for the 65 trial investigators. Effect of Reduced Exposure to Vasopressors on 90-Day Mortality in Older Critically Ill Patients with Vasodilatory Hypotension. JAMA 323:938-949, 2020. doi:10.1001/jama.2020.0930

6. Chelluri L, Pinsky MR, Donahoe MP, Grenvik A. Long-term outcome of critically ill elderly patients requiring intensive care. JAMA 269: 3119-3123, 1993.

7. Ferrante LE, Pisani MA, Murphy TE, Gahbauer EA, Leo-Summers LS, Gill TM. Functional Trajectories Among Older Persons Before and After Critical Illness. JAMA 175:523–529, 2015. doi:10.1001/jamainternmed.2014.7889

8. 2019 American Geriatrics Society Beers Criteria® Update Expert Panel. American Geriatrics Society 2019 Updated AGS Beers Criteria® for Potentially Inappropriate Medication Use in Older Adults. J Am Geriatrics Soc 67: 674-694, 2019. doi:10.1111/jgs.15767

9. Cook D, Rocker G. Dying with dignity in the intensive care unit. N Engl J Med 370:2506-2514, 2014.

10. WHO Definition of Palliative Care. World Health Organization, World Health Organization, 28 Jan. 2012, www.who.int/cancer/palliative/definition/en/

11. Chelluri L, Mendelsohn AB, Belle SH, Rotondi AJ, Angus DA, Donahoe MP, Sirio CA, Schulz R, Pinsky MR. Hospital costs in patients receiving prolonged mechanical ventilation. Does age have an impact? Crit Care Med 31: 1746-1751, 2003. doi:10.1097/01.CCM.0000063478.91096.7D

COVID-19 IN LONG-TERM CARE

Julia Chabot, MDCM, FRCPC, MSc
Assistant Professor, Faculty of Medicine, McGill University
Philippe Desmarais, MD, FRCPC, MHSc
Assistant Clinical Professor, Faculty of Medicine, Universite de Montreal
Michael Stiffel, MD, FRCPC
Assistant Clinical Professor, Faculty of Medicine, Universite de Sherbrooke

Clinical vignette

Mrs. C is an 89-year-old woman living in a Long-Term-Care (LTC) facility. She is known to suffer from type 2 diabetes and major neurocognitive disorder of moderate intensity (Alzheimer's). Three years ago, she was relocated to an LTC facility closed unit due to behavioural issues; verbal aggressivity and wandering. Her medications include short-acting insulin and quetiapine.

A few days ago, a resident living in the same unit as Mrs. C developed a cough and fever and was isolated. A COVID-19 swab was done on this resident, which turned out to be positive. Ever since, the nursing staff has been closely monitoring Mrs. C. Although she has no fever or cough, the staff has noticed that her appetite has significantly decreased and that she has become more confused than her baseline. She continues to wander on the unit and constantly needs to be reminded to go back into her room.

Physical examination reveals that her blood pressure is 95/60 (her usual is 110/80), her pulse is 105, her respiratory rate is 14 per minute, her oxygen saturation is 95%

on room air and her temperature is 36.7 degrees. She appears tired and her mouth is dry. Her cardiac, respiratory and abdominal examinations are unremarkable.

COVID-19 Disclaimer:

It is important to acknowledge that COVID-19 is a new disease and that our understanding of it is constantly evolving. This text reflects our current understanding of the disease as well as our opinions as geriatricians in accordance with our clinical experience of treating older adults with COVID-19.

Virology of SARS-CoV-2

COVID-19 is a disease caused by a coronavirus which was discovered in 2019: SARS-CoV-2 (severe acute respiratory syndrome coronavirus 2). This novel coronavirus was first described in Wuhan, China, in a cluster of individuals suffering from unexplained pneumonia. On March 11th, 2020, the World Health Organization declared COVID-19 a pandemic.

SARS-CoV-2 is mainly transmitted through droplets and contact. Contact can be direct (direct contact with a contaminated individual) or indirect (contaminated surfaces; fomites). Airborne transmission is also possible in the context of aerosol generating procedures or treatments (endotracheal intubation, for example). To this date, fecal-oral transmission has not been confirmed.

The average incubation period for this virus is 5–6 days. This incubation period may be as great as 14 days, especially in individuals with milder forms of the disease. Typically, symptomatic individuals are contagious for 1 to 3 days prior to onset of symptoms. Asymptomatic individuals can be contagious. It is also known that COVID-19 is more infectious than influenza and carries greater mortality.

Epidemiology of Covid-19

In the province of Quebec (Canada), although individuals aged 80 years and older represent about 20% of total confirmed cases, they represent 73% of the overall mortality. The majority (68%) of deaths happened in long-term care settings. (Based on INSPQ July 2020). These figures are similar in many states and countries around the world. In the USA for example, this percentage varied from 21-81% in different states according to data provided by the Kaiser Family Foundation (May 2020).

Older individuals are at higher risk of morbidity and mortality due to multiple factors, including age (which is a risk factor in itself), as well as multiple comorbidities (diabetes, hypertension, chronic obstructive pulmonary disease, etc.). Individuals living in LTC settings are at a higher risk when compared to the general older population for a variety of reasons; they are vulnerable, frail, and have a higher burden of comorbidities, including dementia. They are also frequently in close proximity to their caregivers and other residents, increasing the risk of transmission.

COVID-19 has been classically described as a respiratory disease with a wide spectrum of clinical presentations (from asymptomatic carriers to critical respiratory failure). Disease severity for COVID-19 is divided into mild, moderate, and severe cases. Mild cases represent the most common trajectory of clinical cases where patients present with only minor symptoms such as a low-grade fever, a dry cough, or headaches. Moderate cases are defined by the presence of marked, persistent fever and respiratory symptoms such as dyspnea, chest pains and productive cough, which suggest the presence of underlying pneumonia. Finally, severe cases are defined by the presence of respiratory distress (e.g., marked tachypnea, desaturation), respiratory failure and shock. Although no data is available for the LTC population, the Chinese Centre for Disease Control and Prevention reported that mild, moderate and severe cases were reported in 81%, 14% and 5% of the total case load, respectively.

Furthermore, it has been well documented that a clinical syndrome can evolve rapidly in at risk groups (including older adults and LTC residents).

Clinical Presentation:

Typical clinical manifestations of COVID-19

The classic clinical presentation associated with COVID-19 is that of a viral syndrome, similar in many regards to influenza (influenza is indeed part of the differential diagnosis). This viral syndrome includes fever, chills, myalgia, lethargy, fatigue and an overall reduced general condition. Patients may also present with headaches, joint pains and non-specific chest pains (secondary to pericardial inflammation). In some patients, specifically those in younger and lower-risk groups, the viral syndrome is the only clinical manifestation of COVID-19.

Respiratory symptoms

Respiratory symptoms usually follow after typical viral syndrome symptoms. These symptoms are variable, and often include a dry cough, and dyspnea. Respiratory symptoms are rarely the initial presentation in COVID-19 patients residing in LTC.

Bacterial pneumonia is a possible complication that must be suspected and treated proactively with the appropriate antibiotic options. Additionally, LTC residents are at higher risk for aspiration pneumonia, for a variety of reasons, including underlying neurocognitive disorders and risk of delirium arising from altered mental states. Therefore, bacterial pneumonia should be included in the differential diagnosis of clinical deterioration for COVID-19 patients, especially in LTC facilities.

Non-respiratory symptoms

Although COVID-19 typically presents with respiratory and viral symptoms, there are unique and unusual elements which must not be ignored. These particularities are even more significant in older adults, where clinical presentation can be, and often is, atypical and even asymptomatic. Early recognition, supportive care and appropriate treatment options are therefore essential.

Gastrointestinal symptoms are also frequently observed, including loss of appetite, nausea and diarrhea, which can lead to a significant risk of dehydration in certain populations. As we learn more about this new condition, additional symptoms—some of which are less typical in other viral syndromes—have been identified; specifically, the loss or decrease in sense of taste and smell.

Neurological symptoms going beyond the cognitive changes observed in delirium or secondary to the electrolyte imbalances arising from dehydration and hypoxia have also been observed. COVID-19 creates a pro-coagulant state with increased risk of thrombosis at various sites. It is therefore important to consider strokes and TIA in the differential diagnosis of acute neurological symptoms and changes.

The pro-coagulant state associated with COVID-19 is not limited to neurological complications. Thromboembolic events may also occur at various sites and must be taken into account in the clinical evaluation of these patients. Pulmonary embolisms would worsen respiratory symptoms and venous thrombosis could be overlooked in the context of myalgia.

Considerations for the geriatric population

It is known that the geriatric population is at high-risk for COVID-19. However, other elements must be taken into account. As previously mentioned, initial symptoms in older adults may present more subtly and atypically (e.g., patients presenting with only loss of appetite), which may in turn delay diagnosis/management. Gastrointestinal symptoms, as well as general fatigue, have been observed in COVID-19 patients, placing LTC residents specifically at higher risk for dehydration. Older patients already have decreased feelings of thirst, and diarrhea combined with any decrease in oral intake will expose them to weight loss and dehydration. Consequently, they may suffer from electrolyte imbalances, renal damage and greater difficulty in controlling certain conditions, such as diabetes with hypoglycemia. It is also important to consider the polypharmacy of patients, as acute illness may affect plasma concentrations of different medications, exposing patients to multiple undesirable and potentially harmful side effects.

Clinical Approach:
General Approach

Screening and diagnosis

In the context of an increasing number of COVID-19 cases, as may be seen during an epidemic or pandemic, a low-suspicion threshold should be set to screen, test, and isolate residents in LTC facilities. This is supported by the fact that the virus can spread quickly through asymptomatic carriers, such as facility workers and visiting family members, and that clinical manifestations of the infection in older adults are frequently atypical or subtle. As for the common manifestations of COVID-19; low-grade fever, new onset of weakness, gait impairment or fall, or increased cognitive deficits (e.g., confusion, delirium) in the absence of a clear etiology, may be sufficient to warrant the ruling out of COVID-19 if cases have been reported in the LTC facility or if there is community transmission.

Screening of residents for carrier status and suspected COVID-19 diagnoses is performed by nasopharyngeal swab which must be tested for the presence of SARS-CoV-2 RNA through RT-PCR. False negative results are not uncommon as the test sensitivity is highly dependent on the use of adequate technique to obtain the sample. If the test result is negative but there is a high suspicion of COVID-19, the test should be repeated 24 to 48 hours following the first test.

While the diagnosis of COVID-19 is primarily based on the identification of virus RNA in nasopharyngeal secretions, other investigations may be suggestive of infection. COVID-19 cases frequently present with lymphopenia and thrombocytopenia on CBC, as well as elevated C-reactive protein, d-dimers, and fibrinogen, these latter markers having prognostic utility. Pulmonary imaging, such as chest X-rays and CT scans, may show findings suggestive of viral pneumonia (i.e., diffuse interstitial infiltrates and bilateral perihilar peribronchial thickening), as well as findings for bacterial superinfection or acute respiratory distress syndrome (ARDS), both conditions being common complications of COVID-19. Investigations should be performed in keeping with available resources at the LTC facility, according to the resident's personal wishes, goals, and objectives (i.e., level of care), and depending on whether results of investigations would alter clinical management.

Strategies for disease transmission prevention and protection of workers and residents

In the context of an epidemic or pandemic episode where a significant proportion of cases occur within one specific region, several strategies should be implemented to prevent an outbreak within LTC facilities. These strategies, which may be recommended or ordered by public health officials, will vary, but usually include:

- Widespread screening of asymptomatic and symptomatic residents and facility workers, especially with regard to new admissions and employees;
- Potential quarantining of residents;
- Reinforcing hand washing, respect of respiratory hygiene/cough etiquette, and donning and doffing of face masks for all facility workers, as well as for residents (when they are not alone in their room);
- Limiting visits to asymptomatic primary caregivers of residents wearing appropriate personal protective equipment;
- Limiting personnel movement and deployment on multiple floors and/ or units;
- Updating resident level of intervention in personal medical charts.

Additionally, in the case of an outbreak within an LTC residence, the following strategies should be implemented to prevent further transmission within the facility:

- Separate floors and/or units for infected and non-infected residents and adoption of appropriate droplet precautions throughout the facility;
- Workers dedicated to specific floors and/or units (i.e., avoid having workers care for infected and non-infected residents within the same shift);
- Limiting the number and duration of interactions with residents to essential visits, as well as maximizing the number of interventions within a single visit. This can be achieved by:

- ○ Simplifying the residents' drug regimen by limiting it to essential drugs only, which may reduce the number of daily visits to their room for drug administration. For instance, drugs prescribed for primary prevention indications may be stopped temporarily (e.g., vitamin D, bisphosphonates);
- ○ Administering drugs to residents during daily mealtime-dedicated visits.

Supportive care

As is often the case with other viral respiratory infections, there is currently no clinically approved curative treatment for COVID-19. Supportive care measures should be provided to infected residents, which include prescribing antipyretic and analgesic drugs for fever and pain, implementing non-pharmacological interventions for persistent and bothersome coughs, ensuring adequate food and liquid intake, and ensuring frequent normal bowel function.

Vaccines

In the United States and Canada, priority in receiving two new mRNA vaccines has been given to the older population and their caregivers. In the first instance, these vaccines have been made available to residents of nursing homes and similar long term care facilities, with recommendations for further priority to be given to all people in the USA aged 65 and older. In Canada, that recommendation begins at 80 years of age and decreases to 70 as supplies of vaccine become available. These vaccines have an efficacy of 94 percent and over in preventing COVID19 disease. The messenger RNA instructs the cell to make only part of the SARS-CoV-2 spike protein (so no disease is caused) which in turn activates the immune response, with production of memory T-lymphocytes and B-lymphocytes. Protein subunit vaccines (containing harmless viral proteins) and vector vaccines that carry genetic SARS-CoV-2 material within a different weakened virus are becoming available as well.

Treatment

Treatment approaches currently may include, with appropriate medical care in acute care settings, the administration of anti-SARS-CoV-2 monoclonal antibodies to affected people 65 years of age and above with comorbidities, with the aim of reducing severe disease.

Hospitalized patients with severe disease may have time to recovery shortened by the use of the antiviral remdesivir.

In patients requiring invasive mechanical ventilation, dexamethasone has been shown to decrease mortality to some extent.

Residents with COVID-19 should be closely monitored for commonly seen complications of the infection, such as bacterial superinfection, ARDS, thromboembolic events (e.g., deep vein thrombosis and pulmonary embolisms), delirium, cachexia, dehydration, and the emergence of immobility syndrome. Risk of bacterial superinfection can be reduced by ensuring proper oral hygiene and appropriate diet (to avoid aspiration in the context of dysphagia). If a bacterial superinfection is suspected, antibiotics should be promptly initiated, such as azithromycin with ceftriaxone. Although not part of common LTC clinical practices, residents suffering from a clinically moderate to severe case of the disease should be prescribed anti-thrombotic prophylaxis, as thromboembolic events are particularly frequent and lethal.

Palliative care

Since older adults residing in LTC facilities usually present with multiple comorbidities and are frail, mortality due COVID-19 is unsurprisingly high, especially considering that the disease can evolve quickly toward respiratory distress and death. Despite the extraordinary precautions and strategies necessary to reduce the risk of contamination, appropriate palliative care can be achieved within an LTC facility and every medical team has the capacity to provide adequate end-of-life care. In cases where palliative care is chosen, interventions should be implemented to actively ensure the resident's physical and mental well-being.

All unnecessary IV accesses, tubes, and cannulae may be discontinued, but a subcutaneous access should be kept for easy administration of medication. Respiratory distress protocol to alleviate terminal symptoms should be prescribed the moment that end-of-life care is chosen by the resident and his or her family, as respiratory distress may occur dramatically quickly with the disease. Given their potent analgesic properties, opioids should be prescribed to treat tachypnea, aiming for a breathing rate below 24/min. Antipsychotics and benzodiazepines may be prescribed for agitation and anxiety. Nausea and vomiting may be addressed with diphenhydramine or ondansetron. Haloperidol may also be used for nausea, as well as agitation. Constipation should be aggressively treated with laxatives in order to avoid abdominal discomfort.

If possible, families should be allowed to visit for humanitarian reasons. It is important for the team to accompany these families, both to provide support but also to ensure the correct use of appropriate personal protective equipment.

When to transfer to an acute care facility

According to the resident's level of care and the disease's evolution, residents presenting with clinically moderate to severe cases of the disease may have to be transferred to an acute care facility in order to receive interventions which cannot be performed within an LTC facility. Examples include respiratory and circulatory failure requiring invasive respiratory support and fluid resuscitation, as well as scenarios where appropriate palliative care cannot be provided locally.

Specific interventions for older adults

Loss of appetite, dehydration, and poor oral intake

COVID-19 is notably associated with anosmia and dysgeusia, which may cause loss of appetite, cachexia, and dehydration in older adults. Additionally, the infection and its associated hyperinflammatory state increase catabolism, which accelerates cachexia and dehydration. To reduce the risk of acute undernutrition and its complications, restricted diets (e.g., low carbohydrates, low salt, and low fat) should be avoided. Nutrition consultants and speech specialists, when available, should be quickly involved as they can design and implement specific interventions which may improve the residents' nutritional state.

Residents should be stimulated and, if needed, assisted when eating and drinking at every meal. Sufficient time should be allotted to meal intake. Dietary supplements may be used (after a meal and not to replace a meal) in order to increase caloric intake. Water pitchers should be provided to residents and hydration should be encouraged at every room visit. While IV fluids are generally to be avoided in LTC facilities, they may be utilized in specific cases.

Immobility syndrome and falls

Immobility syndrome is particularly frequent in older adults with COVID-19, partly as a side-effect of confinement and respiratory isolation measures. Cachexia, sarcopenia, respiratory symptoms (i.e., dyspnea), and hypoactive delirium may also contribute to immobility and falls. IV tubes, oxygen cannula, and Foley catheters may promote immobility and precipitate falls as well. Mobile residents should be encouraged to move about their room as much as possible, to use their walking aid appropriately, and to carry out daily living activities in whatever capacity they can. The use of catheters and tubes should be discontinued if feasible in order to reduce the risk of falls and to promote ambulation. When available, physiotherapists should be involved as they can design personalised exercise programmes. If residents become confined to their bed (i.e., bedridden), adequate therapeutic surfaces should be utilized to reduce the risk of pressure ulcers and residents should be moved in their bed as frequently as possible.

Delirium and behavioural issues

Fever, dehydration and hypoxemia, as well as confinement and isolation, may precipitate delirium in LTC residents. Delirium may also be secondary to another underlying medical problem and should therefore be investigated and treated appropriately. Behavioural issues in the context of delirium or dementia (i.e., Behavioral and Psychological Symptoms of Dementia: BPSD) represent a significant challenge in the context of precautions and strategies seeking to reduce the risk of transmission and contamination. Residents presenting behavioural issues may break droplet precaution and confinement orders. Non-pharmacological interventions (i.e., behavioural approaches) should be favoured, at first, to manage behavioural issues. These include:

- Reminding the resident at every visit of the importance of staying in their room;
- Providing them with cognitive or physical activities to do in their room;
- Putting a "STOP" sign on their door or other visual stimuli to keep them in their room;
- Asking a family member or volunteer to talk to them on the phone frequently.

Another avenue to consider is having a volunteer, in appropriate personal protective equipment, stay near the door of the resident's room, to remind them to stay inside. If these behavioural approaches fail and droplet precaution rules are repetitively broken by an infected resident, the possibility of locking the resident's door, using physical restraints (e.g., an abdominal belt while sitting in a chair), or prescribing pharmacological interventions (e.g., low dose antipsychotics) may be considered, but only as a last resort and after having carefully weighed the risks and benefits of such measures. The resident's family should be informed of these issues and be involved in the decision-making process regarding the measures which should be implemented. The least limiting measure should be selected, its indication and success should be reviewed frequently, and it should be discontinued whenever feasible and appropriate.

Case summary

Mrs. C lives in an LTC facility, on a closed unit. Recently, a resident from her unit was diagnosed with COVID-19 and was isolated in his room. Mrs. C is known to suffer from major neurocognitive disorder of moderate intensity (Alzheimer's), and presents with a clear change from her baseline behaviour and general state; her increased confusion suggests that she is suffering from delirium. It is also important to recognize that delirium can be both hyperactive and hypoactive. Therefore, patients can become either more agitated or lethargic.

She does not present with any viral syndrome or respiratory symptoms but does suffer from a decrease in appetite. Although she is afebrile and saturating well without signs of respiratory distress, she is already showing signs of dehydration (tachycardia and decreased blood pressure).

Considering that a resident on her unit has tested positive for COVID-19, all the residents from this unit, including Mrs. C, should be tested and isolated to prevent the propagation of the virus. It is important to frequently reassess the clinical status of Mrs. C as COVID-19 is a disease which can evolve rapidly. Furthermore, the person in charge of making medical decisions for Mrs. C should be frequently informed of her clinical status and the objectives for her care should be discussed. Other preventative measures, as described above, should be implemented:

- Nutrition and hydration: Mrs. C should be encouraged to eat and drink. She may also benefit from dietary supplements to increase her caloric intake. Considering her tachycardia, IV fluids could be considered.
- Mobility: She should be encouraged to move, to prevent deconditioning all while respecting current isolation measures. (Mrs. C should ambulate in her room.)
- Diabetes: Mrs. C is known to suffer from insulin-dependent diabetes. In the context of her decreased oral intake, her dose of insulin should be adjusted to avoid hypoglycemia.

- Wandering behaviour: As described above, non-pharmacological interventions (i.e., behavioural approaches) should be favoured. Pharmacological measures may be needed, but these should only be undertaken as a last resort.

- Delirium: Mrs. C's cognitive status should be frequently re-evaluated. Her oral intake, sleep, mobility, skin care and elimination should be optimized. If she were to become lethargic, her dose of quetiapine should be decreased.

- Monitoring of respiratory status: As mentioned previously, LTC residents are at high risk of aspiration pneumonia. There is also a risk of bacterial superinfection (pneumonia) with COVID-19. The need for antibiotics should be frequently reassessed.

References:

1. D'Adamo, H., Yoshikawa, T., & Ouslander, J. G. (2020). Coronavirus disease 2019 in geriatrics and long-term care: the ABCDs of COVID-19. *Journal of the American Geriatrics Society, 68*(5), 912-917.

2. https://www.inspq.qc.ca/covid-19/donnees

3. Wu, Z., & McGoogan, J. M. (2020). Characteristics of and important lessons from the coronavirus disease 2019 (COVID-19) outbreak in China: summary of a report of 72,314 cases from the Chinese Centre for Disease Control and Prevention. *Jama, 323*(13), 1239-1242.
   https://www.cdc.gov/coronavirus/2019-ncov/vaccines/different-vaccines.html
   https://www.canada.ca/en/public-health/services/immunization/national-advisory-committee-on-immunization-naci/guidance-prioritization-initial-doses-covid-19-vaccines.html
   https://www.fda.gov/news-events/press-announcements/coronavirus-covid-19-updatefda-authorizes-monoclonal-antibodies-treatment-covid-19
   https://www.nejm.org/doi/full/10.1056/NEJMoa2007764
   https://www.biospace.com/article/releases/government-of-canada-signs-new-agreement-for-a-covid-19-antibody-therapy/#:~:text=Today%252C%2520the%2520Honourable%2520Anita%2520Anand,monoclonal%2520antibody%2520therapy%2520Bamlanivimab%2520(LY%252D
   https://www.canada.ca/en/health-canada/services/drugs-health-products/covid19-industry/drugs-vaccines-treatments/remdesivir-update.html

STROKE PREVENTION IN THE ELDERLY

Liam Durcan, MD, FRCPC, Assistant Professor, Department of Neurology and Neurosurgery, McGill University,

Consultant Neurologist, Stroke Service, McGill University Health Centre

A 74 year-old right-handed woman who had been previously healthy is seen in clinic following her presentation to the emergency department. She relates a history of suddenly losing the ability to speak for 15 minutes on the previous day. She was able to understand all that was said to her during the event. She denied having had any headache or other neurological symptoms. By the time she presented to the emergency department her symptoms had resolved and her neurological exam was normal. Her blood pressure was 160/95.

Brain imaging (a non-contrast CT scan) showed no acute stroke nor hemorrhage. The only abnormality on a carotid doppler done the same day was an 80% stenosis of the right internal carotid artery. ECG revealed normal sinus rhythm.

Her fasting glucose was 6mmol/l and her LDL was 3.8 mmol/l. She is a non-smoker.

The diagnosis of isolated expressive aphasia, due to a transient ischemic attack, was made.

Preamble

Stroke is a leading cause of death and disability. Risk of stroke is age-related and age is the most important non-modifiable risk-factor. Modifiable risk factors for recurrent stroke include hypertension, diabetes, dyslipidemic states, smoking, symptomatic carotid stenosis and atrial fibrillation.

The incidence of stroke increases with age, doubling for each decade after age 55. Among adults ages 35 to 44, the incidence of stroke is 30 to 120 of 100,000 per year, and for those ages 65 to 74, the incidence is 670 to 970 of 100,000 per year.

Stroke risk is further heightened after TIA and minor stroke– observational and risk-stratification studies have shown between 2% and 17% within the first 90 days. In patients who have had a transient ischemic attack, one in five will have a subsequent stroke, heart attack or die within one year, with stroke being the most common outcome.

One of the challenges in stroke prevention in the elderly is the application of evidence-based treatment or investigational recommendations in an age group who have often been excluded from randomized trials on which those recommendations are based. Unlike in younger adults where the evidence for secondary stroke prevention is well established and supported by randomized clinical trial data, evidence is often less clear in older adults.

What is the risk to this patient?

A recent TIA is associated with a significant increase of subsequent stroke. Tools such as the $ABCD_2$ score can give some insight to the degree of that heightened risk as well as risk-stratify patients according to their demographics, vascular risks and clinical presentation.

$ABCD_2$ score		Points
Age > 60 years		1
BP > 140/90 at presentation		1

Clinical features of the TIA
  Speech disturbance without weakness or
  Unilateral weakness
		1
		2

Duration of symptoms
  10-59 minutes
  ≥60 minutes
		1
		2

Diabetes in patient's history		1

Risk of stroke following various ABCD$_2$ scores:

Total Risk	Scores	2 days	7 day	90 days
Low	0-3	1.0	1.2	3.1
Moderate	4-5	4.1	5.9	9.8
High	6-7	8.1	12.0	18

This patient's ABCD2 score is 4—her risk of event recurrence, using this data, is moderate.

What are her risk factors associated with this presentation?

Age, hypertension, and hyperlipidemia.

Hypertension

Following a stroke or transient ischemic attack, blood pressure lowering treatment is recommended to achieve a target of lower than 140/90 mm Hg. For patients who have had a small subcortical stroke, blood pressure lowering treatment is recommended to achieve a systolic target lower than 130 mm Hg. In patients with diabetes, blood pressure lowering treatment is recommended for the prevention of first or recurrent stroke to attain systolic blood pressure targets consistently lower than 130 mm Hg and diastolic blood pressure targets consistently lower than 80 mm Hg.

Reducing blood pressure is more important than the agent used.

Hypertension in the Very Elderly Trial confirmed the benefit of treating hypertension in patients over the age of 80. Patients were randomized to indapamide or placebo with a target BP of 150/90. No significant differences in adverse events—primarily syncopal episodes and falls of any kind–were noted between the treatment and placebo group. The number-needed-to treat (or NNT) at 2 years was 94 for stroke and 40 for mortality. (the NNT is an epidemiological measure of the effectiveness of an intervention. It is the average number of people who need to be treated to prevent one additional bad outcome compared to the control group. The lower the number the more effective the treatment.)

Carotid stenosis is an important and potentially treatable risk factor for recurrent stroke, with the most important determinants of risk being the degree of stenosis and whether the stenosis is symptomatic. The most important initial decision-point is whether the stenosis is symptomatic: an asymptomatic carotid stenosis of greater than 70% carries a per year risk of 1-3 % and current guidelines recommend maximal medical therapy over endarterectomy. This relatively low risk is contrasted with a 28.3 % 3-year risk of symptomatic carotid stenoses of the same degree.

It is also important to note that risk of recurrent ipsilateral stroke in symptomatic stenosis greater than 70% is markedly increased in the period immediately following the TIA or minor stroke—with ipsilateral recurrence risk ranging from 11.5% to 25% at 14 days. Pooled data from the North American Symptomatic Carotid Endarterectomy Trial and the European Carotid Stenosis Trial showed performing carotid endarterectomy within two weeks gave optimum results.

Atrial fibrillation is a cardiac arrhythmia associated with an increased risk of ischemic stroke and peripheral embolization. The arrhythmia is associated with a gradual increase in left atrial volume and can be associated with presence of a thrombus in the left atrial appendage. Patients may have a number of symptoms with atrial fibrillation, but it must be remembered that many patients may experience subclinical atrial fibrillation and that symptoms of palpitations are neither sensitive nor specific for atrial fibrillation.

Non-valvular atrial fibrillation increases stroke risk by a factor of 5 and Valvular atrial fibrillation by a factor of 17. Atrial fibrillation becomes more clinically relevant with age: the attributable risk of stroke from AF is estimated to be 1.5% for those aged 50-59 years, and it approaches 30% for those aged 80-89 years. Women are at a higher risk of stroke due to AF than men. Strokes attributed to atrial fibrillation are more severe and TIAs attributed tend to last longer than those attributed to other etiologies.

The diagnosis of atrial fibrillation is most often made from the electrocardiogram—whether it is a single ECG exam, the 24 or 48-hour evaluation of a Holter monitor or more prolonged cardiac monitoring. The Embrace Study compared 30-day ambulatory monitoring with a 24-hour Holter monitor to detect atrial fibrillation in cryptogenic (unknown cause) stroke . The 30-day monitoring arm detected atrial fibrillation in 16.1% compared to 3.2% in the group investigated with 24-hour Holter.

Clinical scores—such as the $CHADS_2$ score and CHA_2DS_2-VASc Score–have been developed to help predict the risk of stroke and systemic embolism in patients with AF, in order to determine whether that risk is sufficient to warrant the bleeding risks associated with anticoagulant therapy. In a patient who presents with stroke or TIA and is found to be in atrial fibrillation, the ischemic event alone carries enough value in these scoring systems to warrant anticoagulation.

Hyperlipidemia- many observational studies have described the relationship between lipid abnormalities and elevated stroke risk, implicated in both intracranial and extracranial atherosclerosis. The pivotal study showing benefit of lipid lowering regimes in stroke prevention was the SPACL study, which randomized patients to atorvastatin 80 mg or placebo. The treatment group had an absolute risk reduction of 2.2% for a number-needed to treat of 45 to prevent one stroke at 5 years.

Diabetes

Through mechanisms such as accelerated atherosclerosis and endothelial dysfunction, diabetes increases not only the risk for stroke, but is also associated with increased post-stroke mortality and poorer clinical outcomes for survivors. Most recently, GLP-1 agonists have shown to have a modest benefit in prevention of stroke in Type II diabetics. (Absolute risk reduction of 0.81% or NNT of 125)

Smoking

Cigarette smoking is associated with an approximate doubling of stroke risk. A recent study has also shown a dose–response relationship for the risk, with an odds ratio ranging from 1.46 for those smoking <11 cigarettes per day to 5.66 for those smoking 40+ cigarettes per day, indicating that while cessation is the ultimate goal, reduction of amount smoked can confer an important risk reduction.

What would be an appropriate initial intervention and further investigations?

As the patient has presented more than a day after her event and has no residual deficits, **she is not candidate for acute revascularization therapies** (intravenous tPA or endovascular thrombectomy).

Tempo of Assessment and Intervention—The EXPRESS Study prospectively looked at 90-day recurrent stroke rates in patients seen in clinic before and after an expedited assessment program was put into place. The establishment of expedited assessment (with a reduction of median time to evaluation of 3 days to 1 day) resulted in an Absolute Risk Reduction of recurrent stroke at 90-days of 8.2%.

The combination of low-dose aspirin and clopidogrel (Plavix) has been found to reduce the risk of recurrent stroke and disability compared with aspirin alone when started as soon as possible after a high-risk transient ischemic attack (TIA) or minor ischemic stroke without persistent disabling neurologic deficit and continued for 10 to 21 days.

Three randomized controlled trials comparing dual antiplatelet therapy with aspirin monotherapy in more than 10,000 patients provided evidence that dual therapy decreased nonfatal recurrent strokes (number needed to treat [NNT] = 53). Dual anti-platelet therapy had no effect on all-cause mortality or the incidence of myocardial infarction or recurrent TIA, and had some associated harms of minor (number needed to harm [NNH] = 143) and moderate to major (NNH = 500) extracranial bleeding.

As the patient is hypertensive and is neurologically stable, **antihypertensive medication** can be started. The choice of agent may be influenced by a number of other health variables or patient preferences.

A more conservative approach is often indicated in patients with an acute and persistent neurological deficit as they may be depending on elevated blood pressure to maintain cerebral perfusion to potentially endangered brain tissue. Often, antihypertensives may be held for 48 to 72 hours following a stroke, assuming the elevated BP is not causing end-organ damage elsewhere.

Cholesterol-lowering agents–Statins are started after stroke, with many stroke specialists using dosages in higher range (Atorvastatin 40-80 mg daily) to achieve a reduction of LDL below 2 mmol/l.

Investigations

TTE

Transthoracic echocardiographic evaluation is recommended for most stroke patients, primarily to investigate the conditions associated with Atrial fibrillation and to assess valvular structures, which may influence the type of antithrombotic agent used.

Holter

Paroxysmal AF may not be detected on serial ECGs or short-term cardiac monitoring. In cases of acute cerebral ischemia where the diagnosis of atrial fibrillation is not already made, a 24- or 48-hour Holter monitor is indicated. If these investigations are negative but atrial fibrillation is still clinically suspected (cryptogenic stroke, no evidence of large vessel atherosclerosis, increased Left atrial volume on TTE, excessive number of premature atrial beats: e.g. >500 per 24 hrs of monitoring) ambulatory cardiac monitoring for 30 days is suggested.

Education

All patients are counselled on lifestyle changes that have positive effects on reducing stroke recurrence. As well, a key part of any initial assessment is ensuring the patient understands the symptoms of stroke, to be better able to present immediately should they experience recurrent symptoms.

Resolution of the clinical vignette.

The patient remained asymptomatic. At 21 days post-event, Plavix was stopped and low-dose (81 mg daily) enteric-coated Aspirin was continued. The patient was started on atorvastatin 40 mg daily and perindopril 4 mg/ indapamide 1.25 mg daily. Her Hemoglobin A1c was not elevated.

In this case, the carotid stenosis, although greater than 60%, is in the right Internal Carotid Artery and the patient's stroke is localized to an area supplied by the left carotid artery. The right carotid stenosis is an **asymptomatic stenosis** and best managed medically. Endarterectomy is not indicated.

The patient had a trans-thoracic echocardiogram that showed slightly increased left atrial volume without structural abnormality of the valves. A 48-hour Holter monitor did not detect atrial fibrillation but did show greater than 1500 premature atrial beats per 24 hours. A 30-day implanted device revealed prolonged episodes of atrial fibrillation. The patient was started on Apixaban 5 mg BID. Aspirin was stopped.

References:

1. Dual Antiplatelet Therapy for High-Risk TIA and Minor Stroke: BMJ Rapid Recommendation *BMJ*. December 2018;363:k5130

2. Atrial Fibrillation in Cryptogenic Stroke. Gladstone D, et al. N Engl J Med 2014; 370:2467-2477

3. Validation and refinement of scores to predict very early stroke risk after transient ischaemic attack. Johnston SC et al. Lancet. 2007 27;369(9558):283-92.

4. Effect of urgent treatment of transient ischaemic attack and minor stroke on early recurrent stroke (EXPRESS study): a prospective population-based sequential comparison. Rothwell et al. Volume 370, Issue 9596, 20–26 October 2007, Pages 1432-1442.

5. Smoking and Risk of Ischemic Stroke in Young Men. Janina Markidan et al. Stroke. 2018;49:1276–1278

ADVANCES IN CARDIAC CARE FOR OLDER PERSONS

P. David Myerowitz, MD, FACS, FACC, Former Karl P. Klassen Professor and
Chairman Thoracic and Cardiovascular Surgery The Ohio State University

Introduction

Heart failure (Decreased or Preserved Ejection Fraction) and Hypertension

    Definitions and Medical Therapy

    Cardiac Resynchronization Therapy (CRT) / Implantable Cardioverter Defibrillator (ICD)

    Heart Transplantation and Mechanical Pumps

Coronary Artery Disease

Valve Disease

  Aortic Valve Disease

  Mitral Valve Disease

  Tricuspid Valve Disease

Arrhythmia – Atrial Fibrillation

  Medical Therapy and Cardioversion

  Ablation

    Pulmonary Vein Isolation

    AV Node Ablation + Pacemaker

Watchman Device for Stroke Prevention in Atrial Fibrillation

Palliative Cardiac Care

Advances in Cardiac Care for Older Persons

Many of the advances in cardiac care in the last two decades have focused on minimally invasive procedures especially aimed at the elderly and vulnerable. This chapter will attempt to chronicle these treatments, mainly surgical and invasive cardiological, but also some new drug therapies that have proven especially advantageous to the older cardiology patient. For the purpose of this chapter I will use age 65 – 84 as elderly and over 85 as very elderly. Since new procedures, devices and drugs are continuously added to the clinician's armamentarium, this chapter is not meant to be comprehensive. Nor is it written for cardiac care physicians. Rather it is a plain language description of the latest advances in cardiac care available to older patients designed to improve both length and quality of life.

Since the concept of frailty was discussed in an earlier chapter, I will not repeat the discussion. Although there are objective measures, such as the Charlson Comorbidity Index, for most of my career as a cardiac surgeon, the concept of frailty was more a subjective assessment, i.e. you'll know it when you see it. That said, my first heart transplant in 1984 was in a man over 50 years old which at that time was pushing the age limit (he survived over ten years to see multiple grandchildren born). I also remember a blind, formerly active 90 year old man confined to his bed with severe aortic stenosis whom I was pushed to operate on in the 1980s and whose family sent me a picture ten years later of him celebrating his 100th birthday. In my opinion, age alone should not definitively rule out most if not all available options for cardiac care.

In fact, there is a quarterly journal, Journal of Geriatric Cardiology, devoted to the care of the older patient with cardiovascular disease.

Heart failure (Decreased or Preserved Ejection Fraction) and Hypertension
Definitions and Medical Therapy

Heart failure occurs when the heart is unable to pump enough blood to keep up with the oxygen demands of the body. Some of the typical symptoms include shortness of breath, fatigue, peripheral edema (swelling of the legs), persistent cough, rapid weight gain and confusion. The common measurement used to define this condition and which is easily obtained by a noninvasive test called an echocardiogram is the ejection fraction, the percentage of the volume of blood in the left ventricle (the heart's main pumping chamber) that is ejected with each heartbeat. Normally this is greater than 50%. A value below 40% is consistent with heart failure and is labeled heart failure with reduced ejection fraction (HFrEF).

The New York Heart Association for classification of heart failure describes four categories based on severity of symptoms: Class I is no symptoms with no limitation of activity; Class II is symptoms on normal activity with slight limitation of activity; Class III is marked limitation of activity with symptoms on less than normal activity; and Class IV is symptoms on any activity with inability to perform any activity. Roughly one third of patients are in Class I, a third in Class II and a third in Class III and IV.

Studies show that 1 – 5% of the population have chronic heart failure and 50% of these heart failure patients are over 75 years of age. Eighty-five percent of first-time hospitalizations for heart failure are over 65 and 60% are over 75 years old with one-third of these patients dying within 6 months of diagnosis.

Fifty percent of patients and increasing in frequency comprise a second group of patients with heart failure with preserved ejection fraction (HFpEF). These patients have characteristic symptoms of heart failure but a normal ejection fraction. This diagnosis can also be made by echocardiogram and most likely results from stiffness of the muscle of the left ventricle. I will first discuss heart failure with reduced ejection fraction.

The mainstay of treatment for HFrEF is drug therapy and perhaps the most commonly used categories of drugs are the angiotensin-converting enzyme inhibitors (ACE inhibitors) and angiotensin receptor blockers (ARBs) that block the release of substances that cause narrowing of blood vessels. There are many affordable brand-name and generic versions of these drugs available. By dilating peripheral blood vessels the workload of the heart is reduced, much like opening a nozzle on the end of a hose reduces the workload on a water pump. Unfortunately, multicenter studies show that these drugs are vastly underutilized, especially in the older population, and when used are given in much lower doses than recommended.

High blood pressure, hypertension, commonly accompanies heart failure in the elderly. The target for systolic blood pressure (upper number) however has been a moving target for those heart councils recommending treatment. While 120 / 80 (mm.Hg.) is the classic normal blood pressure, treatment for decades was recommended for blood pressures over 130 systolic and 90 diastolic, with numbers in-between these two levels termed pre-hypertension. Recently the recommendation for target systolic pressure was lowered to 120; however, management in the elderly remains controversial. While the diastolic pressure (lower number) target remains the same, in the elderly a systolic of 130 seems realistic with a level of 150 in those over 80 to avoid the complications of sudden drops in blood pressure leading to syncope and falls.

A newer combination drug, angiotensin receptor blocker – neprilysin inhibitor (brand name in United States Entresto) has been shown to be even more effective in the treatment of HFrEF and should be used in patients who have a suboptimal response to the above drugs. Though somewhat more complicated in its action, the neprilysin inhibitor increases the activity of substances that block the retention of sodium, a common problem in heart failure patients.

Another commonly used category of drugs used in heart failure are diuretics which prevent fluid retention, presenting as fluid in the lungs as well as peripheral edema or swelling of the legs. Leg edema in the elderly may also be caused by venous insufficiency, poor nutrition with low protein levels in the blood and adverse drug effects (e.g. use of calcium channel blockers), resulting in frequent misdiagnosis especially in the very elderly. A recent blood test, B-type natriuretic peptide, is significantly elevated in heart failure and may be useful to confirm or rule out the diagnosis. Hydrochlorothiazide and spironolactone are commonly used affordable diuretics that are also effective in treating hypertension and HFrEF. With refractory or acute fluid retention, furosemide (brand name Lasix) is extremely effective in eliminating fluid retention demonstrated by sudden weight gain, but frequently causes a potentially dangerous lowering of potassium in the blood which can lead to heart rhythm disturbances.

Low dose beta blockers such as carvedilol and metoprolol are also commonly used to treat both heart failure and hypertension. If tolerated, a heart rate target of less than 70 should be achieved.

Side effects may occur with any of these drugs and include elevated blood potassium causing heart rhythm abnormalities and kidney dysfunction with ACE inhibitors, spironolactone and ARBs; vertigo, asthma-like bronchial constriction, depression and cognitive impairment with beta blockers; and low blood sodium with kidney failure and delirium for diuretics. These drugs must be monitored carefully as new drugs are added or their doses increased to prevent hypotension (low blood pressure). Orthostatic hypotension – a drop in blood pressure when one stands from sitting or lying down – is common, but may be transient and respond to temporary cessation of a drug followed by a more gradual increase in dose to allow accommodation. Bradycardia or a slow heart rate is a common side effect of all beta blockers. Heart rates of 60 to 70 are usually well tolerated.

Ancillary office personnel should do regular checks inquiring as to shortness of breath, dizziness or falls and patients should be instructed on regular two or three times-a-day home monitoring of blood pressure using an automated device and daily weight. Most automated blood pressure cuffs (Many cuffs are accurate and easy to use) also provide heart rate and store measurements for later review by caregivers. Patients should be instructed to report a rapid change up or down in weight, blood pressure or heart rate, especially if accompanied by dizziness.

In very elderly patients and all older patients with frailty demonstrated by muscle wasting, poor appetite, depression, lack of exercise and comorbidities such as diabetes and renal insufficiency all of these drugs must be used with extra caution. Drug levels tend to be higher in this population at the same doses as younger patients.

Multicenter studies have shown that these drugs, though highly effective, are not prescribed for many heart failure patients, especially the elderly, and, even if ordered, are not given in recommended dosages. With careful monitoring, these drugs can and should be prescribed for the older patient with symptomatic heart failure with reduced ejection fraction and/or hypertension.

The incidence of heart failure with preserved ejection fraction is increasing in the elderly and now represents half of all patients with heart failure. Nonetheless, this group of heart failure patients is less well understood and has no effective therapy. Echocardiographic studies frequently demonstrate diastolic dysfunction or stiffening of the left ventricle.

Treatment of associated conditions such as coronary artery disease and hypertension should be addressed. However, despite treatment regimens similar to heart failure with reduced ejection fraction, little gains have been achieved in reducing mortality, the need for re-hospitalization or improving symptoms and quality of life as has been accomplished with HFrEF. Nonetheless, the same drugs discussed above should be tried in these patients in hopes of achieving some improvement.

No discussion of the treatment of heart failure in the older person would be complete without a discussion of end of life care. Hospitalizations are frequent, and at some point, options for additional therapy run out. Since most adults with heart failure die in a hospital, palliative care at home may be appropriate treatment for this cohort in an attempt to improve quality of life and reduce costs associated with repeat hospitalizations.

Cardiac Resynchronization Therapy (CRT) / Intracardiac Defibrillator (ICD)

Nearly a century ago, researchers found that heart rhythm abnormalities led to impaired heart function. Eighty years later, in the 1990s, heart failure patients with electrical conduction abnormalities on their electrocardiogram (ECG), specifically a left bundle branch block (LBBB) producing delayed contraction between the right and left ventricles, showed significant improvement in ejection fraction when a pacemaker was used to correct this abnormality. Not all patients show improvement with a third not responding at all.

The technique involves the transvenous insertion of electrodes into the right atrium, right ventricle and a third electrode through the coronary sinus into a vein on the back of the left ventricle. Initiation of contraction begins with sensing of an electrical impulse in the right atrium followed by simultaneous firing of the right ventricle and left ventricle electrodes so their contractions occur simultaneously. This provides optimal filling of the left ventricle and, in two thirds of patients, reduction in symptoms and improvement in heart function. The addition of defibrillator function to the device also reduces the incidence of sudden death.

All heart failure patients in Class III or IV heart failure with the likelihood of significant survival who demonstrate a left bundle branch block on ECG should be considered for a CRT pacemaker insertion.

Heart Transplantation and Mechanical Pumps

As I mentioned in my introduction, in its early years, heart transplantation was restricted to the young - under age 50 - with no other organ dysfunction. The number of donors per year has struggled to keep up with an expanding pool of recipients including the elderly resulting in longer waiting lists and the search for alternative solutions. Comparing 2008 to 2018, the percent of adult heart transplant recipients over the age of 65 increased from 13.9% to 22.2% in the United States. In absolute numbers, 660 heart transplants were performed in 2018 in people over the age of 65. The push for this expansion came as multiple single center studies showed similar survival rates in the elderly as in younger than 65 recipients. At the same time, the percent of adults receiving a heart transplant for coronary artery disease decreased while the percent performed for cardiomyopathy increased, most likely the result of improved treatment of coronary artery disease as well as the increase in end stage heart failure patients.

Part of the explanation is the expanded donor pool during this time which until 2010 had been stagnant at about 2500 a year. But in the second half of the last decade, numbers jumped to 3500 perhaps partly as a result of expanding acceptable criteria for donors and older population growth. These new criteria included increasing donor age to 65; accepting Hepatitis C positive donors and then treating the hepatitis with a newly discovered, expensive but very effective treatment in the recipient; and accepting marginal hearts requiring corrective procedures (such as coronary bypass or valve repair) or a period of mechanical support for recovery of function. Many of these marginal donor organs were used in older recipients with good results.

The technique of heart transplantation has basically not changed since first performed in the late 1960s. The results, however, have greatly improved with current one, three, and five year survival at 90%, 85% and 80% respectively.

Much of the improved survival is a result of safer and more effective immunosuppressive drugs such as cyclosporine and more recently tacrolimus and mycophenolate mofetil/mycophenolic acid. These drugs have reduced the frequency and severity of acute rejections and possibly chronic rejection as demonstrated by diffuse coronary artery vasculopathy, a common cause of late mortality. They have also allowed the more aggressive and early tapering of corticosteroids, another immunosuppressive mainstay which has severe side effects. These newer drugs are especially important in the older recipient in whom the side effects of corticosteroid therapy such as hypertension and diabetes are more frequent.

Other factors leading to improved survival, with heart transplants performed since 2000 experiencing a median survival of 12 years, include better preservation of donor hearts and mechanical devices used pretransplant to stabilize and improve multi-organ dysfunction in severely ill recipients. These pumps have developed along two distinct pathways, ventricular assist devices (VADs) and total artificial hearts (TAHs). A VAD is attached to the patient's existing heart while a TAH replaces the heart. Most patients can be managed with a single left-sided VAD since the predominant problem is left ventricular dysfunction and a single VAD connected to the apex of the left ventricle with outflow to the ascending aorta is able to pump the entire cardiac output to the systemic circulation. If there is additional right ventricular dysfunction, either an additional right sided VAD may be implanted or, if available, a TAH can be implanted. Currently available TAHs are more complicated to insert and, of course, eliminate any chance for native heart recovery and removal.

Mechanical pumps have been effectively used as a bridge to transplantation for almost 40 years. Unlike earlier pulsatile pumps, more recent models are continuous flow (the patients do not have a pulse), use floating blades to propel the blood and require less anticoagulation than earlier models. Patients on transplant waiting lists who are failing medical therapy can be supported for months or years while multi-organ failure is reversed and they are stabilized prior to transplantation. They can be discharged to home with much improved quality of life awaiting a suitable donor. The poster child for an older person with this therapy is former Vice-president Dick Cheney. He underwent implantation of a VAD at age 69, appeared in a television interview while on the device and subsequently, at age 71, underwent a successful heart transplant in 2012.

The next stage of development of particular importance to those heart failure patients over 65 is the use of VADs or total heart replacement with a mechanical pump as destination therapy, rather than as a bridge to transplant . Most patients only require support of the left ventricle which can be accomplished with a VAD. For those with damage to both the right and left ventricles, a total artificial heart may be necessary. In fact, I wrongly predicted shortly after I started our heart transplant and mechanical pump/ artificial heart program at The Ohio State University in 1986 that heart transplantation would be obsolete in 10 years, replaced by mechanical pumps. With vast improvements in technology, we are finally getting closer. Recent studies show two-year survival in these critically ill terminal heart failure patients receiving destination therapy with a VAD of 50 – 80 %, making this option viable. Over 10,000 patients worldwide have undergone implantation of a HeartMate II VAD.

Unfortunately, it is estimated that 300,000 patients would benefit from implantation of a VAD for end stage heart failure. Obviously, the cost, estimated at $200,000 to $300,000 an implant would be prohibitive. How this technology will be applied to the thousands of terminal heart failure patients over 65 remains in question.

Coronary Artery Disease

Heart attacks and angina (crushing chest pain usually described as a weight on the chest rather than sharp pain and frequently confused with indigestion) occur when one or more of the three major arteries or their branches on the surface of the heart (coronary arteries) suffer restricted flow or blockage. The average age at presentation with acute coronary syndrome, a constellation of symptoms occurring during a heart attack (ACS) is 65 for males and 72 for females, the delay in the latter being perhaps due to the protective effects of estrogen in earlier life. Two thirds of myocardial infarctions, heart attacks, occur in those over 65 years of age and 85% of the mortality in ACS is in the Medicare population.

Age impacts not only the risk of cardiovascular events (heart attacks, strokes and peripheral vascular disease), but also the selection of treatment and the outcomes and complications of therapy. Older patients tend to have more complex disease of the arteries as well as more comorbidities including hypertension, heart failure, heart rhythm abnormalities, anemia and kidney failure which contribute to the risk of the use of blood thinners or the recommendation for invasive therapy.

ACS presents differently in the elderly than it does in those under 65 years of age. Chest pain, the hallmark of heart attack occurs in less than half of those over 85 compared with over three quarters of those under 65 years of age. Older patients more frequently exhibit shortness of breath, profuse sweating, nausea and vomiting and syncope. Because of muscle stiffness and frequent diffuse disease of all three major coronary arteries, the older patient frequently is diagnosed with heart failure which delays appropriate interventions designed to limit heart muscle damage from a heart attack.

Once a diagnosis of ACS is made, two treatment options exist if the event is less than 12 hours old: clot busting drugs given intravenously or an invasive procedure. Most often for the last decade the invasive procedure in this acute setting is percutaneous coronary intervention (PCI) which is done in the catheterization laboratory by a cardiologist. Under sedation, a tube is threaded from the groin or arm into the artery or arteries exhibiting blockage, a balloon inflated to open the narrowing and a metal cage or stent placed to keep the artery from closing again. The options of types of stents (bare metal, drug eluting and absorbable) and manufacturers is beyond the scope of this chapter and each design has its specific application; however, drug eluting stents seem to have the best results and widest application at the time of this writing. Occasionally the anatomy is unfavorable and the only option is coronary artery bypass surgery (CABG) where veins from the leg or an artery from the chest wall or both are used to bypass the blockage by providing a new route for oxygen rich blood to flow beyond the obstruction.

These same two options apply to patients with angina or episodic heart failure but who do not present with an impending heart attack. The debate over which procedure is superior in this elective setting, percutaneous coronary intervention vs. coronary artery bypass graft surgery is never ending and constantly evolving and to some extent depends on the aggressiveness of the catheterization laboratory cardiologist. PCI is now used for virtually all categories of coronary artery disease including left main coronary artery disease – obstruction of the main artery supplying most of the left ventricle – a subcategory of anatomy that used to be reserved for surgery. Recent studies suggest that diabetics, including elderly diabetics, have better outcomes with

CABG than PCI. Indeed, older patients with complex multivessel disease may be better served with surgery than with a difficult PCI.

As with all invasive procedures in the elderly, careful consideration of comorbid conditions such as kidney failure, previous stroke, dementia, frailty and biological as well as chronological age should be considered when deciding which or if invasive therapy is indicated.

After either invasive therapy, a cardiac rehabilitation program with monitored increasing exercise should be recommended. This is especially important in the elderly where in addition to improved cardiovascular performance, the patient may benefit from improved physical fitness, balance, muscle strength and instruction in fall prevention.

In addition, medical therapy if not already in place should be instituted to reduce the likelihood of recurrent disease. All patients should be treated with high dose cholesterol lowering or statin drug therapy. If the blood pressure is elevated or not already treated, the drugs already discussed for the treatment of hypertension should be instituted. Low dose beta blocker as well as aspirin if no bleeding contraindication should also be instituted. However, doses should be adjusted for kidney function and begun judiciously with increases based on tolerance. Frequent visits or calls as drugs are adjusted are required and a cardiac rehab facility is another venue that can oversee these changes. The risk of side effects from drugs increases from around 10% with two medications to nearly 40% with four and over 80% with seven or more.

Valve Disease

Aortic Valve Disease

As with coronary disease in the 1970s, the treatment of valve disease has undergone a revolution in the last decade due to development of new minimally invasive technology. The aortic valve controls the unidirectional flow of blood from the left ventricle to the aorta (major artery taking oxygen rich blood to the body). Calcific aortic stenosis, a degenerative disease of this valve mainly in older patients affects around 5% of people over 65 and is moderate to severe in half of those. Up to half of these patients are asymptomatic, yet once they develop symptoms, expected survival is less than 3 years. Because many of these asymptomatic patients have other comorbid conditions or a high frailty index, in the past up to half of them received no further evaluation and were not referred for surgery. There is no effective medical therapy option for aortic stenosis as it is a fixed blockage preventing blood from leaving the left ventricle. With the advent of Transcatheter Aortic Valve Replacement (TAVR), this has all changed.

TAVR was first performed in 2002 in France. Originally designated for use only in older patients deemed inoperable by the usual open surgical technique, the FDA (Food and Drug Administration) approved them for use in 2011. Currently they are FDA approved for use in all patients and offered routinely to older patients instead of the open surgical procedure.

The procedure is performed under awake sedation and local anesthesia usually through an artery in the groin, where a 5-6mm. catheter or tube containing the collapsed valve is threaded up and through the aortic valve. The metal cage or stent containing the valve is released and expanded opening the native valve and allowing the artificial valve leaflets attached to the stent to expand and function. The stents are metal and the leaflets are composed of preserved pericardium (the sack that surrounds the heart) from cows or pigs. Once expanded the new valve provides instantaneous relief of the obstruction. This improved opening allows improved blood flow to the body, reduced strain and workload on the left ventricle of the heart and improvement in symptoms.

Two manufacturers (Edwards and Medtronic) supply most of the valves currently used. They produce different versions of their valves and of its insertion technology both aspects of which continue to be refined. Smaller catheters make insertion easier and less risky for vascular complications. At first Edwards relied on balloon expansion of the stent containing the three semilunar valve leaflets fashioned from preserved bovine pericardium and Medtronic a self-expanding stent. Currently, Edwards has both technologies available in different models.

Surgical valve replacement under direct vision offers some advantages over this much less invasive technique including thorough removal of calcium deposits on the valve which crumble much like dried dirt, assurance that the openings of both coronary arteries aren't obstructed, avoidance of the heart's electrical conducting system and assurance that there are no leaks around the valve. Coronary obstruction is a rare complication with a properly seated TAVR and newer models can be repositioned if this occurs. There continue to be issues post-procedure with paravalvular leaks (leaks occurring between the stented valve and the heart tissue) and heart block requiring a pacemaker. These are troubling problems which may limit the extension of the TAVR valve to a population that would also be amenable with low risk for surgical replacement.

The lack of the ability to debride calcium deposits from the valve tissue resulting in embolization (breaking off and causing strokes or damage to other organs) seems to have been at least partially resolved by new technology. Many centers now insert a second catheter with nets that deploy in the arteries to the brain or in the aorta above the valve to protect the entire body. Embolized chunks of calcium are captured in the nets and retrieved when the nets are closed and the catheter is withdrawn. This new technology seems to be effective.

Another long term issue which may limit the use of these valves in younger patients (those under 65) and perhaps even the elderly is the durability of the valve tissue. Although surgically implanted pericardial valves have been used for decades with good long-term results, the different stresses on the pericardial tissue within a metal stent may have an impact. At 5 year follow-up in one trial comparing the two different TAVR technologies, there were no significant differences between the balloon expandable and self-expanding valves in one thousand patients, half of these high risk patients were dead and half of those deaths were of cardiovascular causes. Deterioration of the valve tissue was more common in the balloon expandable valves and must be watched closely for further acceleration which would frustrate, in my opinion, those who optimistically assert that TAVR will be the procedure of choice in the future. There have been recent studies comparing surgical valve replacement with TAVR that have shown comparable or superior results with TAVR, but I remain somewhat skeptical. In older patients with limited life expectancy, TAVR is the procedure of choice. Even in those who are likely to survive for more than 10 years, if structural valve deterioration occurs, a second TAVR can be placed inside the original one (valve in valve procedure) expanding the indications for this procedure.

Mitral Valve Disease

The mitral valve is the one way valve between the upper left heart chamber or left atrium (LA) which receives oxygen rich blood from the lungs and the lower left heart muscular pumping chamber or left ventricle (LV) which pumps the oxygen rich blood to the body. The valve has two leaflets and a number of fibrous chords (chordae tendineae) which attach the free edge of the leaflets to the papillary muscles in the wall of the left ventricle. When the valve is closed it resembles a flat parachute. When functioning properly, this valve opens to allow blood to fill the left ventricle from the atrium and then closes when the left ventricle squeezes preventing blood from leaking back into the left atrium and the lungs. Diseases affecting the mitral valve produce stenosis (blockage, MS), regurgitation (leakage, MR) or both. For simplicity I will deal with the pure forms of stenosis and regurgitation.

Mitral stenosis is at this time a surgical disease with no approved catheter-based treatment yet available. One cause, rheumatic heart disease, is rare in developed countries due to the rapid diagnosis and treatment of streptococcal infections which, when left untreated, lead to rheumatic disease and valve calcification. As discussed in the aortic valve section, stenosis may also be caused by calcific degeneration. In either case the valve is treated by open or, in select centers, robotic / minimally invasive procedures. If the valve is pliable, a commissurotomy may be performed using a scalped to divide the fused leaflets and supporting structures of the valve. In most instances the valve is too heavily diseased and is replaced by a mechanical valve in younger patients or a biological valve in the elderly.

It is likely in the near future that transcatheter mitral valve replacement will become more accepted. Major stumbling blocks are the difficulty in gaining access to the mitral valve and past problems with rapid degeneration of biological valves in the mitral position. Exposure can only be obtained by either punching a hole in the atrial septum (the tissue dividing the right and left sided upper chambers of the heart) or by surgically exposing the apex of the left ventricle and opening a hole in that location. That said, several companies are working on this technology which will enter mainstream therapy, especially in the elderly, soon.

Mitral regurgitation (MR) may be primary or secondary. Primary mitral regurgitation may be caused by non-calcific degeneration of the valve tissue, stretching of the opening to which the leaflets attach (annulus) and lengthening or tearing of the supporting cords (which attach the leaflets to the heart muscle in the left ventricle and keep the valve from prolapsing into the left atrium). The degeneration of the valve tissue is termed myxomatous degeneration. The physiological abnormality is mitral valve prolapse where the leaflets upon closure do not adjust to the annulus or coapt, but travel into the left atrium allowing blood to leak backwards. This results in greater work for the left ventricle muscle and may produce high pressure over time in the lungs. If left untreated, the result is heart failure with a dilated left atrium and left ventricle. This process may take years to decades. Earlier intervention regardless of symptoms may prevent these changes. If surgery is delayed due to age and lack of symptoms, careful follow-up is required to allow consideration of intervention (especially with newer catheter-based techniques to be described) before irreversible damage has occurred.

Surgical intervention with valve repair has been the gold standard for three decades. Removing redundant parts of leaflets, placing Gortex sutures to replace torn cords and placing a cloth covered ring to cinch up the annulus (the fibrous ring to which the leaflets are attached) is performed in various combinations to accomplish a competent valve in most patients. Some centers now do these repairs using minimally (small incisions) invasive or robotic techniques. All require cardiopulmonary bypass. If repair is not possible, valve replacement is performed.

Secondary (or functional) mitral regurgitation occurs when the valve leaks secondary to dilatation of the left ventricle and atrium but the valve tissue itself is normal. The dilatation stretches the annulus so the leaflets though normal in size fail to coapt. Once a patient has severe symptoms, valve repair or replacement fails to improve survival and, in some cases, may make symptoms worse by placing a greater workload on the left ventricle. A new device, the Mitra Clip, is approved for both primary and secondary MR. The cloth covered metal clip is inserted through a catheter which punctures the inter-atrial septum. The clip grasps and approximates the middle section of the two leaflets of the mitral valve thus decreasing the amount of leakage. For primary MR the need for reoperation within a year for 20% or more of patients is too high compared to surgical repair for younger patients. However, in high risk older patients it would seem to be worth a try. For secondary MR, the advantage of Mitra Clip over medical therapy alone is controversial. Two studies with a mean patient age of 70 recently showed improved survival and reduced hospitalization for heart failure in one and not the other. A third study including both primary and secondary MR patients with a mean age of 80 compared valve repair to Mitra Clip with significantly better results with surgery.

This technology will continue to improve (there is already a newer version of the Mitra Clip). Other devices including annular rings that can be implanted through a catheter and further improvements in the technique and devices for transcatheter mitral valve replacement will also occur. While all catheter based technologies hold the promise of quicker recovery, less pain and lower risk in high risk patients, surgical techniques of mitral valve repair have proven themselves effective and long lasting in all age groups for thirty years. In the end, the patient regardless of age, should be presented all options. A healthy 70 year old might not want to risk a repeat operation at age 80 when a surgical valve repair has a proven long term excellent result.

Tricuspid Valve Disease

The tricuspid valve is the right heart equivalent of the mitral valve on the left, a one way valve separating the right ventricle (lower pumping chamber) from the right atrium that receives the blood returning to the heart from all the veins in the body. Although tricuspid regurgitation (TR) is estimated to afflict 1.6 million people in the United States, corrective surgery is performed less than 500 times a year. The leakage is almost always secondary to left sided muscle or valve disease resulting in heart failure. With heart failure the pressure in the left ventricle is elevated and this pressure elevation backs up into the left atrium. The elevated pressure in the left atrium is transmitted back into the vessels in the lungs (pulmonary hypertension) and the right atrium with secondary dilatation of the right ventricle and tricuspid annulus.

Despite the few surgeries currently performed, I believe, because of the ease of access to the tricuspid valve and annulus through a major neck or groin vein, that this technology will be used more often in the future. There are at least two other leaflet coaptation devices like the Mitra Clip in development as well as seven or more transcatheter annuloplasty rings. Once proven on the right side with easier access, I believe many of the annuloplasty devices designed to cinch the annulus tighter and reduce leakage will be reconfigured for use on the left side or mitral annulus. As of this writing there is not enough information to warrant a positive recommendation for routine use of any of these devices with perhaps the exception of the Mitra Clip on the tricuspid valve.

Arrhythmia – Atrial Fibrillation

It is estimated that 75% of patients exhibiting this rhythm are between the ages of 65 and 85 years. Up to 10% of those over 80 years of age will exhibit atrial fibrillation with a four to five times greater risk of stroke.

With newer home monitoring devices being advertised daily (Kardia, Apple watch) that can detect this abnormal rhythm, and because of the serious and debilitating complication of stroke which frequently accompanies it, there is increased awareness of treatment to eliminate atrial fibrillation.

The normal heart rhythm is called sinus rhythm where the electrical stimuli that trigger contraction of the heart (right and left atria followed by right and left ventricle) progresses in an orderly fashion. The stimulus begins in the SA node, an area of specialized tissue in the right atrium with spontaneous automaticity (firing off an electrical stimulus at a rate of 60 – 80 beats per minute) that is also influenced to increase or decrease that rate by both the nervous system (sympathetic and para-sympathetic) and hormonal influences. Examples of these effects are the increase in heart rate when frightened or during exercise. The subsequent contraction of the right and left atria tops off the preceding passive filling of the left and right ventricles by adding up to an additional 20% to the volume of blood in these chambers. The stimulus then travels to the AV Node at the top of the interventricular septum, the muscle separating the left and right ventricles, from which It spreads to both ventricles to initiate an orderly contraction of these two pumping chambers.

In atrial fibrillation, the right atrium is bombarded with fast recurrent stimuli originating spontaneously from the areas where the pulmonary veins enter the left atria. Instead of an orderly contraction, the atria quiver sending a barrage of stimuli to the AV node, only some of which are conducted through this area to stimulate contraction of the ventricles. In addition to not fulfilling their role of topping off the ventricles, the sluggish flow of blood in the atria allow clots to form in finger like out-pouchings (atrial appendages) off of the main body of the atria which can then break loose and in the case of the left atrium go to the brain causing a stroke. Physiologically this rhythm can reduce the cardiac output (the amount of blood the heart pumps) by 20%. The heart rate at which the ventricles pump is frequently quite rapid (100-175 beats per minute at rest) which can result in a drop in blood pressure, light headedness and syncope. Patients may exhibit symptoms of their heart pounding rapidly (palpitations), shortness of breath, fatigue and chest pain.

Medical Therapy and Cardioversion

When first diagnosed, patients with non-valvular atrial fibrillation of recent onset frequently present with severe symptoms of low cardiac output and low blood pressure due to the drop in filling of the left ventricle and the rapid heart rate. Depending on severity of symptoms, chemical cardioversion with medications may be tried over hours to a few days, or, if severely symptomatic, electrical cardioversion in the ER is feasible. Commonly, a dose or two of a calcium channel blocker drug, e.g. cardizem will frequently convert to sinus rhythm. If successful, maintenance drug therapy with any number of drugs may be used. If not, electrical cardioversion should be attempted after performing a trans-esophageal echocardiogram (TEE) to rule out a clot in the left atrium or appendage. If present, cardioversion is delayed and full anticoagulation is started. Awake sedation is used since the procedure is painful.

After successful cardioversion, maintenance drug therapy depending on which drug is tolerated and anticoagulation with a non-warfarin drug (NOAC – novel oral anticoagulant) in the elderly is recommended, although in practice up to 50% of elderly patients are not placed on anticoagulation due to the fear of falls resulting in bleeding into the brain (intracerebral hemorrhage). NOACs have been shown to be as effective as warfarin (the previously used anticoagulant) with a lower bleeding risk.

One alternative to cardioversion is to leave the patient in the abnormal rhythm and use drugs to control the heart rate. A target heart rate of less than 80 at rest and less than 110 with moderate exercise should be set. Although a number of drugs singly or in combination have been used, beta blockers are the first line drug. An intravenous form of the drug can be started in symptomatic patients who are not candidates for cardioversion and subsequent oral doses should be gradually increased until therapeutic. Other drugs can be added or substituted if needed including calcium channel blockers such as cardizem. Digoxin may also be used although some have cautioned that it may increase mortality. The evidence for this is unclear especially in light of its use for over a century.

Ablation – Pulmonary Vein Isolation

The aim of pulmonary vein isolation is to return the patient to sinus rhythm. This is accomplished by interrupting the pathways from the openings of the pulmonary veins from which signals are transmitted to the atria by creating physical barriers of scar tissue by either balloon cryoablation (cold) or radiofrequency (heat). In addition to isolating the pulmonary vein openings, additional sites of origin within the left atrium may require ablation. The success rate regardless of age appears to be 70 - 80%. The main complications are perforation due to full-thickness penetration into the pericardium with tamponade, pulmonary vein narrowing due to excessive scarring and stroke. The frequency of these complications does not seem to be age related and varies in different series from 0 – 10%.

Post procedure anticoagulation is required for at least three to six months at which time if the patient has maintained sinus rhythm therapy may be discontinued. As with cardioversion, with the increased risk of warfarin anticoagulation in the elderly the newer drugs (NOACs) with a better safety profile are preferred.

In patients undergoing open heart surgery for coronary or valvular heart disease and who are in atrial fibrillation or have been in and out of this rhythm, pulmonary vein isolation combined with left atrial appendage exclusion may be added expeditiously with little increased risk.

Ablation – AV Node Ablation and Pacemaker

Another alternative for rate control, though less desirable, is AV node ablation with the mandatory insertion of a permanent pacemaker. AV node ablation produces complete heart block by completely interfering with any electrical conduction from the atria to the ventricles. This makes the patients 100% dependent on a pacemaker while leaving the atria in most cases in fibrillation. The incidence of heart failure is more than double that with pulmonary vein isolation and afflicts more than half the patients treated with this strategy. In addition, over time right ventricular pacing may further compromise cardiac function although these effects may be improved with the use of biventricular pacing (synchronizing the contraction of the right and left ventricles with wires in each ventricle) or atrial sensing in the third of patients who convert to sinus rhythm (a wire in the right atrium senses a stimulus and then fires a stimulus to the ventricle, much as a normal heart beat).

In order of desirability, in the setting of acute onset atrial fibrillation an attempt at medical or electrical cardioversion should be attempted. If unsuccessful or if atrial fibrillation recurs more than once or twice (except in the very frail elderly or those with limited survival potential) pulmonary vein isolation should be attempted once or twice. If that is unsuccessful, rate control first with medical therapy and as a last resort with AV node ablation and pacemaker should be used. NOACs unless absolutely contraindicated should be used for anticoagulation in those in whom a rate control strategy is adopted and at least for 3 – 6 months in those undergoing pulmonary vein isolation.

Watchman Device for Stroke Prevention in Atrial Fibrillation

Surgical closure of the left atrial appendage either from the outside by over-sewing or applying a clip to the base of this thumb-like outpouching off the left atrium or by use of a purse string suture excluding its opening from inside the left atrium during mitral valve surgery has been used by some for 70 years. Unfortunately, there is no good data to prove the effectiveness of this additional procedure. I routinely excluded the left atrial appendage from inside in all mitral valve surgeries in patients with a history of atrial fibrillation since it made sense (the left atrial appendage is the site of stroke causing emboli in up to two thirds of patients in atrial fibrillation) and added less than five minutes to the procedure. There is currently a large randomized multi-center study to answer the question. However, especially in atrial fibrillation patients with a contraindication to anticoagulation one would assume this simple procedure would be of benefit.

A catheter-based technique has been introduced recently to simulate internal closure of the appendage. The Watchman device is an umbrella shaped metal expandable stent with a fabric covering that is deployed inside the opening of the left atrial appendage excluding it from the circulation. Studies have shown that this device reduces the risk of stroke to the same level that oral anticoagulation does. However, there are significant, frequent complications with this technique including dislodgement, leakage of blood into the pericardium (the sac surrounding the heart) and stroke. Therefore, although I believe that surgical closure will prove to be a useful adjunct in open heart surgery, further experience with the Watchman with further reduction in complications will be necessary before it can be a first-line therapy.

Palliative Cardiac Care

While palliative or hospice care has been well defined for cancer patients, such treatment for end stage heart failure or valvular heart disease has only recently being recognized especially for the elderly. Not only do these patients suffer the common symptoms of heart disease including shortness of breath, fatigue and fluid accumulation in the periphery(edema) and abdomen (ascites), but they also exhibit pain, nausea, anxiety and depression. While heart transplant and /or permanent ventricular assist devices may be applicable to some, many patients may either not be a candidate for such therapy or may not be willing to subject themselves to the demands of such therapy. The topic of palliative care is rarely included in cardiology journals or national meetings and is not routinely part of cardiology training programs.

Prognosis in end stage cardiac disease is more variable than with cancer with many patients' survival extending for months to over a year with exacerbations and remissions. Medicare approval for some home therapies such as inotropes (intravenous infusions of drugs to improve heart function) frequently are not approved and hospice level care at home and in extended care facilities may require repeat certification. Functional status may decline for prolonged periods of time requiring long periods of support for patients and caregivers. Prolonged psychosocial support both inpatient and at home is required.

Many of the medical and catheter-based therapies discussed in this chapter may also be applied in the palliative setting. Only after a thorough discussion with the patient and caregivers outlining all reasonable options based on both the patient's age and functional status should a course of action be undertaken. As with all palliative care, quality of life is important and, I believe, especially in the uncertain prognostic arena of end stage heart failure should take precedence over quantity.

Suggested Additional Readings

Jankowska, EA,Vitale, C, et.al. Drug therapy in elderly heart failure patients. Eur Heart J Suppl 2019; Dec 21(Suppl L):L8-L11

Leyva, F, Nisam, S, et.al. 20 Years of Cardiac Resyncrhonization Therapy. J AmColl Cardiol 2014; 64:1047-58

Stehlik, J, Kobashigawa,J, et.al. Honoring 50 Years of Clinical Heart Transplantation in Circulation In-depth State-of-the-Art Review. Circulation 2018; 137:71-87

Daneshvar, DA, Czer, LSC, et.al. Heart transplantation in the elderly: Why cardiac transplantation does not need to be limited to younger patients but can be safely performed in patients above 65 years of age. Ann Transplant 2010; 15(4):110-19

Abdel-Wahab, M, Neumann, FJ, et.al. 5-year Outcomes After TAVR With Balloon-Expandable Versus Self-Expanding Valves: Results From the CHOICE Randomized Clinical Trial. JACC Cardiovasc Interv 2020; 13(9):1071-82

Shah, M, Jorde, UP Percutaneous Mitral Valve Interventions (Repair): Current Indications and Future Perspectives. Front Cardiovasc Med 2019; 6: 88-123

Kapa, SK, Bala, R Ablation of Atrial Fibrillation in the Elderly: Current Evidence and Evolving Trends. J Atr Fibrillation 2011; 4(2): 341-53

Holmes, DR Jr., Kar, S et.al. Prospective Randomized Evaluation of the Watchman Left Atrial Appendage Closure Device in Patients with Atrial Fibrillation Versus Long-Term Warfarin Therapy: The PREVAIL Trial. J Am Coll Cardiol 2014; 64(1): 1-12

Sepheri, A, Beggs, T, et.al. The impact of frailty on outcomes after cardiac surgery: A systematic review. J Thorac Cardiovasc Surg 2014; 148(31): 3110-17

Teuteberg, JJ, Teuteberg WG Palliative Care for Patients with Heart Failure. www.acc.org/ latest-in-cardiology/articles/2016/02/11/08/02/ palliative-care-for-patients-with-heart-failure

HOW TO MANAGE TYPE 2 DIABETES IN FRAIL ELDERLY PATIENTS

Dr. Young-Sang Kim, MD, PhD
Associate Professor, Department of Family Medicine,
CHA Bundang Medical Center, CHA University.

José A. Morais, MD, FRCPC
Professor, Faculty of Medicine, Director, Division of Geriatric Medicine, Lead,
Dementia Education Program, McGill University, Co-Director, Quebec Network for Research on Aging

Clinical Vignette

Mrs. Sweet is an 86 year old widow. She was admitted with a hip fracture consecutive to a fall. She is known for type 2 diabetes of 15 years duration. She also has a history of hypertension, dyslipidemia, coronary artery disease and arthritis. She uses a walker to ambulate but has no memory issues. Her medications include glyburide 5 mg bid, metformin 500 mg bid, perindopril 4 mg die, metoprolol 25 mg bid, ASA 80 mg die, atorvastatin 10 mg die and acetaminophen 500 mg tid, on needed basis. She has a good appetite. Her body mass index (BMI) is 31 kg/m^2 and her BP is 140/90 mmHg, sitting. According to the results of initial laboratory tests, the concentration of morning fasting blood glucose was 9 mmol/L, hemoglobin A1c level 9.2 %, creatinine clearance 55 mL/min/1.73m^2 and the concentration of LDL-cholesterol 3 mmol/L. What could be the objectives in treating type 2 diabetes in this frail patient?

Background

Type 2 diabetes (T2D) is highly prevalent in older adults afflicting 25% of those > 75 years old, which is double that of a middle-aged population. In long-term care settings, these figures reach 1/3 of residents who carry a very high comorbidity burden. Unfortunately, in the community, only half of the individuals are aware of the diagnosis and therefore cannot benefit from lifestyle advice and treatments available to reduce the morbidities associated with this medical condition. The reason for a high percentage of elderly people with T2D is that aging is associated with adipose tissue accumulation especially intraabdominally, sedentary lifestyle, low-grade inflammation, abnormal secretion of insulin and the effects of certain drugs. T2D increases the risk of micro and macro vascular complications that contribute to an acceleration of the manifestations of aging and predispose the elderly to geriatric syndromes. In more advanced age, T2D is associated with decreased weight, loss of independence, falls, cognitive impairment and depression. It has been estimated that T2D by these complications increases the risk of hospitalization in acute care by 43% and placement in long-term care by more than 52%. This population has particular characteristics, including a great heterogeneity of insulin secretion according to body composition. It has been found that in older adults with BMI < 27 kg/m^2, the main mechanism contributing to hyperglycemia is defective insulin secretion whereas in those with BMI > 27 kg/m^2 it is insulin resistance. These characteristics are good to keep in mind to guide in the selection of the most appropriate antidiabetic medications.

Risk of hypoglycemia

Another important aspect to consider in this population is their propensity to develop hypoglycemia. The rate of emergency room visits for hypoglycemia has been estimated at 54 vs 19/1000 diabetic visits in those ≥75 y compared with those 45-64 y. Hypoglycemia tends to be less perceived in older adults with T2D as both autonomic (e.g., sweat) and neuroglycopenic (e.g., slowness of thought) symptoms of hypoglycemia are vague in older patients, especially in those who are frail. These frail patients also are more frequently malnourished. Therefore, in the frail elderly with T2D, it is more important to prevent hypoglycemia than to control hyperglycemia intensively. Hypoglycemia itself carries detrimental consequences including cardiovascular disease, fall, fracture, physical deconditioning, and progressive neuroglycopenia (psychomotor slowness). Of interest, frailty has been found to be a better predictor of complications and death in older adults with diabetes than chronological age or burden of comorbidity. When treating older adults with diabetes one has to keep in mind the objectives presented in Table 1 that are relevant to this population. Further, the determination of the presence of frailty is of utmost importance as vigorous older adults with T2D should be treated similarly to middle-aged individuals whereas those with frailty required special consideration.

Table 1. General treatment objectives
Maintain adequate caloric intake
Set appropriate A1C targets
Avoid hypoglycemia
Consider kidney function of the elderly patient
Consider the cardiovascular health risk of the elderly patient
Maintenance of quality of life

Assessment of frailty

Frailty is the manifestation of impairment in multiple organ systems that results in increased susceptibility to poor health outcomes and reduced physical function. Please refer to the chapter on frailty of this book for further information on this syndrome. The most used definitions of frailty include the Frailty Phenotype and the Frailty Index. The Former is based on five criteria that include shrinking (i.e., weight loss), weakness (i.e., loss of muscle strength), exhaustion, slowness (i.e., decreased walking speed) and low levels of physical activity. Having > 3 criteria defines frailty, having 1-2 criteria is consider pre-frailty and none is a normal state. The Frailty Index is calculated based on the deficit of any variable one wishes to apply to assess frailty with a minimum of ten to be included. Frailty is considered when a quarter of the variables show a deficit. These and other methods of assessing frailty requiring measurements can be cumbersome in a busy clinical practice. The Clinical Frailty Scale is a frequently employed tool that can overcome this limitation by simply recognizing a patient's vulnerability. The CFS uses clinical descriptors and pictographs that provide clinicians with an easily applicable tool to stratify older adults according to level of vulnerability. It ranges from very fit (stage 1) to terminally ill (stage 9), in which the first 3 stages are considered non-frail or functionally independent, stage 4-7 as frail with increasing dependency, whereas stage 8-9 individuals are totally dependent, which implies that they are disabled and therefore more than frail. A patient suffering from dementia is, by definition, classified as being frail.

Suggested hemoglobin A1c targets, blood pressure and lipids outcomes

In the frail elderly with T2D, since it is difficult to maintain adequate caloric intake and to avoid hypoglycemia, clinicians need to set appropriate hemoglobin A1c targets and to re-evaluate the patients on a regular basis. As presented in Table 2, these targets are slightly different between national or international societies according to the criteria retained to ascertain frailty, but all societies propose less stringent A1C targets to prevent hypoglycemia. While the target for most adults with T2D is below 7.0%, for functionally dependent patients it is better to aim at 7.1-8.0%. For those patients clearly considered as frail, the target should be further eased to <8.5%, whereas for end-of-life patients one should aim at avoiding symptomatic hyperglycemia with no hypoglycemia.

Table 2. Recommendations for clinical outcomes for older adults with type 2 diabetes

Outcome	Diabetes Canada	American Diabetes Association	International Diabetes Federation
A1C	Functionally independent: ≤ 7.0% Functionally dependent: 7.1–8.0% Frail and/or dementia: 7.1–8.5% End of life: A1C measurement not recommended. Avoid symptomatic hyperglycemia and any hypoglycemia.	Healthy: <7.5% Complex/Intermediate: <8.0% Very Complex/Poor Health: <8.5%	Functionally independent: 7.0%–7.5% Functionally dependent: 7.0%–8.0% Sub-level frail: <8.5% Sub-level dementia: <8.5% End of life: avoid symptomatic hyperglycemia
Blood Pressure	Functionally independent with life expectancy >10 years: <130/80 mmHg Functionally dependent, orthostasis or limited life expectancy: individualize BP targets	Healthy: <140/80 mmHg Complex/Intermediate: <140/80 mmHg Very Complex/Poor Health: <150/90 mmHg	Functionally independent: <140/90 mmHg Functionally dependent: <140/90 mmHg Sub-level frail: <150/90 mmHg Sub-level dementia: <140/90 mmHg End of life: strict BP control may not be necessary
LDL-C	<2.0 mmol/L or >50% reduction from baseline	<1.8 mmol/L	<2.0 mmol/L and adjusted based on CV

A1C: glycated hemoglobin; BP: blood pressure; CV: cardiovascular; LDL-C: low density lipoprotein cholesterol. Adapted from Diabetes Canada

As for blood pressure control (Table 2), the Canadian guidelines are the most stringent, aiming at values < 130/80 mmHg until a person with diabetes becomes dependent. Both the ADA and the IDF guidelines are more liberal by setting the goal for BP control to < 140/80-90 mmHg and comprising intermediary stages with acceptable BP up to 150/90 mmHg, depending on the severity of the functional impairment. Finally, recommendations for lipid control are an LDL-C value < 2 mmol/L, with the exception of the ADA that recommends <1.8 mmol/L.

Pharmacotherapy in the frail older adult with type 2 diabetes

In frail older people with T2D, sulfonylureas should be used with caution and some products avoided (e.g., glyburide) because the risk of hypoglycemia increases substantially with age. Hence, some classes of antidiabetic medications with low risk of hypoglycemia are preferred to them. Available oral agents include biguanides such as metformin, dipeptidyl peptidase -4 inhibitors (DPPi-4), and if used carefully, insulin secretagogues such as meglitinides, and the sulfonylureas gliclazide and glimepiride. DPPi-4 should be used over sulfonylureas as second line therapy to metformin, because of a lower risk of hypoglycemia. To use sulfonylureas in older persons, the initial doses should be started at the half of those commonly used for younger people, then the doses could be increased slowly. Gliclazide, gliclazide MR and glimepiride should be used instead of glyburide, as they have evidences of lower frequency of hypoglycemic events than glyburide. Meglitinides (Repaglinide, Nateglinide) may also be used instead of glyburide to reduce the risk of hypoglycemia, keeping in mind that they have a rapid onset of action with a short duration. In those patients with erratic eating behavior, one should offer the meglitinide after having been assured that the patient has eaten half of her/his meal.

In frail persons, some other classes of medications are to be avoided. These include thiazolidinediones (TZDs) due to the concern of fluid retention and heart failure. Sodium-glucose co-transporter protein -2 (SGLT-2) inhibitors carry a risk of dehydration with hypotension and urinary tract infections. Alpha-glucosidase inhibitors commonly cause enteric symptoms and possibility reduce appetite. Among the parenteral agents, insulin can be used with careful monitoring, but glucagon-like peptide -1 (GLP-1) receptor agonists are not recommended due to suppression of appetite.

Or note, decreased serum albumin is commonly observed in persons with severe malnutrition, in cancer, heart failure, and other systemic illness. If the albumin-bound drugs decrease in circulation, this implies that the free portion is elevated and so is the risk of adverse or toxic effects. In the presence of malnutrition, due to concerns with adverse effects, some anti-diabetic medications including repaglinide, gliclazide, and glimepiride should be discontinued.

Reduced Kidney Function

Reduced kidney function is common in the frail elderly. When the kidney function is impaired, one needs to avoid certain antidiabetic medications, and to make dosage adjustments according to the kidney function impairment. A key value of estimated glomerular filtration rate (eGFR) to retain is 30 ml/min/1.73 m² as several antidiabetic medications are required to be stopped. These include metformin (risk of lactic acidosis), sulfonylureas, and most GLP-1 analogues, except for liraglutide. DPPi-4 are safe, except for saxagliptine when eGFR is < 15 but all require dose adjustments when eGRF is below 50-60. In a non-frail patient and although not recommended, liraglutide can be used without dose adjustment when eGFR > 15 mL/min/1.73 m². In patients with an eGFR < 60, dapagliflozin is not recommended, and when an eGFR is below 45, the other SGLT-2 inhibitors also need to be avoided or used only with caution. Due to a concern of fluid retention, TZDs are less preferred in patients with chronic kidney disease.

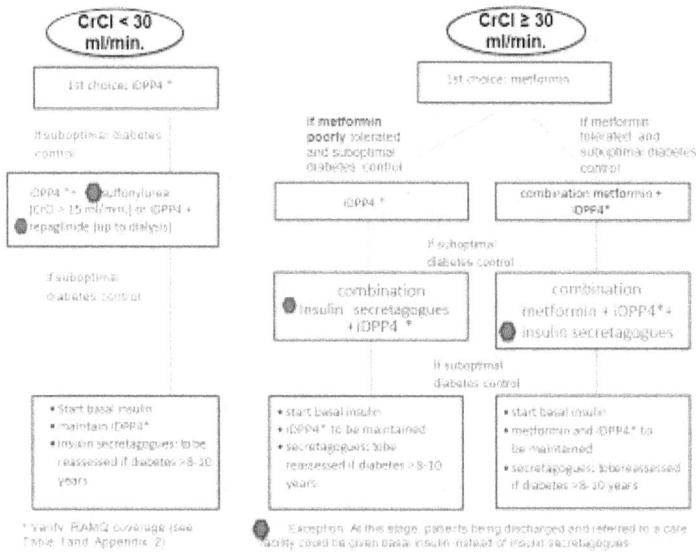

Figure 1. Drug treatment algorithm in the elderly diabetic based on renal function

Figure 1 presents a guide to select safe antidiabetic classes for frail older adults with T2D in the presence of kidney dysfunction. When the eGFR is less than 30, DPPi-4 are recommended as the initial choice, then one can progress to insulin therapy or to the insulin secretaguogue, repaglinide that is safe in kidney failure. When the eGFR is greater than 30, metformin should be used as the first choice, then one can add or change to DPPi-4. If glucose control requires further adjustments, insulin secretagogues (except glyburide) and sub-cutaneous insulin may be used consecutively.

Remarks about cardiovascular safety and heart failure

In older diabetic patients with clinical cardiovascular disease and with an eGFR >30 mL/min/1.73 m^2, clinicians can choose or add an agent with demonstrated cardiovascular outcome benefit to reduce the risk of major cardiovascular events. Among the DPPi-4 which are preferred in the frail elderly with T2D, all have demonstrated to be cardiovascular safe, from the ischemic heart perspective.

As for congested heart failure, each 1% increase in hemoglobin A1c is associated with 8% increased risk of heart failure. Anti-diabetic treatment has been expected to lower the risk of the complication of heart failure in diabetic patients. However, rosiglitazone and other TZDs are known to precipitate congestive heart failure in susceptible patients. Among the DPPi-4 inhibitors, saxagliptin significantly increased the risk of hospitalization for heart failure in post-hoc analyses of SAVOR-TIMI 53 study. Alogliptin, sitagliptin, and linagliptin were confirmed not to increase the risk of hospitalization for heart failure.

To treat the older patient with T2D and heart failure, clinicians should approach heart failure in the same way as in a patient without diabetes. Concurrently with the diabetes treatment and unless contraindicated, clinicians need to carefully use inhibitors of the renin angiotensin aldosterone system or the combination of sacubitril/valsartan, known to increase the B-type natriuretic hormone. TZDs and saxagliptin need to be avoided.

Insulin

If oral agents are contraindicated or glucose control is suboptimal, insulin is an inevitable choice in the frail elderly with T2D. Insulin types are roughly classified into bolus and basal insulins. Bolus insulins are rapid-acting analogues and regular human insulins, which are usually used at prandial time. Basal insulins are long-acting analogues and intermediate-acting human insulins, administered once or twice a day.

Because of the high risk of hypoglycemia, insulin should be used with caution. In fact, insulin is the second leading cause of emergency visits for adverse drug events.

The frequency of dosages needs to be minimized in patients with a high prevalence of cognitive disorders, dexterity problems (e.g., arthritis, neuropathy, and movement disorders), vision problems, irregular eating patterns, and so on. In many instances, a system of surveillance or assistance to administer insulin needs to be put in place to help maintaining the older person safely at home. These involve use of pens, providing daily pre-filled syringes or having a nurse visiting on daily basis. Patients whose clock drawing ability is deficient are at risk of having problems with insulin regimen.

Insulin may be used temporarily in short-term geriatric care units. Insulin use is required in diabetic patients who have erratic eating patterns, have to remain fasting, or are suffering from an acute episode leading to uncontrolled glycaemia. In these cases, insulin treatment should not be based on a sliding scale. Instead, a morning dose of long-acting basal insulin analogue needs to be calculated. Patients in whom oral agents are no longer effective would be candidates for a permanent insulin regimen. When adding basal insulin to oral agents, insulin secretagogues are not recommended, and the combination of DPPi-4 with basal insulin should be preferred. If insulin therapy is the sole anti-diabetic treatment, a regimen of long-acting basal insulin analogue combined with fast-acting bolus insulin analogue is the best choice.

Resolution of the clinical case

Soon after her admission, we should plan to improve the diabetic treatment of Mrs. Sweet. The initial target of hemoglobin A1c should be 7-8% since she is moderately frail as evidenced by using a walker. Her renal function is slightly below normal and therefore there is no contraindication to raise the dosage of metformin. We would increase metformin to 850 mg bid. Meanwhile, glyburide should not be used in a frail elderly, because of the concern of hypoglycemia, and in her case one could hypothesize that it may be related to the fall. Hence, we should stop glyburide. At this point, there are two options in the selection of an oral agent. The first option would be to start gliclazide MR 30 mg PO die for a week, and then increase to 60 mg PO die if no adverse event occurs, including hypoglycemia. The second option is to switch the sulfonylureas all together to a DPPi-4. For this purpose, we could choose sitagliptin 100 mg PO die instead of glyburide. After 3 months on a stable dose and good control based on an A1C at the target value above, the oral anti-diabetic regimen could be simplified into Janumet 50/850 mg bid or Janumet XR 50/1,000 mg die.

The BP control is appropriate for her age and functional capacity level. There is room to improve the lipid values by increasing atorvastatin to 20 mg die. No attempt should be made to reduce caloric intake in this patient. During her stay in the hospital or rehabilitation, one should evaluate the gastric or digestive tolerance of higher metformin doses, the stability of blood glucose level, and the presence of muscle symptoms possibly caused by the higher dose of atorvastatin. There is also an opportunity to teach her how to monitor blood glucose with capillary measurements, and how to recognize and manage the symptoms of hypoglycemia. Eventually, one should be able to discharge her and plan the next outpatient visit. We should ask her to measure and record capillary blood glucose at home twice a day on a cycle of morning with once at lunch time, next day at supper and the following day at night time, and to restart the cycle. Eventually, if glucose values are very stable, the intensity of monitoring can be reduced to twice a week at different times of the day. Recommendation to ambulate using the walker should be made to prevent further falls. Finally, the patient should be referred to home care services and advised to receive influenza vaccination.

Conclusion

The approach to the frail elderly patient with T2D is different in several ways from that of an older robust patient or a middle-aged person. Optimized strategies are required to cope with the more frequent hypoglycemia, reduced kidney function, poor appetite, comorbidities and shorter life expectancy. In the frail elderly, the above mentioned situations and the frequently encountered cognitive deficits compel the physician to allow a less tight hemoglobin A1c control and to define a more personalized approach. The diet doesn't need to be controlled, suffice to adherence to a healthy diet plan. The simplest drug regimen should be proposed to facilitate patients' compliance.

References

1. Lee PG, Halter JB: The Pathophysiology of Hyperglycemia in Older Adults: Clinical considerations. *Diabetes Care* 2017, 40(4):444-452.
2. Bremer JP, Jauch-Chara K, Hallschmid M, Schmid S, Schultes B: Hypoglycemia unawareness in older compared with middle-aged patients with type 2 diabetes. *Diabetes Care* 2009, 32(8):1513-1517.
3. Moorhouse P, Rockwood K: Frailty and its quantitative clinical evaluation. *J R Coll Physicians Edinb* 2012, 42(4):333-340.
4. Meneilly GS, Berard LD, Cheng AYY, Lin PJ, MacCallum L, Tsuyuki RT, Yale JF, Nasseri N, Richard JF, Goldin L *et al*: Insights Into the Current

Management of Older Adults With Type 2 Diabetes in the Ontario Primary Care Setting. *Can J Diabetes* 2018, 42(1):23-30.

5. American Geriatrics Society Beers Criteria Update Expert Panel. American Geriatrics Society 2015 Updated Beers Criteria for Potentially Inappropriate Medication Use in Older Adults. J Am Geriatr Soc 2015, 63(11):2227-2246.

CANCER IN OLDER ADULTS

Doreen Wan-Chow-Wah, MD, FRCPC
Assistant Professor, Faculty of Medicine, Division of Geriatric Medicine, McGill University and McGill
University Health Centre

Clinical vignette

An 87 year old woman living in a seniors' residence is referred by the oromaxillofacial surgeon to assess suitability for surgery for a squamous cell carcinoma of the tongue which will involve a resection under general anesthesia. Her comorbidities include hypertension, diabetes mellitus type 2, gastroesophageal reflux disease, osteoarthritis, and osteoporosis. Her medications include amlodipine 7.5 mg qd, acetaminophen 650 mg TID, lorazepam 1 mg qHS, metformin 500 mg TID, ECASA 80 mg qd, pantoprazole 40 mg qd, vitamin D 10 000 units qweek, calcium 500 mg qd, and alendronate 70 mg qweek. She is an ex-smoker, and denies alcohol consumption or recreational drugs.

She is independent for her activities of daily living and the residence provides meals and medications. Her daughter assists her with her finances. She uses no walking aids, and does not drive. She has lost 10 lbs over the last 6 months, unintentionally. She is a retired seamstress with an elementary school level of education.

On examination, BP 133/81, pulse 64, weight 61.9 kg, BMI 23, grip strength 24 kg (normal for her gender and BMI), gait speed 0.74 meter/second (normal is ≥ 1meter/ second). Her general physical examination was unremarkable. MMSE Folstein was 23/30. Her creatinine clearance was calculated as 55 ml/min, and the rest of her blood test results were within normal limits.

1. Epidemiology of cancer in older adults

Geriatric Oncology is a relatively young subspecialty. Originally well established in the United States and Europe, it has been developing in Canada over the past 10 years, starting with the Geriatric Oncology clinic established at the Segal Cancer Center of the Jewish General Hospital in Montreal. Since then, other centers across Canada followed, recognizing the unique needs of older cancer patients.

Aging is the number one risk factor for developing cancer. With the growth and aging of the population, we are seeing an increasing cancer burden. Cancer is the leading cause of mortality in the country, surpassing cardiovascular disease. 44% of new cancer cases are diagnosed in patients aged ≥ 70, and 62 % of deaths due to cancer occur in those aged ≥ 70. Lung, colorectal, prostate and breast cancers are the most common cancers diagnosed in the older population. Half of all newly diagnosed lung and colorectal cancer cases will occur in those aged 70 and older. More deaths from breast cancer occur in those ≥ 80 than any other age group.

2. Particularities of older patients with cancer

The elderly constitute a heterogeneous population, meaning that a group of 80 year old individuals will differ significantly in terms of their health and functional status, as compared to a group of 40 year old adults. With aging comes various physiological changes (increased fat, decreased muscle mass, decreased renal function and hepatic metabolism) that impact cancer and its treatment. There are age-based disparities in the provision of cancer care. We know that the elderly are understaged, under-treated, and overall receive suboptimal care. A certain proportion of patients are also overtreated, and suffer the consequences of treatment toxicities which impact significantly on their quality of life.

Important questions to ask ourselves are: will the patient die WITH or FROM the cancer, will they suffer from the cancer, will they tolerate the treatments, and are there factors (medical, functional, social) which may interfere with the cancer treatment but are potentially reversible. Because the elderly are underrepresented in clinical trials, there is a lack of guidelines on how to best treat this population.

Older patients may be socially isolated or have limited social support which increases their vulnerability. Some patients are caregivers for their spouse. Many suffer from various degrees of cognitive impairment which has important implications on their ability to adhere to treatments (e.g. medication adherence) and recognize side effects of treatments. Seemingly trivial logistical issues such as transportation to and from medical appointments can actually be significant barriers to older patients receiving adequate cancer treatments.

3. Determining fitness for cancer treatments

Patients may undergo one or more of the following treatment modalities: surgery, chemotherapy, radiotherapy, and, increasingly, targeted treatments that can involve immunotherapy (See: Glossary: Cancer, Immunotherapy, Checkpoint Inhibitor, Receptor Site, T Cells, Vaccine). Cancer treatments can be administered with curative or palliative intent. Alternatively, patients may also be referred to palliative care to receive end-of-life care and adequate management of symptoms. Guidelines put forth by scientific organizations such as SIOG (International Society of Geriatric Oncology) and the NCCN (National Comprehensive Cancer Network) recommend a comprehensive geriatric assessment (CGA) for patients aged 70 years and older for whom chemotherapy is considered. Studies have confirmed the usefulness of the CGA in oncology. A CGA can help detect impairment not identified on routine history or physical examination, predict severe treatment-related toxicity, predict overall survival in a variety of tumors and treatment settings, and influence treatment choice and intensity. Treatment must be tailored to patients' health and functional status rather than their chronological age.

Given oncologists' busy practice, it has been proposed that older cancer patients should first be screened for potential vulnerabilities, and that those who screen positive should subsequently be referred for a comprehensive geriatric assessment.

There exists several screening tools to choose from; the G8 (Oncodage) and Vulnerable Elders Survey (VES-13) have been well validated in geriatric oncology.

In the Geriatric Oncology Clinic, the following domains are evaluated as part of a comprehensive geriatric assessment (CGA): comorbidities, medications, functional status, mood, cognition, nutritional status, social support, life expectancy and patient's goals. We describe a patient's functional status based on their ability to perform activities of daily living (ADLs) and instrumental activities of daily living (IADLs). Cognitive screening tools such as the Mini-Cog (3 word delayed recall + clock drawing), Mini mental state examination (MMSE), and/or Montreal Cognitive Assessment test (MoCA) are used to evaluate cognitive function. In order to better detect potential vulnerability, we also measure grip strength and gait speed which are sensitive markers of frailty.

3a. Polypharmacy

About 1/3 of community dwelling older adults take ≥ 5 prescription drugs. A study looking at the prevalence of polypharmacy and inappropriate drug use in ambulatory older adults with cancer found that 41% of seniors took more than 5 medications, 43% took more than 10 medications, and 51% took potentially inappropriate medications. Taking multiple medications increases the risk of drug-drug interactions and drug-disease interactions.

Older patients with cancer often already take multiple prescribed drugs for pre-existing comorbidities. The addition of cancer treatments such as chemotherapy or molecularly targeted therapies and their potential side effects and/or toxicities constitute an added challenge. Certain chemotherapy drugs such as taxanes or platinum agents can cause painful peripheral neuropathy. Aromatase inhibitors prescribed for hormone receptor positive breast cancer decrease bone mineral density and can cause arthralgias and myalgias, which can be debilitating in older women. Many systemic cancer treatments, as well as radiotherapy, can cause significant fatigue which interfere with daily function.

Another potential side effect of cancer treatments is "chemo brain" which is now referred to as cancer and/or cancer therapy-related cognitive changes. Cognitive changes are not solely related to getting chemotherapy. They can occur after receiving a cancer diagnosis, or after surgery or radiotherapy (particularly but not restricted to the brain). The exact pathophysiology remains unclear but the cognitive impacts are described as difficulties in concentration, multitasking, attention and short-term memory amongst others. The evolution of these cognitive changes is also unknown; they may resolve after the cancer treatment ends, or may persist over a more prolonged period.

Patients are also often prescribed supportive therapies in conjunction with their chemotherapy to minimize side effects. Supportive drugs such as antiemetics and potent steroids such as dexamethasone can cause unwanted side effects, or interact with pre-existing conditions (drug-disease interactions). For example, prochlorperazine (Stemetil) use on a regular basis can lead to extrapyramidal side effects, causing parkinsonism. Dexamethasone (Decadron) in diabetic patients can cause significant hyperglycemia requiring adjustments of oral hypoglycemic agents or insulin.

It is important to frequently re-evaluate medications at each medical visit. Given the potential for one's health condition to change especially while undergoing cancer treatments, prescription drugs which may have been appropriate prior to the cancer diagnosis may actually be detrimental as the patient's health changes along their cancer care trajectory. For example, antihypertensives in the context of dehydration will further lower blood pressure and cause orthostatic hypotension and subsequent falls. In another scenario, a diabetic patient taking Gliclazide may become hypoglycemic if their oral intake decreases significantly because of chemotherapy-induced nausea and vomiting. Hypoglycemia can lead to mental status changes, weakness, and even syncope and falls if severe.

3b. Life expectancy

It is possible to estimate one's life expectancy, based on the number and severity of comorbidities and functional status (degree of autonomy); these are stronger predictors than age alone. A patient with severe congestive heart failure, severe obstructive lung disease, end stage renal disease or who is very dependent for their basic activities of daily living will have a life expectancy much below average; on the other hand, a patient with few comorbidities who is autonomous in their daily activities will have a life expectancy much above average.

There exists a useful online prognostic tool called eprognosis (www.eprognosis.org) which was developed to help clinicians estimate their patients' mortality risk based on various indices. Knowing a patient's life expectancy can assist in the treatment decision-making process. The CARG (Cancer and Aging Research Group) predictive chemotherapy toxicity tool can help clinicians estimate a patient's risk of developing toxicity from chemotherapy. It has shown that factors such as age >72, a gastrointestinal or genitourinary cancer, standard chemotherapy dose, polychemotherapy, decreased hemoglobin (<11g/dL in males and <10 g/dL in females), decreased creatinine clearance (<34 ml/min), impaired hearing, falls in the past 6 months, requiring help to take medications, inability to walk one block, and limitations in social activities, increase the risk of toxicity from chemotherapy.

4. **Goals of care and advanced care planning**

When facing a potentially fatal disease like cancer, the goal of treatment is often to cure and prolong survival. However, for many older adults, the most important reason to undergo treatment is preservation or improvement of quality of life. Older patients favor quality of life over quantity, and wish to maintain their independence. It is important for clinicians to establish early on in the therapeutic relationship the goals of care of the older patient and whether they have discussed advanced care planning which involves expressing their wishes based on their values and ensure they have a designated substitute decision-maker in case of incapacity. It is imperative to determine "what matters most" to the patient.

Resolution of the clinical vignette

The comprehensive geriatric assessment revealed that our 87 year old patient with a squamous cell carcinoma of the tongue has certain frailty markers including cognitive impairment (Major Neurocognitive Disorder), diminished gait speed and weight loss. She has a 59% risk of mortality at 4 years according to the Lee index (eprognosis.org). Given her baseline dementia, she is at a higher risk for post-op delirium and therefore, preventative measures for delirium should be implemented such as early mobilization and reorientation, early removal of IV's and catheters, adequate pain control, avoidance of anticholinergic drugs, ensuring adequate bladder and bowel hygiene. Particularly in her case, one must not forget to represcribe her regular nighttime dose of lorazepam to prevent withdrawal symptoms and delirium. At a later stage one could consider a tapering of this medication. Despite the frailty markers, we recommended to proceed with the surgery since not having the surgery would translate into further morbidity and limited life expectancy. Knowing the information obtained from the CGA allows the treating team to put measures in place to prevent delirium as well as post-op complications and deconditioning.

References

1. Canadian Cancer Society - Canadian cancer statistics 2016
2. Walter LC and Covinsky KE. Cancer screening in elderly patients: A framework for individualized decision making. *JAMA 2001; 285: 2750-2756.*
3. Extermann M. Basic assessment of the older cancer patient. Current Treatment Options in Oncology 2011: 12; 276-285
4. Hurria A. Predicting chemotherapy toxicity in older adults with cancer: A prospective multicenter study. JCO 2011; 29: 3457-3465.
5. Nightingale G et al. Evaluation of a pharmacist-led medication assessment used to identify prevalence of and associations with polypharmacy and potentially inappropriate medication use among ambulatory senior adults with cancer. JCO 2015; 33 (15):1453-1459.
6. www.SIOG.org

CANCER SCREENING IN THE OLDER ADULT

Catalina Hernandez-Torres MD, FRCP(C)
Geriatric Oncology, Ottawa Hospital Cancer Center

Tina Hsu, MD, FRCP(C)
Assistant Professor, Division of Medical Oncology, University of Ottawa

Clinical Vignette

Mrs. Smith is a 77-year-old female who has a past medical history of hypertension, diabetes, coronary artery disease and osteoarthritis. She presents to her family doctor for her regular follow up visit. Her medications include hydrochlorothiazide, metformin, metoprolol, aspirin, acetaminophen as needed. She reports overall doing well with no new significant concerns. She continues to live by herself, and she is independent for all her instrumental activities of daily living. She wants to discuss with her family physician whether she should continue to have cancer screening for breast and colon cancer. She has two close friends who were recently diagnosed with cancer. One friend was diagnosed with early breast cancer and another one with colorectal cancer. She has had regular mammograms with no prior abnormalities; the last mammogram was 3 years ago. She also had screening for colorectal cancer with fecal occult blood testing that was negative 4 years ago. She does not have any family history of cancer.

Introduction

Cancer is a common diagnosis and age is a major risk factor. When diagnosed late, it can be associated with significant morbidity and mortality. Older adults are often diagnosed at more advanced stages. Furthermore, older adults are more likely to be under-treated when diagnosed, which can result in worse outcomes in some older patients. The role of cancer screening in older adults, however, is controversial. This chapter provides an approach to cancer screening in older adults, in particular for breast, colorectal, lung, prostate and cervical cancer.

Considerations in Cancer Screening

Early diagnosis of cancer through cancer screening before a patient becomes symptomatic can improve morbidity and mortality associated with cancer. As per the World Health organization (WHO), "Screening refers to the use of simple tests across an apparently healthy population to identify individuals who have risk factors or early stages of disease, but do not yet have symptoms". For a screening test to be beneficial several criteria must be met (Table 1).

Table 1: Characteristics of an effective screening test (adapted from the World Health Organization)		
Disease characteristics	Screening Test characteristics	Diagnostic and treatment characteristic
• Prevalent disease • Natural history well understood • Long time between the presence of risk factors or subclinical disease and overt disease • Early intervention improves clinical and public health outcomes	• High sensitivity and specificity • Simple, reliable and affordable test • Acceptable to patient and staff	• Access and availability to diagnostic facilities • Accessible and effective treatment options • Cost-effective and sustainable treatment • The benefit of treatment outweighs the harm

The benefit of screening can be expressed as the number of subjects needed to be screened over a period of time to prevent one death associated with the specific disease. This is known as the number needed to screen (NNS). The larger the benefit, defined as the absolute risk reduction (ARR), the smaller the number needed to screen to prevent one death. The NNS is the inverse of the ARR, which is calculated by subtracting the mortality associated with non-screened population (CER) event rate from the screened population event rate (SER) (Equation 1). The NNS also depends on the prevalence of the disease in the screened population.

AAR: Absolute risk reduction. SER: Screened Event Rate. CER: Control Event Rate.

Screening and early detection can also be associated with negative outcomes or risks. Risks associated with screening include:

- False positives: a test result that indicates that a disease is present when there is no disease, leading to unnecessary investigations and anxiety
- False negatives: a negative test result when the person has the disease. This results in false reassurance and can delay treatment.
- Overdiagnosis: the diagnosis of a disease that will never cause symptoms or death. Overdiagnosis results in patients receiving treatment that they otherwise did not need (overtreatment) and/or psychological distress from diagnosis of disease

For example, out of 1000 adults screened for lung cancer with low dose CT, only three will benefit from screening (i.e. not die from lung cancer due to screening). However, seven will be diagnosed with lung cancer that would not have affected their life expectancy (overdiagnosis leading to overtreatment). Furthermore, 351 will require further testing that ultimately reveals no cancer (false positives), of which three will have major complications from invasive testing, and one will die from invasive testing.

The implementation of cancer screening has resulted in earlier diagnosis of cancer and improved outcomes for some cancers. However, an understanding of its potential risks is important to help individualize the decision of whether to initiate or stop screening.

Cancer Screening Recommendations

Both Canada and the United States have organizations that issue clinical practice guidelines for preventive health care. Table 2 provides a summary of current cancer screening guidelines in Canada and the United States. Recommendations are based on a systematic review of scientific evidence from which consensus recommendations are developed. However, older adults, over the age of 75, are rarely included in the studies upon which these guidelines are based. Although these guidelines provide specific ages when screening for cancer should be discontinued, data to decide at what age to discontinue screening is limited. For this reason, a discussion with those older adults interested in continuing screening about the benefits and harms of screening is recommended.

Table 2 also has links to patient decision aids that illustrate the performance of each screening test demonstrating how many patients benefit and are harmed by the test.

Table 2: Summary screening recommendations from the Canadian Task Force on Preventive Health Care and the United States Preventive Services Task Force

Cancer	Screening modality/ frequency	Age to start screening	Age to consider stopping screening	Comments
Breast cancer	Screening Mammography every 2 years	50 years old	74 years old	Breast Cancer 1000- Patient Tool*
Colorectal cancer	Stool based tests: gFOBT and FIT every year (Canada and U.S.) Direct visualization tests: Flexible sigmoidoscopy every 5 (Canada) to 10 years (U.S.) or Colonoscopy every 10 years (U.S.) or CT Colonography every 5 years (U.S.)	50 years old	75 years old	Colorectal screening Decision Aid Tool*
Lung cancer	Low-dose CT scan for high-risk patients Canada: Annually for up to 3 years U.S.: Every year	55 years old	Canada: 75 years old U.S.: 80 years old, has not smoked in the last 15 years, or develops a health problem that limits life expectancy	For patients at high risk of lung cancer (30 pack-year smoking history who currently smoke or quit less than 15 years ago) Lung cancer 1000 -person Tool*
Prostate cancer	PSA - no routine screening schedule.	Do not routinely screen at any age	Do not routinely screen at any age	U.S.: Individualized decision starting at age 55 Prostate Cancer Screening 1000-Person Tool*
Cervical cancer	Pap smear Cervical cytology every 3 years (Canada and U.S.) or hrHPV testing every 5 years in women age 30-65 (U.S.)	Canada: 25 years old U.S.: 21 years old	Canada: 70 (if the last 3 Pap test for the last 10 years were negative) U.S.: 65 (if adequate prior screening)	Adequate prior screening: 3 consecutive normal cytologies or 2 consecutive normal hrHPV tests. Cervical screening clinician algorithm. Cervical screening FAQ*

gFOBT: guaiac fecal occult blood test; FIT: Fecal Immunochemical Test; PSA: Prostate Specific Antigen; CT: computed tomography; hrHPV: high risk Human Papillomavirus

* Decision aid screening tools from CTFPHC available online at https://canadian-taskforce.ca/tools-resources/

Factors to consider when discussing screening for cancer in older adults.

Cancer screening decisions in older adults are complex, and screening guidelines provide only a baseline to initiate these conversations and ultimately make shared decisions with patients. This section provides a general approach to cancer screening in older adults (Figure 1).

Figure 1: Approach to cancer screening in older adults.

Cancer Risk Assessment

Reviewing prior screening history may play a role in deciding if screening should be considered in older adults. For instance, in cervical cancer, a one-time screening is recommended for women 65 and over that have incomplete, or no prior screening for cervical cancer, as data shows that most women aged 65 and over who are diagnosed with cervical cancer did not have prior appropriate cervical cancer screening. Similarly, some studies suggest that older adults who benefit most from colorectal screening are those who have never had any prior screening.

The information provided in this chapter pertains to cancer screening for those at average risk of breast, colorectal, cervical or prostate cancer. Lung cancer is the only cancer screening program focused on patients at high risk, defined as patients with a 30 pack-year smoking history who currently smoke or who quit less than 15 years ago. If patients have a prior history of any of these malignancies, extensive family history or recent abnormal screening tests results, these recommendations do not apply. Recommendations for these patients are beyond the scope of this chapter.

Life expectancy

There is often a lag period between the detection of cancer through screening and when it results in a cancer death. For this reason, life expectancy, more so than absolute age, is important to consider when deciding about the benefits of continuing cancer screening. Studies of breast and colorectal cancer have demonstrated that this lag time is approximately 10 years. For instance, it takes about 10 years before one death from colorectal cancer was prevented for 1000 patients screened.

Many different factors influence life expectancy, including current age, the year a person was born, gender, comorbidities, function, social supports, economic status and geographical location. To improve a physician's ability to prognosticate life expectancy, multiple tools can be used . The following are two examples of prognostic tools in clinical practice:

- Life tables: These graphs provide median life expectancy by age group, gender and health status for the United States population (Figure 2). The quartiles differentiate subjects' overall health status. For instance, the upper percentile includes subjects with above average fitness for their age group.
- E-prognosis: Web-based tool that estimates life expectancy based on an evidence-based questionnaire that includes patient factors including health behaviours, comorbidities and functional status. Available free of charge at https://eprognosis.ucsf.edu.

Figure 2A and 2B: Life expectancy for older adults based on age, gender, and health calculated from the 2015 Life Tables in the United States. Adapted using the same calculation method from Walker et al.

Treatment Options

Benefit from screening presumes that a patient will be willing and able to undergo treatment for an early diagnosed cancer. Treatment options include surgical intervention, radiation therapy and/or systemic therapy. The type of surgical procedure and its inherent risks are greatly dependent on the tumour type. In breast cancer, lumpectomy and mastectomy are standard management options and are considered low risk for cardiac complications. In women with multiple comorbidities, resection of the breast tumour can sometimes be done under local anesthetic depending on the size and location of the tumour. On the other hand, resection of a colonic or thoracic malignancy can be much riskier and may not be feasible or palatable in patients who are frail. For lung cancer, a rise in the use of stereotactic radiotherapy has expanded treatment options for patients with early stage non-small cell lung cancers with improvements in primary tumour control and overall survival in patients who are medically inoperable.

Given that the early detection of an asymptomatic malignancy is only potentially beneficial if a patient is eligible and willing to undergo treatment, consideration of patient willingness and fitness to undergo treatment is important when considering whether to continue with screening.

Patients' Values and Preferences

The decision about whether to continue cancer screening in older adults is challenging due to the increased risk of developing cancer with aging, increased risk of death due to non-cancer causes, and lack of knowledge about the benefits and harms of screening in older adults. In this context, personal values and individual preference need to be considered even more when deciding whether to continue screening for cancer as patients age.

Ideally, screening decisions should be made within the primary care setting where there is an established patient – primary care provider relationship. The primary care physician often has a sense of the patients' values and preference and can establish rapport to discuss the benefits and risks of screening in the context of each patient's health status. For some patients, screening provides peace of mind; for others, it can cause increased anxiety.

Patients tend to focus on the benefits of screening, that provide a sense of reassurance when the test is negative. However, they tend to be less well versed in the harms associated with cancer screening. This leads to an overestimation of benefit and underestimation of risk. When cancer screening is framed in terms of increasing harms in relation to decreasing benefit instead of citing the guideline recommendations cut off age as the reason to discontinue screening, most older adults find this approach acceptable, and it promotes the patient- physician relationship. Thus, a discussion that includes the benefits but also the limitations/risks associated with cancer screening to help older adults make an informed decision is essential.

Decision Aid Tools

To better understand the uncertainty and trade-offs of cancer screening, patient decision aids have been developed. Decisions aids can be pamphlets, videos or web-based tools that outline the benefits and harms of a specific health care decision, in this case, cancer screening. These decision aids have shown to increase patients' knowledge of the decision at hand and help patients have an active role in decision making with a more accurate perception of benefits and harms. In turn, decisions aids also help patients make decisions that are better aligned with their values.

Decisions aids developed by the CTFPHC (Table 2) provide an excellent tool to use with patients in clinic for a balanced discussion about cancer screening. Another decision tool for breast cancer and colorectal cancer screening is available on the e-prognosis website (http://cancerscreening.eprognosis.org/). It uses specific data about the patient's overall health to provide an estimate of the benefits and harms of screening. Figure 3 is an example of the breast cancer screening results provided for the case discussed at the beginning of this chapter using this tool.

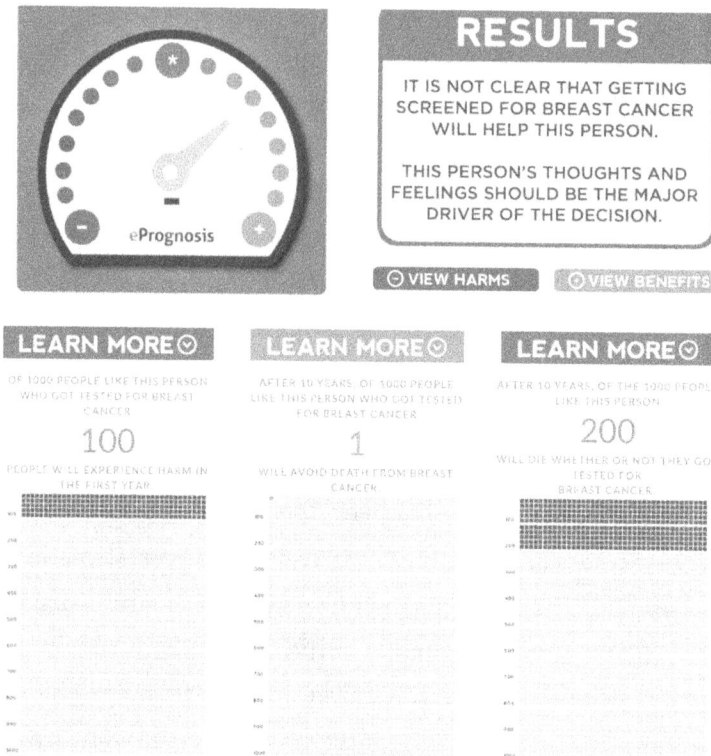

Figure 3. E-Prognosis tool results sample for breast cancer screening in a 77-year-old female with minimal comorbidities (reproduced with permission from E-Prognosis).

Screening for Breast Cancer in Older Adults

Breast cancer is one of the most common cancers diagnosed, with a peak incidence occurring in those 80-84. This age group of women, however, has been generally excluded from trials about screening. Thus, despite the higher prevalence, there remains an uncertainty about whether screening in this population will result in improved outcomes, specifically survival.

The discovery of an abnormality on mammography typically results in a call back for further imaging, including compression mammogram views and targeted ultrasound, to better characterize these findings. If the lesion still appears suspicious, then a biopsy is arranged. Even if testing ultimately rules out the presence of cancer, indicating a false-positive result, these tests can result in anxiety about the possibility of cancer and pain related to biopsies. For older women, the burden of screening may be increased due to difficulties with mobility and transportation. Many studies have shown that the risk of false positives increases with more frequent (annual) screening compared to biennial screening. Thus, a recommendation of screening mammography no more than every two years would be suggested in those women who continue screening beyond the age of 74. This is consistent with the updated American and Canadian preventive screening guidelines.

The greatest potential harm of breast cancer screening in older women relates to the possibility of over-diagnosis and over-treatment of breast cancers that are ultimately not life limiting. The factors that increase over-diagnosis and over-treatment are decreasing life expectancy and a higher prevalence of slower growing disease. As a result, women may undergo treatment, typically surgery, for clinically asymptomatic tumours that are unlikely to affect their outcomes.

Standard treatment of breast cancer and pre-cancerous lesions, such as ductal carcinoma in situ (DCIS), involves surgical resection, either in the form of lumpectomy or mastectomy. Sampling of the axilla is also often conducted to help with prognosis and subsequent treatment decisions. In general, these surgeries are considered low risk surgeries and, depending on the location of the tumour and the patient's comorbidities, can sometimes even be done under local anesthetic. For this reason, many older women will still be offered and receive surgical intervention when diagnosed with breast cancer. However, this strategy can still expose women to a potentially unnecessary procedure and the risks inherent with any surgery. A prior retrospective study suggested that the odds of post-operative complications increased with age (OR 1.85 in patients over the age of 85) and multiple comorbidities (OR 1.71). However, overall survival was not adversely affected by experiencing post-operative complications. Those women with hormone sensitive breast cancers, who are not candidates for surgery or who refuse, can be considered for primary treatment with anti-estrogen agents such as tamoxifen or aromatase inhibitors. However, outcomes with these agents alone are not as robust as with surgery and thus patients with a life expectancy of more than two years should be strongly considered for surgery.

It is important to note that under-treatment of older women with breast cancer is also common. Several studies indicate that older women are more likely to be treated with surgery alone and less likely to receive radiation or systemic treatments. In those patients, age 80 and above, in whom under-treatment is common, this can result in poorer breast cancer outcomes, including increased death from breast cancer.

Although there are no firm recommendations in women age 75 and older, it is reasonable to continue screening every two years in women with a life expectancy of at least ten years who would be willing to undergo surgical resection. In those women with shorter estimated life expectancies, a discussion about the uncertainty of benefits and potential harms of screening is important. In these cases, patient preferences and values play a significant role in deciding whether to continue to undergo screening.

Screening for Colorectal Cancer in Older Adults

More than half of all new cases of colorectal cancer are diagnosed in those 70 and over. There are several screening methods shown to decrease mortality from colorectal cancer, ranging from less invasive testing such as fecal occult blood testing and fecal immunochemical testing to more invasive tests such as sigmoidoscopy. Although several organizations recommend colonoscopy as a method to screen for colon cancer, it has not been prospectively shown to decrease mortality from colon cancer. These studies have been completed, but the results have yet to be reported.

In older adults, several factors need to be considered, including the potential benefits and harms from screening, and eligibility and willingness to undergo treatment. Colon cancers develop over a 10-15-year period from pre-malignant lesions. Thus, removal of pre-cancerous lesions (polyps) results in a decreased risk of colon cancer. Prior studies suggest that a life expectancy of ten years is warranted to benefit from colon cancer screening. Thus, patients with a shorter life expectancy may be less likely to benefit.

Despite the higher incidence of colorectal cancer in those 70 and over, there appears to be a smaller benefit from screening overall potentially due to a decrease in life expectancy. One study reported that although there was a higher prevalence of colorectal cancer detected using colonoscopy in those age 80 and over compared to those 50-54 (28.6% vs. 13.8%), that on average there was a smaller improvement in life expectancy (0.13 years vs. 0.85 years) in older versus younger patients undergoing colonoscopy screening.

Although the absolute risk of complications is low, invasive testing with sigmoidoscopy and colonoscopy risks increased with age and comorbidities. Complications of colonoscopy include bleeding and perforation. This is even higher in those patients who have a polypectomy. Older adults with comorbidities that limit their mobility may also find the procedure and preparation more challenging. There are also higher risks related to the sedation given for colonoscopy in older compared to younger patients, including the potential of delirium. Given the higher risk of significant adverse events with invasive testing, older adults who choose to continue screening should undergo stool-based testing with fecal occult blood testing or fecal immunochemical testing. However, patients should be aware that positive test warrants further testing with colonoscopy and should be willing and able to do so.

Lastly, patients should be aware of potential treatment recommendations if an asymptomatic malignant lesion is found. The standard treatment for colonic tumours is surgical resection, typically a hemicolectomy. The intent is to completely remove the tumor and to allow for nodal sampling, which influences prognosis and subsequent treatment decisions. In general, there are higher risks of surgical complications and mortality in older adults. There is a progressively increased rate of post-operative mortality with each decade of increasing age starting from age 65 onwards with those aged 75-84 experiencing a 3.2 times higher risk of postoperative mortality compared to those <65 years of age. Notably, however, the range of reported rates of complication varied greatly from lows of 0-5% and highs of 15-48.9%, suggesting that patient selection is key. Improvement in post-operative mortality has however, been reported with time, with the greatest improvements seen in patients age 85 and over. This may be related to the greater use of laparoscopic procedures. Emergency or urgent need for surgical intervention is strongly associated with higher peri-operative risk in older adults. Overall, careful patient assessment and selection and planned elective surgeries may help mitigate some of the morbidity and mortality associated with colorectal surgery in this older population.

In early superficial cancers, there is a growing use of endoscopic submucosal dissection. Very few studies have looked at these outcomes and safety in older adults. However, some retrospective observational studies suggest that it can be performed safely, with a perforation rate of 3.1%. Overall, however, further studies are needed to better characterize which patients are ideal for these less invasive procedures and to characterize their long-term outcomes compared to more extensive surgery.

Resection of colon cancer can result in a cure for 85-90% of patients with stage I/II cancer and 40-50% cure in those with stage III (lymph node involvement). Although chemotherapy after surgery is considered standard of care in those with stage III disease, this can be decided on an individual basis with patients after surgery and an unwillingness or inability to undergo chemotherapy should not be a preclusion to definitive treatment of colon cancer or a decision to undergo screening.

Given the above considerations, patient input is very important in the decision to offer or discontinue screening for colon cancer in patients over the age of 75. While the

CTFPHC recommends against screening in adults age 75 and over, the United States Preventive Services Task Force (USPTF) recommends that in adults age 76 to 85, an individualized decision about colorectal screening be made taking in account patients overall health and prior screening history.

Lung Cancer Screening in Older Adults

Lung cancer is the leading cause of cancer death in North America. About 80% of people diagnosed with lung cancer have non-curable disease at the time of diagnosis and most lung cancers when untreated are rapidly fatal. The median age for a diagnosis of lung cancer is 70 years old, affecting older adults disproportionately. Smoking is a well-known risk factor for lung cancer. Lung cancer screening should be offered only to those who are at high risk of developing lung cancer. At the same time, lung cancer differs from other solid malignancies by being known to be often an aggressive cancer that can cause significant morbidity and mortality in a short period of time.

The National Lung Screening Trial (NLST) was the first randomized study to show a benefit to lung cancer screening. This study compared low dose computed tomography (CT) or chest x-ray annually for three years in patients 55 to 74 who had a smoking history of at least 30 pack years or who had quit within the previous 15 years. This study showed a 20% relative reduction in mortality from lung cancer, with a number needed to screen of 320 to prevent one lung cancer death.

Lung cancer screening carries a high risk of false positive results. In the NLST trial, any nodule greater than 4 mm was considered a positive screening result and required further testing. After three years of yearly low dose CTs, 39% of study participants had positive findings, of those finding 95% were falsely positive. However, false positive results were ruled out by using serial CT scans to avoid unnecessary invasive investigations with thoracic biopsies. More recent data suggest that in the NLST trial about 18% lung cancer detected by low dose CT would otherwise not lead to significant morbidity or mortality and thus represent an overdiagnosis.

Extrapolating the finding of the NLST trial to older adults have been controversial as only 8.8% of patients in the NSLT trial were 70 and older. The incidence rate of lung cancer diagnosis was 2.2% in patients 65 and over; however, there was no benefit in mortality in the analysis restricted to patients 65 and over. Guideline recommendation to screen older adults comes from statistical modeling designed to determine the least invasive screening program to prevent the highest percentage of cancer related mortality. However, as most lung cancer cases occur in patients 70 years and older and due to the high morbidity and mortality associated with lung cancer, some guidelines recommend low dose CT screening that extends to patients beyond the age of those included in the NLST trial. The US Preventive Task Force recommends screening patients aged 55 to 80 until patients have quit smoking for more than 15 years or until the patient develops a health problem that will limit their life expectancy or the ability to undergo curative treatment.

Finally, considerations for lung cancer screening should include discussions about diagnostic test (lung biopsy) and treatment options that need to be considered if lung cancer is diagnosed. Treatment of early stage lung cancer typically includes surgical resection. This can range from a wedge resection, lobectomy, or on occasion a pneumonectomy. Increasingly video-assisted thoracic surgery (VATS), rather than a thoracotomy, is being used, which can result in faster recovery and decreased hospitalization. Both of these procedures typically require patients to have adequate lung function to allow resection of the affected lung. There has also been a rise in the use of stereotactic radiotherapy in patients with early stage non-small cell lung cancers with improvements in primary tumour control and overall survival in medically inoperable patients. Patients thus need to be willing and able to proceed with surgery or radiotherapy to benefit from lung cancer screening.

Prostate Cancer Screening in Older Adults

Prostate cancer is the most common cancer affecting men over age 70 and older, and the third leading cause of cancer related deaths. The rate of high-risk prostate cancer increases with age, and older adults are less likely to receive local therapy once a diagnosis is made. Despite this, prostate cancer screening is controversial for all age groups as the harms of screening outweigh the benefits.

The main reason for this is due to the poor test characteristics of prostate specific antigen (PSA) as a screening test. PSA has an estimated sensitivity of 21% for detecting any prostate cancer, meaning that of 100 people with prostate cancer 79 will have a false negative test result. Also, the specificity of the test is poor. The positive predictive value is only 30%, meaning that only 3 out of 10 men with an elevated PSA are diagnosed with prostate cancer. Abnormal PSA values lead to further diagnostic work up with a prostate biopsy. Short term risk of prostate biopsies includes anxiety, pain, hematuria, infection and hospital admission in up to 7% of patients.

Because of the indolent natural history of many prostate cancers, an estimated 40-60% of screen detected prostate cancers are felt to be an overdiagnosis, in which the diagnosis of prostate cancer will never cause symptoms or death. The rate of overdiagnosis in prostate cancer is directly correlated to the age of diagnosis. Consequently, older adults are at increased risk of experiencing harm from prostate cancer screening. Overdiagnosis leads to psychological distress and unnecessary treatments. Primary treatment of prostate cancer can include either prostatectomy or radical radiotherapy plus or minus androgen deprivation therapy. Adverse effects of treatment with prostatectomy and radiotherapy include bowel dysfunction, urinary incontinence, erectile dysfunction and premature death, particularly in older men with poor functional status. Because a large proportion of prostate cancers are felt to be an overdiagnosis, current practice guidelines recommend active surveillance for men with clinically localized low risk prostate cancer to minimize overtreatment in prostate cancer. This means curative intent treatment is deferred until there is evidence of disease progression. Even in the absence of treatment, however, diagnosis of a non-significant cancer can lead to undue anxiety.

In conclusion, PSA screening for prostate cancer should not be routinely performed in patients of any age and particularly in older adults in whom the harms of screening can significantly affect their quality of life without improving prostate cancer related morbidity and mortality.

Cervical Cancer Screening in Older adults.

One third of cervical cancer deaths occur in women age 65 and older. For average risk women, leading professional organizations recommend cervical cancer screening be discontinued in women 70 and older if they have had three consecutive negative cytologies in the last ten years. Nevertheless, many women approach age 65 without adequate screening for cervical cancer and catch up screening may be needed to achieve adequate negative screening history.

Organized screening has reduced the incident rates of cervical cancer. Screening methods include Pap test and HPV testing either alone or in combination. Both tests require a gynecological exam with a speculum. A Pap test looks for abnormal cells in the cervix, and the HPV test detects HPV DNA viruses that could lead to cervical cancer. The risks associated with cervical cancer screening include a 14.4% rate of false positive cytology that resulted in unnecessary diagnostic tests and treatments. If cytology is abnormal, further testing with repeat cytology followed by colposcopy is required. This testing can lead to significant anxiety and discomfort in patients. For older post menopausal women, the vaginal exam may be more uncomfortable given the hormonal changes associated with aging.

Cervical cancer is treated with a radical hysterectomy with pelvic lymph node dissection or pelvic external beam radiation therapy (EBRT). Depending on the stage of the cancer at diagnosis, EBRT is sometimes combined with chemotherapy or brachytherapy (localized radiation delivered directly to the cervix). Patients who have lymph node involvement or positive margins following surgery are also treated with EBRT and chemotherapy with or without brachytherapy. Data regarding risks of these treatments, specifically in older women, is unclear. However, older women are more likely to be treated with radiation rather than surgery. Those who do undergo surgery are less likely to have a lymph node dissection.

In summary, for women 70 and older who had a documented history of negative cervical cancer screening with 3 consecutive Pap test and/or HPV tests in the last 10 years, there is no evidence to support further screening. However, for older women who have never been screened a discussion about one-time screening may be considered.

Resolution of the clinical vignette

Mrs. Smith's health history was reviewed, and physical examination, including a normal breast exam, was completed. Using the e-prognosis tool (mortality risk for Lee Index), her median life expectancy was estimated to be 17.7-21.1 years with a ten-year mortality risk of 15-23%. In the context of her life expectancy, her physician decides it is reasonable to discuss the pros and cons of continuing cancer screening.

Mrs. Smith is provided with information regarding the benefits and harms of cancer screening, for breast and colorectal using e-prognosis tool (Figure 3). After reviewing the data, she decides to continue with mammogram screening at this time given her overall good health and the fact that she would be willing to undergo treatment if needed.

For colorectal cancer, she decides against colorectal screening as she does not feel that she would be willing to undergo colonoscopy if stool based testing was positive. She is educated on the signs and symptoms associated with colorectal cancer, including change in bowel habits and melena or hematochezia.

Given Mrs. Smith was not a smoker, lung cancer screening was not indicated. Further review of her history shows that she had 3 consecutive cytology results for cervical cancer screening that were normal. Thus, further cervical cancer screening is not recommended.

Conclusion

Cancer screening in older adults is a complex process that requires knowledge of the natural history of the specific malignancy, life expectancy estimates and understanding of a patient's values and preferences. It is reasonable to consider ongoing screening in those who are fit with a life expectancy of at least 10 years who are willing and able to undergo cancer treatment if a cancer diagnosis is confirmed.

Reference

1. Bibbins-Domingo K, Grossman DC, Curry SJ, et al. Screening for Colorectal Cancer: US Preventive Services Task Force Recommendation Statement. JAMA. 2016;315(23):2564-2575. doi:10.1001/jama.2016.5989

2. Curry SJ, Krist AH, Owens DK, et al. Screening for Cervical Cancer: US Preventive Services Task Force Recommendation Statement. JAMA 2018;320(7):674–86.

3. Fenton JJ, Weyrich MS, Durbin S, Liu Y, Bang H, Melnikow J. Prostate-Specific Antigen–Based Screening for Prostate Cancer: Evidence Report and Systematic Review for the US Preventive Services Task Force. JAMA 2018;319(18):1914–31.4. Walter LC, Covinsky KE. Cancer Screening in Elderly Patients: A Framework for Individualized Decision Making. *JAMA.* 2001;285(21):2750-2756. doi:10.1001/jama.285.21.2750

4. Lee SJ, Boscardin WJ, Stijacic-Cenzer I, Conell-Price J, O'Brien S, Walter LC. Time lag to benefit after screening for breast and colorectal cancer: meta-analysis of survival data from the United States, Sweden, United Kingdom, and Denmark. BMJ. 2013;346:e8441. doi:10.1136/bmj.e8441

5. Moyer VA, U.S. Preventive Services Task Force. Screening for lung cancer: U.S. Preventive Services Task Force recommendation statement. Ann Intern Med. 2014;160(5):330-338. doi:10.7326/M13-2771

6. National Lung Screening Trial Research Team, Aberle DR, Adams AM, et al. Reduced lung-cancer mortality with low-dose computed tomographic screening. N Engl J Med. 2011;365(5):395-409. doi:10.1056/NEJMoa1102873

7. Siu AL, U.S. Preventive Services Task Force. Screening for Breast Cancer: U.S. Preventive Services Task Force Recommendation Statement. Ann Intern Med. 2016;164(4):279-296. doi:10.7326/M15-2886

8. Walter LC, Covinsky KE. Cancer Screening in Elderly Patients: A Framework for Individualized Decision Making. JAMA. 2001;285(21):2750-2756. doi:10.1001/jama.285.21.2750

9. Walter LC, Schonberg MA. Screening Mammography in Older Women: A Review. JAMA. 2014;311(13):1336-1347. doi:10.1001/jama.2014.2834

10. Wilson JMG, Jungner G. Principles and Practice of Screening for Disease. World Health Organization; 1968.

PSYCHO ONCOLOGY: LIVING WITH THE FEAR OF DEATH

Norman Straker MD, DLFAPA
Clinical Professor Weill Cornell, Department of Psychiatry
Consultant, Sloan Kettering Cancer Center, Division of Behavioral Science

Psycho oncology is a subspecialty of psychiatry that specifically addresses the emotional and psychiatric care of cancer patients and their families. While cancer is no longer a death sentence, and much more frequently a treatable or chronic disease, the emotional experience of carrying a cancer diagnosis for some patients is terrifying and the most difficult part of the disease. However, many doctors and patients are inclined to avoid any discussion about their anxieties about cancer and their fears of dying.

My education as a medical student, intern, resident, and psychoanalyst left out the problem of how to help patients face death and how one can have a dialogue with a patient dealing with the patient's concerns about dying. In fact, to a large extent my experience is that for the most part the problem of avoiding the patient's concerns about dying is still true to the present time.

The longstanding avoidance of helping patients manage their fears and concerns about dying, because of the discomfort of the doctor or therapist should no longer be accepted.

Psychotherapy with patients facing death requires a deep personal involvement in the patient's life and the angst that is facing all of us. It is a daunting task. The intimate connection with the dying person is an essential part of the therapeutic process. Usually the therapist is the singular person with whom the patient shares their daily suffering and their concerns about dying.

A wall of silence usually surrounds the patient and the family about such matters. The patient often wants to be remembered as stoic and brave and does not want to be a burden to the family. The family worries that any discussion with the patient about their declining health will lead to the patient feeling hopeless, and that he or she is dying. The therapist's openness to such discussions lessens the patient's aloneness and isolation and can be extremely helpful.

To some degree depending on the personality of the oncologist, he or she may be involved to a greater or lesser degree in some of the same issues, although to a more limited extent. For some oncologists, however, the acknowledgement that the treatments are no longer working is experienced as a personal failure and is hard to accept. This denial may delay a referral for palliative or hospice care.

It has been my good fortune to benefit from some research on the natural defenses against death anxiety known as terror management. (Solomon 2011) These natural defenses include the individual's life achievements that will live on after a patient dies and an elevated self-esteem. I have incorporated and modified this research to lessen a patient's anxiety about dying. While dying, patients tell their life story, which they tend to do naturally. I suggest validating their achievements and attempting to find aspects of their life that can be complemented as contributing to the greater good. This will raise their self-esteem.

The availability of these interventions has helped me and others feel more comfortable and competent with patients facing imminent death. It has allowed for a detailed dialogue about patients' concerns about dying and death.

A more detailed account of my psychotherapeutic work with cancer patients who survived and those who died, along with detailed case presentations, is available in the bibliography that follows.

Psychiatric Disorders in Cancer Patients

Some psychiatric disorders in the cancer setting are responses to the cancer illness, while others are preexisting conditions that may be exacerbated by the cancer illness. Recent studies have observed that adjustment disorder, major depression, delirium, and anxiety disorders occur in between 10% and 34% of cancer patients. (Zabora AJ 2001 Roth AJ 1998, Zabora JR 2012)

Adjustment disorder is characterized by severe anxiety or depressive symptoms in response to a life stressor and causes undue interference with occupational, social, or school functioning. An initial diagnosis of adjustment disorder may be the beginning stages of a more severe anxiety or depressive disorder. (Li, M., 2012)

Anxiety disorders can be associated with the diagnosis and treatment of cancer or can be related to preexisting chronic anxiety exacerbated during treatment. (Noyes R,1998) The diagnosis of anxiety in cancer patients must be distinguished from medical problems such as inadequate pain control, delirium, steroids, respiratory distress from hypoxia or pulmonary embolism, withdrawal from alcohol, benzodiazepines, and narcotics, or akathisia (see Glossary).

Panic disorders and certain medical phobias can worsen in the medical setting (Miller, K., 2006) and can make medical treatment more difficult. Post-traumatic stress disorder (PTSD) is a specific type of anxiety disorder which can be caused by a life-threatening illness, like cancer. The prevalence of PTSD in cancer patients ranges from 5% to 19% (Rustad, J.K., 2012)

The diagnosis of depression in cancer patients can be difficult, because the physical symptoms of depression and cancer, and the symptoms caused by cancer treatment often overlap. Identification of dysphoric mood, apathy, crying, anhedonia (see Glossary), feelings of helplessness, hopelessness, decreased self-esteem, guilt, social withdrawal, and thoughts of "wishing for death" or suicidal ideation are the hallmarks of depression.(Synderman, D., 2009) Higher prevalence of depression in cancer patients is associated with a physical impairment, advanced stages of illness, inadequately controlled pain, and poor social support (Massie, M.J.,1998) Patients with pancreatic, oropharyngeal, gastric, and lung cancers also have higher rates of depression, (Li, M., 2012.) A few chemotherapeutic agents, such as prednisone, dexamethasone, vincristine, vinblastine, procarbazine, asparaginase, tamoxifen, interferon, and interleukin- 2, produce depressive symptoms. Depressive symptoms can also be produced by metabolic, nutritional, and endocrine disorders, such as electrolyte abnormalities; deficiencies of folate or vitamin B12; and hypothyroidism, hyperthyroidism, or adrenal insufficiency. (Hall RC 1978)

Cancer patients are two times more likely to commit suicide than individuals in the general population. (Synderman, D., 2009) Those at a higher risk for suicide are those with a poor prognosis, advanced stage of illness, a psychiatric history or a history of substance abuse, previous suicide attempts or a family history of suicide. (Breitbart, W., 1989, Zweig, R. A., 1993, Dubovsky, SL, 1978, Murphy GE 1977) and those with lung, stomach, pharyngeal, or laryngeal cancers. (Syderman D 2009)

Delirium presents with restlessness, confusion, disorientation and needs to be differentiated from anxiety. The initial management of delirium requires correction of the underlying medical or physiological causes and a reevaluation of the necessity of all medications that can cause mental status changes. Important nonpharmacologic interventions include providing a safe and supportive environment for patient, staff, and family.(See Chapter: How to diagnose and manage delirium: Haibin Yin)

Symptoms of Cancer and their Relationship to Psychiatric Disorders

Pain, fatigue, insomnia, sexual dysfunction, including side effects from chemotherapy, radiation, pain meds and symptoms of the disease contribute to psychiatric disorders and need to be differentiated from psychiatric disorders.

Uncontrolled pain often interferes with sleep, can cause insomnia and contributes to psychiatric symptoms. Steroids often interfere with sleep and can cause psychiatric disorders. (Howell D 2014). Sexual dysfunction and infertility can be the result of irradiation, surgery, and chemotherapy, or can be concomitant with a psychiatric disorder. (Desimore M 2014)

Bibliography

Breitbart W. Suicide in cancer patients. (1989) In: Holland J, Rowland J, eds. Handbook of Psycho-Oncology: Psychological Care of the Patient with Cancer. New York: Oxford University Press;:291-299

Bukberg, J., and **Straker, N** (1982) The Psychiatric Consultant and the Ambivalent Surgical Patient with Cancer. Psychosomatics, October

Desimone M, Spriggs E, Gass JS, Carson SA, Krychman ML, Dizon DS. (2014) Sexual dysfunction in female cancer survivors. J Clin Oncol.; 37:101-106.

DieTrill, M., and **Straker, N**. (1993) Psychological Adaptation to Facial Disfigurement in a Female Head and Neck Cancer Patient PsychoOncology Issue #4,

Dubovsky SL. (1978) Averting suicide in terminally ill patients. Psychosomatics.;19: 113-115.

Hall RC, Popkin MK, Devaul RA, Faillace LA, Stickney SK (1978.) Physical illness presenting as psychiatric disease. Arch Gen Psychiatry.; 35:1315-1320.

Howell D, Oliver TK, Keller-Olaman S, et al. (2014) Sleep disturbance in adults with can- cer: a systematic review of evidence for best practices in assessment and management for clinical practice. Ann Oncol.; 25 :791-800.

Kissane DW, Clarke DM, (2001) Demoralization syndrome—a relevant psychiatric diagnosis for palliative care. J Palliat Care.; 17:12-21.

Li M, Fitzgerald P, Rodin G (2012.) Evidence- based treatment of depression in patients with cancer. J Clin Oncol.; 30:1187- 1196.

Massie M.J., Holland J. C., Straker N., (1989) Psychotherapeutic Interventions in Holland J.C., and Rowland E.D.S., Handbook of Psycho oncology NY Oxford Press

Miller K, Massie MJ. (2006) Depression and anxiety. Cancer J. 12:388-39734

Mount BF, Boston PH 2007 Healing Connections, On Moving from Suffering to a Sense of Well-being J of Pain Symptom Management Apr 33 (4)372-88

Murphy GE. (1977) Suicide and attempted suicide. Hosp Pract. ; 12:73-81.

Noyes R, Holt C, Massie M. Anxiety disorders (1998). In: Holland J, ed. Psycho oncology. New York: Oxford

Pao M, Kazak AE (2009) Anxiety and depression. In: Weiner LS, Pao M, Kazak AE, Kupst MJ, Patenaude AF, eds. Quick Reference for Pediatric Oncology Clinicians: The Psychiatric and Psychological Dimensions of Pediatric Cancer Symptom Management. Charlottesville, VA: IPOS Press;

Robinson Burney S. Kissane DW Brooker J Burney S (2015) A Systematic review of the demoralization syndrome in individuals with progressive disease and cancer: a decade of research. J Pain Symptom Manage.; 49:595-610.

Rustad JK, David D, Currier MB. (2012) Cancer and post-traumatic stress disorder: diagnosis, pathogenesis and treatment considerations. Palliat Support Care.; 10:213- 223.

Solomon S. Greenberg J, Pyszczynski T., 2015 The worm at the core, on the role of life in death Random House

Straker N, & Drazen R., (1990) On the Edge of Being, When Doctors Confront Cancer video presentation on (www.international psychoanalysis.net)

Straker N 1998 Psychodynamic psychotherapy for cancer patients J of Psychotherapy Practice and Research 7,11-9

Straker N (2005) The Courage to Survive, Facing the Loss of Your Soul -mate video presentation (www. International psychoanalysis.net

Straker N (2008) Dynamic psychotherapy for cancer patients and their spouses, Psychiatric Times 8(9)119-21

Straker N. (2011) The Courage to Survive, Facing the loss of your soul-mate Palliative and Supportive Care 9)2)

Straker N (2013) "Facing Cancer and the Fear of Death, a Psychoanalytic Perspective on Treatment" Roman and Littlefield

Straker, N. (2019). Psychodynamic Psychiatry for Cancer Patients, Survivorship accepted for Sept publication Psychodynamic Psychiatry

Straker, N (2019) Psychodynamic Psychotherapy: The Treatment of Cancer Patients Who Die accepted for Sept publication Psychodynamic Psychiatry

Snyderman D, Wynn D (2009). Depression in cancer patients. Prim Care.; 36:703-719.

Zweig RA, Hinrichsen GA. (1993) Factors associated with suicide attempts by depressed older adults: a prospective study. Am J Psychiatry. 150:1687-1692.

INCONTINENCE IN OLDER ADULTS

Samer Shamout MD, MSc
Fellow, Division of Urology, McGill University

Lysanne Campeau, MDCM, PhD, FRCS(C)
Assistant Professor of Surgery, Division of Urology, McGill University
Division of Urology, Department of Surgery, Jewish General Hospital, McGill University, Montreal, Quebec, Canada

Clinical vignette

An 83-year-old man with Alzheimer disease is being cared for at home. During the past 2 months, his wife has noticed that it is increasingly difficult for him to make it to the restroom in time to urinate. He has stopped telling her when he needs to use the restroom, and she is unable to direct him to the restroom in the house quick enough. This is causing significant caregiver stress. His wife believes his cognition has begun to worsen during the past 6 months, and she is considering placing him in a nursing home. His medication list includes terazosin 2 mg at bedtime, aspirin 81 mg daily, donepezil 10 mg at bedtime, lisinopril 5 mg daily, and venlafaxine extended release 75 mg daily. His Mini-Mental State Examination score is 15/30, and his Geriatric Depression Scale is 3/15. Standing blood pressure is 110/70 mm Hg.

The urinary incontinence is a significant problem for this patient and his caregiver, and should be addressed with appropriate workup and management plan.

Why is urinary incontinence a remarkable clinical condition in elderly population?

Urinary incontinence (UI), is a common and undertreated condition of morbidity in Canada and worldwide, with peak prevalence in the geriatric population. Approximately, 3.3 million (10%) Canadians experience urinary incontinence, of whom 30 to 60% are over 65 years old. The prevalence of incontinence increases noticeably with age, affecting 19% of women and 10% of men above 60 years old. Urinary incontinence (UI), is defined as the complaint of involuntary leakage of urine.

The cost of UI in this population extends beyond monetary costs. It has a substantial negative impact on physical, psychological and health related quality of life. Moreover, UI has a great economic burden on society and on the healthcare system. It has been linked to many other critical health risks, including increased risk of hospitalization, frailty, fractures, functional disability and depression. The social implications of incontinence include diminished self-esteem, restriction of social and sexual activities and increased caregiver burden.

Unfortunately, elderly individuals encounter several obstacles in obtaining treatment for their problems. UI is rarely discussed by patients, many of whom are less likely to seek healthcare for this condition as they assume that UI is a part of aging process and there is no existing successful treatment.

What are the risk factors for UI?

The etiology of UI among the geriatric population is different and often multifactorial. As people age, physiological and functional changes in the lower urinary tract may contribute to the loss of continence in this population. Frail elderly people may have multiple comorbid medical illnesses, lifestyle, and medication changes that can cause or predispose to UI. Therefore, the evaluation and management of UI in older adults should be multidisciplinary with comprehensive understanding of the multidimensional concept of continence.

Risk factors for UI in women include changes related to anatomy, previous childbirth, hysterectomy, and menopause. Loss of estrogen at menopause and changes in the pelvic connective tissue support may explain higher prevalence of UI in postmenopausal women. On the other side, factors associated with UI in men include prostatic enlargement or prostate surgery. Despite surgical advances, UI is frequently observed following prostate surgery, with reported estimates ranging from 6% to nearly 70%.

Multiple other conditions are also associated with UI in the frail elderly population. These include:

- Uncontrolled comorbid medical conditions that predispose to polyuria or increased nighttime urine production (e.g., congestive heart failure, peripheral venous insufficiency, diabetes mellitus, sleep apnea)
- Conditions resulting in impaired mobility and/ or cognition (e.g., stroke, Parkinson's disease, degenerative joint disease, dementia)
- Constipation and fecal impaction that may contribute to double incontinence (urinary and fecal)
- Mental and cognitive disorders e.g., depression and dementia
- Medications: diuretics, calcium channel blockers, prostaglandin inhibitors, alpha-adrenoceptor blockers, selective serotonin reuptake inhibitors, cholinesterase inhibitors, opioid analgesics, psychotropic drugs and systemic hormone replacement therapy.
- Environmental factors e.g., inaccessible toilets or unavailable caregivers for toileting assistance.

In general, it is challenging to distinguish a single etiology responsible in the vast majority of geriatric population, as more often several factors interact. The above possible causes of reversible UI can be summarised in a mnemonic DIAPPERS (Delirium, Infection, Atrophic vaginitis, Psychological, Pharmacologic, Excess urine output, Restricted mobility and Stool impaction).

How is the diagnosis of UI made?

There are different types of UI in elderly population: urgency urinary incontinence (UUI) (involuntary loss of urine associated with urgency), stress urinary incontinence SUI (involuntary loss of urine on effort or physical exertion, or on sneezing/coughing), and mixed UI (a combination of SUI and UUI). A concomitant related condition which is associated with UUI is called overactive bladder syndrome (OAB), defined as urinary urgency, usually accompanied by frequency and nocturia, with or without urgency UI, in the absence of urinary tract infection or other obvious pathology. Other distinct entities are nocturia (frequent nocturnal micturition), and 'functional' incontinence (incontinence caused by either physical or cognitive impairment, with no identifiable lower urinary tract disorder), all being associated with extensive patient and caregiver burden.

Table 1: Common types of Urinary Incontinence				
Overactive bladder	Stress UI	Mixed UI	Impaired Bladder Emptying	Functional incontinence
Urinary urgency, with or without urgency incontinence often with urinary frequency and nocturia	Urinary loss in association with exertion such as coughing, laughing or lifting	Symptoms of both urgency incontinence and exertional incontinence (take a careful history as urgency or precipitancy is often reported by women with stress UI only)	Incomplete emptying is not well reported by men, but more so by women. A large post-void residual volume without symptoms (recurrent UTI, frequency, dribble, upper tract involvement) does not need treatment (a 250-ml residual volume may be acceptable in older people)	Incontinence unrelated to an underlying disorder or lower urinary tract function, perhaps related to either physical or cognitive impairment
Modified from Urinary incontinence in older adults. *Medicine.* 2017;45(1):23-27.				

How should patients be investigated ?

(see appendix for grading)

Unlike urinary incontinence evaluation in younger adults, frail older persons often require a comprehensive approach. The basic evaluation should primarily emphasize identification of transient and established causes of UI, assess the patient's environment and existing support, the degree of bother to the patient, and recognize other less common but serious entities that may trigger incontinence. The primary step is active screening for UI in the geriatric population, as more than 50% of elderly patients do not report their urinary symptoms to their health care providers. This could be due to numerous reasons, including social embarrassment, coping with symptoms, or misunderstanding that UI is a part of aging process and nothing can be done to improve this condition **(grade A)**. The patient history is often the most important element in recognizing the type, severity, and burden of incontinence for those patients. Commonly, clinical evaluation requires numerous office visits for frail older individuals in order to perform the necessary tests and to avoid additional assessment in patients who respond to ordinary measures.

History

The history should identify treatable, potentially reversible comorbid conditions, functional and cognitive impairment, and current medications that can cause or exacerbate UI in frail older people **(grade B)**. The mnemonic DIAPPERS has been commonly utilized to remember these conditions. The basic assessment must include an evaluation of the frequency and duration of symptoms, associated factors or events, precipitating and influential factors, and any measures of control that have already been used. During the history, account should be taken of the patient's medical and surgical history (ie, bowel, menstrual, obstetric, and sexual history), and risk factors which helps recognize possible influencing factors on symptoms. Furthermore, fluid/volume status, symptom severity, accessibility to toilets and social support, patient's and caregivers' expectations for UI care, should be explicitly explored **(grade B)**. It is also essential to consider the patient's likely level of cooperation, overall prognosis and life expectancy **(grade C)**.

In frail elderly people with bothersome nocturia, the treating physician should focus on detecting any potential triggering factors, including sleep apnea, nocturnal polyuria, and conditions associated with elevated post void residual (PVR). A complete and precise bladder diary (frequency-volume chart) of a minimum 3 days' duration can be a useful tool in the assessment of individuals with nocturia **(grade C)**. However, this may not always be feasible for all patients and caregivers.

Physical examination

The initial step is to perform a relevant pelvic or genital and rectal examination to evaluate for vaginal\genital atrophy, pelvic organ prolapse, prostate nodules or masses, sphincter tone, faecal impaction and the presence of a distended bladder or a pelvic mass. The initial physical examination should also include cognitive and functional assessments as well as examination for relevant neurological conditions (e.g. Parkinson's disease, stroke, spinal stenosis, and cauda equina syndrome) to rule out potential comorbid illnesses, which can directly influence continence status.

TABLE 2: Recommendation for initial evaluation of older adults with urinary incontinence[*]
Recommendations
Assess, treat and re-assess potentially treatable conditions (DIAPPERS)
Medical History
Evaluate treatment expectations regarding the continence paradigm
Physical examination including cognition, functional assessment, neurological and rectal examinations
Urine analysis
* Modified from 2012 update: guidelines for adult urinary incontinence collaborative consensus document for the canadian urological association. Can Urol Assoc J. 2012;6(5):354-363.

Useful tools for the diagnosis of UI

Basic investigations

- Dipstick urinalysis is recommended as an initial UI assessment, it helps to identify urinary tract infections as well as other abnormalities such as hematuria, pyuria, and/or bacteruria. All patients should be screened for haematuria **(grade C)**, while persistent pattern should prompt further evaluation, including upper tract imaging and cystoscopy.
- Measurement of the post-void residual volume is considered fundamental to an initial UI assessment to investigate for incomplete bladder emptying in frail older patients with long standing diabetes mellitus, previous history of urinary retention, recurrent urinary tract infections, medications known to decrease detrusor contractility (e.g., anticholinergics), severe constipation, complex neurologic disease, as well as persistent or deteriorating UI despite treatment **(grade C)**.
- Bladder diaries recording details of fluid intake, voiding times, and volumes are an appropriate assessment tool which help determine UI type, severity, and circumstances. A minimum of three days diary is recommended.
- Serum electrolytes, creatinine, and glucose maybe required if there is concern for renal impairment or in older adults with polyuria.

Specialist investigation

- Routine multichannel urodynamics testing is not necessary, but possibly warranted when diagnostic uncertainty may impact treatment decision, in patients who have not experienced significant improvement in symptoms despite prior therapy, and for patients considering invasive treatment. Urodynamic evaluation in frail older persons is safe, feasible, and reproducible.
- More invasive investigation such as cystourethroscopy is a potential diagnostic tool used in outpatient urology settings, indicated in the presence of hematuria or otherwise unexplained pelvic pain.

What are the interventions to reverse UI?

Before recommending a therapeutic intervention, it is crucial to determine the factors contributing to UI in the specific case presentation (review the mnemonic DIAPPERS). In the frail elderly patient, initial management is based first on the precise diagnosis of the type of UI experienced by the patient, severity of symptoms and bother, expectations and concerns of the patient and their caregiver(s). Treatment preferences, the level of cooperation, and the overall prognosis and life expectancy should also be considered. Below is an algorithm with an approach to treatment of UI.

Modified from 2012 update: guidelines for adult urinary incontinence collaborative consensus document for the Canadian Urological Association. *Can Urol Assoc J.* 2012;6(5):354-363.

Abbreviation: UI: urinary incontinence; BOO: bladder outlet obstruction; DHIC: detrusor hyperactivity with impaired contractility; UTI: urinary tract infection; CIC: clean intermittent catheterization.

Conservative and behavioral treatment strategies are useful in the broad management of UI **(grade C)**. lifestyle modifications and behavioral interventions that may be helpful include:

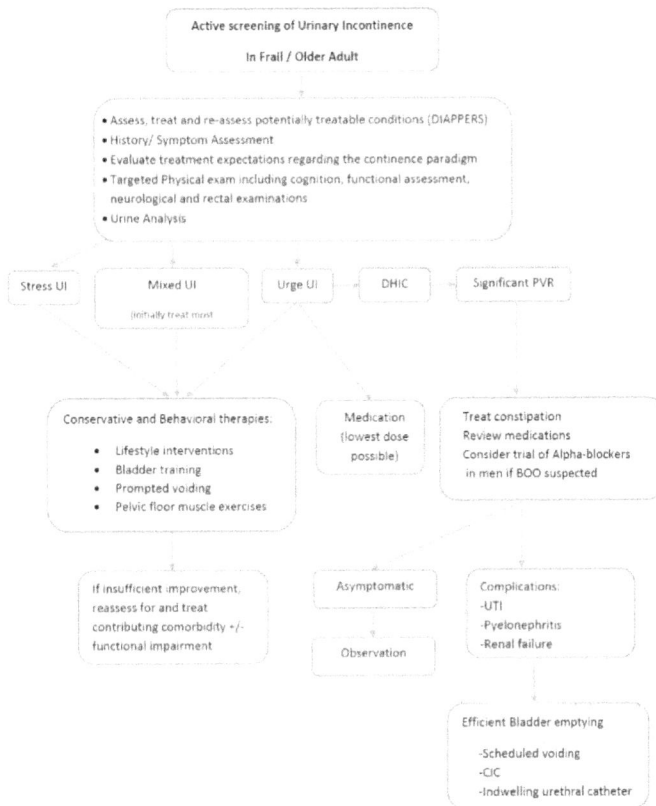

- Avoiding excess fluid intake, caffeinated drinks, and alcohol.
- Weight loss has been shown to be beneficial in reducing UI in morbidly obese women.

- Bladder training for capable patients and prompt voiding for frail and cognitively impaired individuals **(grade B).**
- Pelvic muscle exercises may be considered, but evidence on their effectiveness are deficient **(grade C)**.
- Adjunctive management considerations for the geriatric population involve appropriate continence products and devices, along with proper skin hygiene and breakdown prevention of the external genitalia, and perineum.

Pharmacotherapy does not cure UI, but is often considered for symptomatic relief particularly in UUI. In the elderly population, any drug treatment should be started very carefully due to several factors, which include: polypharmacy, drug-drug interactions, impact on cognitive function, high potential for adverse events in this patient population. Additionally, it should be started with a low dose regimen and titrated gradually with regular assessment of clinical benefits and side effects. Table 3 summarizes recommendations for pharmacologic therapy in the geriatric population with urinary incontinence.

TABLE 3: Summary of Age-related pharmacokinetics changes, and their potential effect on urinary incontinence drugs		
Parameter	**Age-related changes**	**Potentially Affected UI Medications**
Absorption	Minimal quantitative change despite delayed gastric emptying	Extended-release formulations
	Decrease subcutaneous fat	Topical preparations
Distribution	Decrease in lean body mass leads to: -Longer half-life of lipophilic agents -Higher serum concentration of hydrophilic agents	Tricyclic antidepressants
	low protein binding in older adults with low albumin level, give rise to greater concentration of free drug molecules	Tolterodine
Metabolism (hepatic)	Decreased oxidation/reduction reactions No change in hepatic glycosylation	Tricyclic antidepressants
	Decreased Hepatic blood flow and hepatic mass: less first-pass effect and increased serum level of un-metabolized drug	Oxybutynin, tolterodine, solifenacin, darifenacin
	Stereoselective selectivity in metabolism (hypothetical)	Enantiomers
	Cytochrome P450	Oxybutynin, tolterodine, solifenacin, darifenacin, mirabegron, 5-hydroxymethyl tolterodine
Excretion (renal)	Decrease in renal clearance (-GFR)	**Tolterodine, fesoterodine**
Modified from "CUA guideline on adult overactive bladder." *Canadian Urological Association Journal* 11.5 (2017): E142. Abbreviation: GFR = glomerular filtration rate		

These interventions should be individually tailored; and in certain patients a combination of the above approaches may be utilized. However, compliance may be a concern with some forms of therapy. Ultimately, consideration of specialist referral is recommended for older adults with hematuria, pelvic pain, complex neurologic disease, prior pelvic surgery, and a response to initial management that is insufficient. Identifying incontinence is the most important step. Nowadays, various therapeutic interventions are available for this prevalent geriatric problem, but the first priority should be directed to encourage elderly people to discuss their urinary symptoms with health care provider(s).

Many older people will require continence products (pads and protective garments). However, these products should be offered following a proper assessment and management plan or as a short-term relief until definitive diagnosis is explored. Indwelling urethral catheters or intermittent catheterization may be necessary for older adults with a significant PVR and impaired bladder emptying. It should be reserved when medical or surgical treatment is not possible and should not be considered as a replacement approach for nursing care of older adults with incontinence.

Summary

UI is a highly prevalent condition in the geriatric population and is associated with considerable patient, caregiver, and healthcare system burden. It represents a geriatric condition with multiple risk factors and modifiers that include age-related changes, potentially comorbid conditions, medications, and functional impairments. Active screening for UI among frail older people is strongly recommended. A comprehensive initial evaluation requires assessment of potentially reversible conditions and impairments, as well as detailed history, physical exam, and urinalysis.

UI management in this population involves a multidisciplinary and stepwise approach progressing from lifestyle and behavioral modifications, pharmacotherapy to more invasive treatment strategies, as needed.

Appendix a- Grade of recommendation·	
Grade	Nature of recommendations
A	Based on clinical studies of good quality and consistency addressing the specific recommendations and including at least one randomised trial
B	Based on well-conducted clinical studies but without randomised clinical trials
C	Made despite the absence of directly applicable clinical studies of good quality
D	Evidence inconsistent/inconclusive (no recommendation possible) or the evidence indicates that the drug should not be recommended
* Modified from 2012 update: guidelines for adult urinary incontinence collaborative consensus document for the canadian urological association. Can Urol Assoc J. 2012;6(5):354-363.	

References[1-6]

1. Bettez M, Tu le M, Carlson K, et al. 2012 update: guidelines for adult urinary incontinence collaborative consensus document for the canadian urological association. *Can Urol Assoc J.* 2012; 6 (5): 354-363.
2. Thuroff JW, Abrams P, Andersson KE, et al. EAU guidelines on urinary incontinence. *Eur Urol.* 2011; 59 (3): 387-400.
3. Shaw C, Wagg A. Urinary incontinence in older adults. *Medicine.* 2017; 45 (1): 23-27.
4. Searcy JAR. Geriatric Urinary Incontinence. *Nurs Clin North Am.* 2017; 52 (3): 447-455.
5. Weiss BD. Diagnostic evaluation of urinary incontinence in geriatric patients. *American family physician.* 1998; 57: 2675-2694.
6. Corcos J, Przydacz M, Campeau L, et al. CUA guideline on adult overactive bladder. *Canadian Urological Association Journal.* 2017; 11(5): E142.

POLYPHARMACY AND DEPRESCRIBING IN THE ELDERLY

Louise Mallet, B.Sc.Pharm., Pharm.D., BCGP, FESCP, FOPQ
Professor in clinical pharmacy, Faculty of Pharmacy,
University of Montreal
Pharmacist in geriatrics, McGill University Health Center, Glen site

Clinical vignette

Mrs. D is a 92-year-old woman who lives alone in an upper duplex. She sustained a fall last week. She has two daughters that are involved in her care and visit their mother at least twice a week. Mrs. D needs help with ADLs (Activities of Daily Living) such as washing. She receives private help once a week for bathing. She also has a cleaning person who comes once a week. She still cooks but her daughters bring her meals that can be heated in the microwave. She dresses by herself and goes out with friends twice a month. It is mentioned by the daughters that Mrs. D does not always take her medications as prescribed. They often find pills on the floor when they visit. There are no known allergies

Past medical history is significant for hypertension, diabetes type 2, hypothyroidism, dyslipidemia, insomnia, constipation and a history of falls.

Weight: 50 kg. Height: 165 cm. Patient says she lost 5 kg in past 3 months.

Laboratory results from a week ago disclose (normal values in parenthesis):
- Na: 129 mmol/L (133-143)
- K: 4.4 mmol/L (3.5-5.0)
- Mg: 0.60 mmol/L (0.75-1.25)
- Creatinine: 85 µmol/L (40-85; stable)

- Albumin: 39 g/L (8-50)
- TSH: 9 µU/mL (04-4.4)
- Vitamin B12: 176 pmol/L (> 133)
- HbA1c 6,5% (4.3-6)
- Calculated Cr Cl using Cockcroft/Gault formula: 30 mL/min (>60)
- Blood glucose reported by daughter: between 4 and 7 mmol/L (3.9-11; done once a week at different times during the week)

Her current medication list is as follows:
- Amlodipine 5 mg po daily
- Pantoprazole 40 mg po daily
- Furosemide 40 mg po daily
- Levothyroxine 88 mcg po daily
- Metformin 850 mg po bid
- Atorvastatin 40 mg po daily
- Glyburide 5 mg po bid
- Docusate sodium 100 mg po bid
- Citalopram 20 mg po daily for the past 10 years
- Lorazepam 1 mg po at bedtime, prn
- Acetaminophen (Tylenol PM^{MD}) 1 tablet po at bedtime, prn

Her medications are delivered in vials. She has her own system to organize her medications. She prepares her medications for one week at a time using vials.

This case illustrates the problems with polypharmacy in older patients. This chapter will present a systematic process to optimize the medications prescribed for Mrs. D.

> *"When an elderly patient presents with a status change, unless proven otherwise, it should be assumed to be a medication related problem".*
>
> *Jerry Gurwitz M.D.*

What is polypharmacy?

Polypharmacy is common in the elderly. However, there is no standard definition for polypharmacy. The World Health Organization (WHO) defines polypharmacy as multiple medicines for chronic use at the same time, usually more than 4 medications. Some authors have defined polypharmacy as "the prescription of more medications than clinically indicated, use of unnecessary drug, use of ineffective medication, the

presence of therapeutic duplications or the concurrent use of 2 to 9 different therapeutic agents. Excessive polypharmacy is defined as the concurrent use of at least 10
medications in older adults.

Polypharmacy has been associated with decreased physical and social functioning, increased risk of falls, delirium, decreased adherence to medication, higher costs,
emergency room visits, hospital admissions, nursing home placement and death.

In Canada, 20% percent of older adults aged 65 to 74 take 10 medications or
more per day. This percentage increases to 32% for those aged 75 to 84 and to 40%
for those≥ 85 years of age. It is reported that 30% of hospitalization in older adults
75 years of age and over are related to medications. (Canadian Institute for Health
Information *2014*)

What is deprescribing?

Deprescribing is the process of stopping an inappropriate medication, supervised by
a health care professional with the goal of managing polypharmacy and improving
outcomes. Inappropriate medications are defined as medications in which risks outweigh benefits. Patient's goals, life expectancy, values, preferences and level of care
should be discussed in the context of deprescribing. The activity of deprescribing
should be part of the continuum of prescribing. It is a patient-centered intervention
which includes patient consent, and close monitoring. Deprescribing encompasses
the process of deciding with the patient which medications can be discontinued,
planning a cessation protocol when needed and monitoring the plan and follow-up.

Which factors should be considered when evaluating medications in the elderly?

Is the patient really taking the medication?

- Ask the patient to bring medications (prescribed, over the counter, vitamins,
  eye drops, natural products, essential oils etc.). Mrs. D has a bottle of Tylenol
  PM[MD] which contains Acetaminophen 500 mg and diphenhydramine 25
  mg. Diphenydramine is an anticholinergic medication which can have an
  impact on her cognition and also cause falls. She has a history of falls and
  sustained a fall last week. She says that she recently bought this product
  as suggested by a friend. She took it once and did not like the feeling of it.

- TSH is elevated. Is Mrs. D taking her levothyroxine correctly? Daughter says that pills are found on the floor on a regular basis when she visits. It is suggested to continue the same dose of levothyroxine for now and repeat TSH in one month.
- Verify which system is used to help take her medication; dispill, dosett or other self-created system. Ask Mrs. D what she does when she forgets to take her medications. Verify with the community pharmacist whether she renews her medication on a regular basis. For example, Mrs. D has a prescription for lorazepam, a benzodiazepine, prescribed "prn" or as needed for sleep. It is important to verify if she takes it every night on a regular basis or say, once a week to avoid the risk of precipitating withdrawal symptoms. Benzodiazepines have been shown to increase the risk of falls, hip fractures, cognitive impairment, delirium, dementia and traffic accidents.
- Ask Mrs D if she knows the indication for each her medications; is she taking all her prescribed medications on a regular basis and if not, the reasons why (side effects, too many medications or forgetting to take them).

What are the current indications for each drug?

- Verify the indication for each medication.
- Verify the presence of a medication cascade. A prescribing cascade is observed when an adverse drug reaction is misinterpreted as a new medical problem. A second medication is prescribed which places the patient at risk of adverse drug reaction or potential drug-drug interactions. This domino effect can go on if not recognized by the health care provider. Some examples of prescribing cascades can be found below.
- Consider discontinuation or tapering the medication if no valid indication.
- Match each medication with a medical problem. For Mrs. D:

Examples of prescribing cascade
Furosemide → urinary incontinence → oxybutynin
Amlodipine → peripheral edema → furosemide
Risperidone → rigidity → levodopa + carbidopa
Ciprofloxacin → hallucination → risperidone
Atorvastatin → leg pains → quinine
Digoxin → nausea/vomiting → metoclopramide
Venlafaxine → hyponatremia → salt supplements

Medications	Medical problems
Amlodipine	Hypertension
Furosemide	Lower leg edema from use of amlodipine? Medication cascade?
Atorvastatin	Hypercholesterolemia ?
Metformin	Diabetes
Glyburide	
Pantoprazole	GI problems?
Levothyroxine	Hypothyroidism
Docusate Sodium	Constipation
Insomnia	Lorazepam, Tylenol PM^{MD}
Citalopram	Depression?

What is Mrs. D's life expectancy and what are her expectations and preferences?

- Discuss with Mrs. D her expectations and preferences in terms of her medications.
- Estimate Mrs. D's life expectancy and objectives of treatment. She has a limited life expectancy between 1,9 and 3,9 years based on published literature.
- Define the therapeutic objective for the use of atorvastatin for Mrs. D. Suggest to discontinue considering her age.
- If a new medication is added, verify the time for benefit before prescribing considering her limited life expectancy.
- Identify medications which may cause harm. For example, use the American Geriatrics Society (AGS) Beers Criteria for potentially inappropriate medication (PIM) use in older adults, to verify which medications are potentially inappropriate.

AGS Beers Criteria for PIM	Reasons
Glyburide	Severe hypoglycemia
Citalopram	Hyponatremia, falls
Lorazepam	Slowness, confusion, falls
Pantoprazole	Use > 8 weeks causes hypomagnesemia, risk of Clostridium difficile infection

Considering pharmacokinetic modifications with aging, which factors should be taken into consideration when evaluating Mrs. D's medication?

Pharmacokinetic changes should be considered when evaluating Mrs. D's medications. With aging, a decrease in renal function is reported. Mrs. D's creatinine clearance calculated using the Cockcroft and Gault formula is 30 mL/min. Medications that are renally excreted should be adjusted. Metformin in this case is contraindicated with a creatinine clearance of less than 30 ml/min. Metabolites of glyburide are also renally excreted and not indicated with a CrCl of less than 50 ml/min due to their accumulation and increased risk of hypoglycemia. Age-related changes with absorption, distribution, metabolism and elimination of medications with normal aging and in the frail elderly are described in the following table.

Age-related changes in pharmacokinetics with normal aging and in the frail elderly

	Age-related changes	Normal Aging	Frail elderly
Absorption	No changes	No clinical impact	⇓
Distribution	Body Fat	⇑volume of distribution for liposoluble drugs Adjust dosage for fat soluble drugs such as antipsychotics, antidepressants, benzodiazepines	⇑⇑
Distribution	Total water	⇓Volume of distribution for water-soluble drugs. Adjust dosage for water-soluble drugs such as diuretics, digoxin, oral hypoglycemic	⇓⇓
	Albumin	⇓Free fraction for drugs that are more than 90% bound to albumin such as phenytoin, valproic acid, warfarin	⇓⇓
Metabolism	Hepatic blood flow	⇓First-pass extraction by the liver for drugs such as verapamil, propranolol.	⇓⇓
	Esterase enzymes	⇓Metabolism of drugs metabolized by esterase enzymes. For ex: decreased metabolism of prodrug-enalapril to enalaprilat	⇓⇓
	Phase I metabolism	⇓Metabolism of drugs metabolized by oxidation reaction	⇓⇓
	Phase II metabolism	No changes with normal aging	⇓Changes in glucoronidation of acetaminophen and clearance of metoclopramide
Elimination	Glomerular filtration rate	⇓Elimination of drugs renally excreted	⇓⇓
	Tubular secretion	⇓Elimination of drugs excreted by tubular secretion such as cimetidine, trimethroprim	⇓⇓
	Serum creatinine	No changes with normal aging	⇓⇓ For low weight patient with decreased muscle mass, decrease in serum creatinine level
	Creatinine clearance	⇓with normal aging	⇓

What are the therapeutic objectives for her diabetes and hypertension?

Considering her life expectancy and level of autonomy, therapeutic objectives for Hb A1c of < 8,5% and glucose level between 5 and 10 mmol/L would be appropriate for this patient to avoid hypoglycemia (cause of falls). Metformin and glyburide can be discontinued with close monitoring of blood glucose. Her daughter can be involved in documenting blood glucose for the next few weeks. If needed, another antidiabetic agent such as an inhibitor of the dipeptidyl peptidase-4 (DPP-4) can be prescribed.

For her hypertension, blood pressure goals should be less than 150/90 without orthostatic hypotension. Evaluation of orthostatic hypotension should therefore be done. If Mrs D has peripheral edema due to her amlodipine and was prescribed furosemide for this problem (medication cascade), these drugs should be discontinued. An angiotensin-converting-enzyme inhibitor should be considered.

Why should drugs with anticholinergic properties be avoided in the elderly?

Studies have shown that medications with anticholinergic properties have been associated with falls, and a decline in functional and cognitive capacity. A withdrawal plan should be implemented when stopping these medications. As discussed, Mrs D is taking Tylenol PM which has acetaminophen and diphenhydramine as active ingredients. This should be stopped and discussion of the treatment of her "insomnia" initiated.

As per Beers Criteria for PIM, the following table illustrates a list of medications with strong anticholinergic drugs that should be avoided in the elderly. The following table illustrates the most common anticholinergic drugs used in clinical practice.

Common drugs with anticholinergic properties as listed in AGS Updated Beers Criteria 2015

Antiemetic	Dimenhydrinate, promethazine
Antihistamines	Chlorpheniramine, cyproheptadine, diphenhydramine, hydroxyzine, meclizine
Antidepressants	Amitriptyline, desipramine, doxepin (>6 mg), nortriptyline, paroxetine
Antimuscarinics	Darifenacin, fesoterodine, oxytubynin, solifenacin, tolterodine, trospium
Antiparkinsonian	Benztropine, trihexyphenidyl
Antipsychotics	Cloxapine, loxapine, olanzapine
Antispasmodics	Atropine (excludes opthalmic), clidinium-chlordiazepoxide, dicyclomine, scopolamine
Skeletal muscle relaxants	Cyclobenzaprine, Methocarbamol, orphenadrine

Which drugs can be discontinued in Mrs D's case?

When the decision is made to implement a drug deprescribing plan, thus discontinuing medications, a plan should be put in place for monitoring and follow-up. This is an on-going re-evaluation. The following table illustrates the problems, drugs, therapeutic objectives and other considerations to evaluate if needed.

- For example, are the treatment goals achieved.
- Can a non pharmacological approach be implemented.
- Determine if you need to taper a medication.
- Supervision of drug discontinuation should be made by one physician. Collaboration can be made with community pharmacist for example to taper a benzodiazepine.

Match problems, drugs and therapeutic objectives

Problems	Current Drugs	Therapeutic objectives	Others
Falls	Tylenol PM	Pain control with acetaminophen alone	Gait evaluation and rehabilitation
Diabetes	Metformin 850 mg po bid Glyburide 5 mg po bid	HbA1c<8,5% Glucose between 5 and 10 mmol/L	
Hypertension	Amlodipine 5 mg daily Furosemide 40 mg daily	SBP < 150 without orthostatic hypotension	Moderate salt intake
Hypothyroidism	Levothyroxine 88 mcg po daily	TSH 0.4 and 4.4	Verify compliance
? GI	Pantoprazole 40 mg po daily	**Clarify indication**	**Discontinue. Suggest looking at www. Deprescribing.org**
? Cholesterol	**Atorvastatin 40 mg po daily**	Discontinue	
Depression	Citalopram 20 mg po daily	No clear indication	Geriatric Depression Scale
Insomnia	Lorazepam 1 mg po at bedtime	Better sleep	Sleep hygiene
Constipation	Docusate sodium 100 mg po bid	Regular bowel movement as per patient	Docusate sodium not effective long term. Change for Lax-a-day 17 g po daily

Conclusion

Evaluating medications in the elderly should be done on a regular basis, in order to modify risk factors to avoid geriatric syndromes such as falls, delirium etc. When prescribing a new medication to an elderly patient, the patient's expectations and preferences, and the objective of treatment according to life expectancy should be included in the discussion.

"It takes one minute to prescribe a medication but years to discontinue it."

Louise Mallet, February 2018.

Suggested reading

1. American Geriatrics Society 2015 Beers Criteria Update Expert Panel (2015) American Geriatrics Society 2015 updated Beers Criteria for potentially inappropriate medication use in older adults. J Am Geriatr Soc 63: 2227-2246

2. Bowles S. Polypharmacy. In: Huang A, Mallet L. ed. Medication-Related Falls in Older People: Causative Factors and Management Strategies. Springer Nature, Switzerland, 2016, p. 41-54.

3. Holmes, H. M. et al. Life expectancies predictions for women and men on the basis of US life tables. Arch Intern Med 2006; 166: 605-609

4. Reeve E, Shakib S, Hendrix I et al. Review of deprescribing processes and development of an evidence-based, patient-centred deprescribing process. Br J Clin Pharmcol 2014; 78: 738-747.

5. Scott IA, Hilmer SN, Reeve E et al. Reducing inappropriate polypharmacy. The process of deprescribing. JAMA Intern Med. 2015; 175: 827-834.

6. Holmes, H. M. et al. Life expectancies predictions for women and men on the basis of US life tables. Arch Intern Med 2006;166: 605-609

7. Mallet L. Pharmacology of Drugs in Aging. In: Huang A, Mallet L. ed. Medication-Related Falls in Older People: Causative Factors and Management Strategies. Springer Nature, Switzerland, 2016, p. 55-66.

8. Rochon P, Gurwitz JH. The prescribing cascade revisited. Lancet 2016; 389: 1778-1780.

AFTER THE MENOPAUSE

Ronald M. Caplan, MD, CM, FACS, FACOG, FRCS(C)
Clinical Associate Professor Emeritus Obstetrics and Gynecology,
Weill Medical College of Cornell University

Clinical vignette

An independent 96 year old woman, living alone with daytime cleaning help, visits her gynecologist for a routine checkup. She has no specific complaints. She never smoked, and rarely drinks a glass of wine.

She stopped menstruating at age 52 and has not bled vaginally since. She does visit her gynecologist once yearly, before her annual trip to her childhood home, Switzerland. She travels alone.

She is well oriented, rational, and aware of her surroundings. She is mobile without the use of any support. Her body habitus is normal, and she stands erect. She sees adequately with corrective lenses.

She does see a cardiologist for a longstanding, right bundle branch block but is not currently on any medication for this. Her only regular medication is Atorvastatin, prescribed by the cardiologist, which keeps her low density lipoprotein (LDL) within normal limits.

Physical examination, including breast and pelvic examination, is normal. Her vital signs are normal.

A complete blood count and blood chemistries are reported as normal. Urinalysis is normal.

Menopause

Menopause means the stopping of the menstrual flow, at an average age of approximately 50. Women do not normally menstruate beyond the age of 55.

The normal function of the ovaries is lost. There is a high density of nerve fibers in postmenopausal ovaries, inferring altered communication. There is diminished output of estrogen and progesterone by the postmenopausal ovary. The pituitary gland puts out increased amounts of follicle stimulating hormone (FSH) and luteinizing hormone (LH). The pituitary gland itself is controlled by the hypothalamus situated at the base of the brain. Gonadotropin Releasing Hormones (GNRH) from the hypothalamus act on the pituitary gland to release FSH and LH in rhythmic fashion.

Increasing wealth of societies, better nutrition, and implementation of public health measures are factors that contribute to the lengthening of the reproductive years. These factors help women to stay healthy longer.

Abnormal bleeding in a woman in the menopausal age group and beyond must always be investigated because of the possibility of abnormal growth, notably of the lining of the uterus.

The symptoms of the menopause vary widely in intensity, type and duration from woman to woman.

Hot flushes, the sudden onset of a feeling of heat and flushing of short duration, are a classic symptom.

There may be night sweats. Other symptoms may include sleeplessness, irritability, lack of concentration, changes in appetite, and headache.

There may be a change in libido, or sexual desire and satisfaction.

Hair may be less lustrous. The skin can lose some of its smoothness and glow.

Osteoporosis and Hormonal Replacement Therapy (HRT)

A big concern for women in the postmenopausal years is osteoporosis, which involves demineralization of the bones. There is a reduction in bone quantity. The supporting fibers of the interior of the bone, the trabeculae, become scanty and thin, leading to a propensity for fractures, and postural abnormalities, including "hump" formation at the level of the thoracic spine, an outward curvature indicative of osteoporotic change with anterior compression of thoracic vertebrae (kyphosis). The process in the spinal column can result in compression fractures of the vertebrae. A woman can end up being shorter as she ages.

Of course, menopause is not the only precursor of osteoporosis, and a lesser, but significant proportion of older men have to deal with osteoporosis as well.

It is important for a woman's longevity and wellbeing that postmenopausal osteoporosis be minimized. As a woman ages, it is increasingly important for her to remain mobile. A hip fracture in an older woman can be particularly devastating. She is temporarily immobilized. The fracture may not heal well at least partially because of the osteoporosis. As well, she is subject to blood clots that can travel through her circulatory system to her heart and lungs: a life threatening pulmonary embolism.

In normal bone, the activity of osteoblasts, cells that form bone, and osteoclasts, which absorb and remove bone, are in balance. Bone resorption can be inhibited by drugs, causing bone density to increase, resulting in stronger bones.

Fair, slim women tend to be more at risk for osteoporosis, although all women should be on guard against it. A healthy lifestyle, including regular aerobic and weight bearing exercise, as well as sports activities, are important. Lean muscle mass is important in itself, and for its impact on bone density. These active skeletal muscles are attached to bone. When the muscle contracts, the bone moves.

More information on exercise can be found in the chapter "Physical Activity as a countermeasure to frailty", by Guy Hajj Boutros and Dr Antony Karelis.

Cigarette smoking should be avoided. Alcoholism is a risk factor for osteoporosis. The diet should be healthful and rich in calcium, which is notably present in milk and milk products. The use of skim milk and skim milk products cuts down on caloric intake. Ideally, three glasses of skim milk a day or the equivalent should be included in the diet. A calcium pill is roughly equivalent to the calcium in one glass of milk. If there is no milk in the diet, three 500 mg calcium tablets may be needed each day. However, too much calcium intake can be associated with kidney stone development.

Vitamin D is important in bone metabolism. An adequate diet should generally supply enough vitamin D, but especially in older persons when the diet might be deficient, daily supplementation with 800 International Units (IU) of vitamin D can be helpful.

More information on diet can be found in the chapter "Could my patient be malnourished?" by Dr. Jose Morais.

A variety of treatment options are available for prevention of osteoporosis, which may also have the beneficial effect of lessening menopausal symptoms, notably "hot flushes".

Watchful waiting can be employed if symptoms are not bothersome, if the diet is nutrient rich including adequate calcium intake, that regular aerobic exercise is enjoyed, and that bone density testing remains normal. However, intake of calcium and vitamin D alone is usually not sufficient to stop bone loss.

Osteoporosis occurs along with decreased estrogen production by the ovaries. Estrogen replacement therapy by itself, however, can lead to cancer, notably endometrial cancer. The endometrium is the lining of the uterus. This undesirable effect is largely obviated by the addition of progesterone, another naturally occurring female sex hormone, to the regimen. Estrogen with progesterone is classic Hormonal Replacement Therapy.

Hormonal Replacement Therapy (HRT).

Estrogen can be taken orally or by skin patch. There are vaginal preparations as well. Oral estrogen is processed in the liver, which can lead to problems in women with liver disease. Conversely, because of passage of oral estrogen through the liver, there can be beneficial effects on cholesterol levels, with low density lipoprotein (LDL) cholesterol being lowered, and high density lipoprotein (HDL) being raised. However, levels of C-reactive protein are raised. C-reactive protein is associated with inflammation, and inflammation can be a contributing factor in heart disease.

With estrogen, with or without progesterone replacement, postmenopausal bleeding can occur, sporadically or cyclically. When postmenopausal bleeding occurs, whether in the presence of HRT or not, it should not be assumed that the bleeding is simply due to HRT or some other benign factor. Postmenopausal bleeding is a classic warning sign of gynecologic malignancy, and that possibility has to be ruled out with appropriate investigation by a gynecologist.

HRT should be individualized, after careful examination, and after the risks and benefits have been explained, as well as the possibility of using other therapy, such as Denosumab, Bisphosphonates or Specific Estrogen Receptor Modulators (SERMS).

Benefits of HRT can include lowering of LDL as explained above, and improvement of vaginal lining atrophy (thinning).

In most women, after four years of use soon after menopause, the risk of hormonal replacement therapy with estrogen and progesterone outweighs any possible benefits. However, in some women, symptoms are persistent, even after the age of 65. Risks include cardiovascular disease, heart disease, thrombosis (blood clots) and stroke, and possibly an increased risk of ovarian cancer with prolonged HRT. HRT can increase the eventual risk of getting breast cancer. There may be an increased risk of cognition impairment and dementia.

The diagnosis of osteoporosis is confirmed by bone density studies. These painless tests are performed with the use of DXA machines (Dual Energy X-ray Absorptiometry) and reported as T-scores.

Osteoporosis can be counteracted by aerobic exercise, calcium and vitamin D intake, HRT, Denosumab, Bisphosphonates, or SERM's. Although statins, other drugs, or "natural" alternatives (which could contain varying amounts of unopposed estrogenic substances) may be helpful in some cases, it is important that these are not taken without proper consultation, and with regard to risks as well as benefits.

Denosumab

Denosumab is a human monoclonal IgG2 antibody. "Monoclonal" refers to the fact that the antibody protein is derived from one clone of cells, all of which are identical. The antibody goes to a specific receptor site. The receptor site is a distinctively shaped area on a cell surface, designed to receive a specific substance. In this case, Denosumab binds to the receptor activator of nuclear factor-kB ligand (RANKL). It inhibits bone resorption by impairing the development, activation, and survival of osteoclasts. Denosumab has become, along with bisphosphonates, a widely used osteoporosis treatment. Its effect on bone turnover is quickly reversible. However, stoppage may result in an increased propensity to fracture, and usage may impact response to infection.

Denosumab has been shown to improve bone mineral density (BMD)more than bisphosphonate treatment at the lumbar spine, total hip, and femoral neck.

Bisphosphonates

These nonhormonal drugs specifically combat osteoporosis. Bisphosphonates selectively adhere to and remain within bone. They act at the level of bone resorbing cells known as osteoclasts, inhibiting their activity by inactivation or by promoting apoptosis (programmed cell death). Less bone is absorbed, so bone remains dense and strong. Bisphosphonates provide persistent antiresorptive effect after discontinuation.

The risk of hip and vertebral fractures in older women is reduced significantly with the use of bisphosphonates.

Specific Estrogen Receptor Modulators (SERM's)

These drugs that bind to estrogen receptors are an alternative to HRT in preventing osteoporosis. However, SERM's do not take away symptoms of the menopause, including hot flushes. Specific SERM's may actually decrease the incidence of breast cancer.

Benign tumors of the uterus (fibroids) may shrink. However, the incidence of endometrial cancer is increased with certain of these drugs. There can be an increased risk of thromboembolism.

Calcitonin

This hormone that inhibits bone resorption tends to be ineffective in early menopause. However, it can have some effect more than ten years after menopause in increasing bone mineral density.

Parathyroid Hormone

The tiny parathyroid glands are situated very close to the thyroid gland in the neck. Parathyroid hormone can be genetically engineered. The hormone promotes bone growth

Growth hormone

Growth hormone output decreases as a woman ages. Theoretically, giving growth hormone to women approximately seventy years of age could lessen the decline in their bone mass, as well as the decline in their muscular strength, while gaining less abdominal fat.

Statins

Statins influence the metabolism of cholesterol by inhibiting cholesterol production in liver cells. This prompts liver cell receptors to remove LDL from the bloodstream so that liver cells get the cholesterol they need for cell function. The primary use for this class of drugs is to reduce the risk of cardiovascular disease. Statins can reduce the risk of thrombosis in veins. Additionally, Statins can reduce the risk of bone fracture. They increase bone formation and bone density and may inhibit bone resorption.

Phytoestrogens

Some natural supplements contain phytoestrogens which are derived from plants. The problem with taking such supplements is that the dosage ingested into the human body is often unregulated and unknown. There is no progesterone to counteract the increased incidence of endometrial cancer.

Phytoestrogens may not improve menopausal symptoms, and do not alleviate hot flashes.

Osteoporosis Genes

An international research team led by Dr. Brent Richards (McGill University) reported in 2018 on genes associated with low bone mineral density (BMD) and fracture risk. It was found that a gene called DAAM2 influences bone density, mineralization, porosity and strength. Five other genes were found to probably be important for BMD and fracture as well.

Cardiovascular Event Risk after Menopause

Cardiovascular disease risk is greater after the menopause. Much of this increase simply goes along with general aging. However, it was noted as far back as the classic Framingham Study that the menopause itself did seem to increase cardiovascular disease risk.

Breast Cancer Screening

In the average risk woman after the menopause, breast examination and mammography may be done yearly, with the possibility of decreasing the frequency to every second year at approximately age 55, if agreed upon by the woman and her physician. The decision to continue mammography past age 75 should be made by each woman in consultation with her physician.

Cervical Cancer Screening:

Women should be tested with cytology (Papanicolaou "PAP" smear) and tested for Human Papilloma Virus (HPV) until age 65. If testing has been negative to that point, it may be stopped by her physician. Women who are now menopausal did not have the benefit of being vaccinated against the HPV virus when they were young: the vaccine was not then available.

Libido and Sexual Function

The frequency of sexual intercourse and sexual satisfaction does not necessarily correlate to the cessation of menses. There is, however, a possible diminution in libido and sexual desire.

This is often compounded by the fact that a male partner may be losing sex drive, having erectile problems (Erectile Dysfunction: ED), and may be incapable of having intercourse or achieving orgasm. Urological examination may detect problems including prostatic enlargement that may require intervention. Sex coaching by a professional counselor may be necessary. Drugs such as tadalafil and sildenafil promote erection. Tadalafil use can counteract benign prostatic hyperplasia.

After menopause, there is a decrease in androgen production from the ovaries and from the adrenal glands. Dehydroepiandrosterone (DHEA), DHEA sulphate (DHEAS), androstenedione, and testosterone are all decreased. Estrogen replacement therapy (HRT) further decreases bioavailable free testosterone because of an increase in sex hormone-binding globulin (SHBG). Decreased testosterone can possibly lead to muscle wasting, depression, loss of energy, and decreased libido, as well as osteoporosis.

A recently FDA approved injectable drug for the treatment of Hypoactive Sexual Desire Disorder (HSDD) in premenopausal women is Vileesi (bremelanotide), which activates melanocortin receptors.

This is in addition to the previously FDA approved, for premenopausal women, oral Addyi (flibanserin) which is a serotonin 1A receptor agonist, and a serotonin 2A receptor antagonist.

Libido can possibly be enhanced by small amounts of testosterone. Giving testosterone to women is not without hazard. Acne, irreversible changes in the voice and male pattern hair growth are possible. The clitoris may enlarge. Oral methyltestosterone can be toxic to the liver. If a preparation that combines estrogen with testosterone is prescribed, there can be an increased incidence of endometrial cancer.

Vaginal Difficulties

After the menopause, the vagina may gradually tighten. This effect can be more pronounced if sexual intercourse is infrequent or absent. The vagina loses elasticity, and much of its lubrication. If intercourse is resumed, it may be painful or even impossible. The lower end of the vulva (area of the vaginal opening) called the fourchette, can tear and bleed. There may also be tears with penile penetration further up the vagina. With regular intercourse and the use of vaginal lubrication when needed, these problems generally do not occur.

In severe cases of vaginal tightening, the gynecologist may prescribe the use of vaginal dilators in graduated sizes.

Hormonal replacement therapy (HRT) with estrogen and progesterone cyclically, or in combination orally, or by skin patch, can keep the vagina supple and lubricated.

Discussion

With our burgeoning population of seniors, the majority of whom are women, the postmenopausal years have become an increasingly significant proportion of life. If the average age of menopause today is approximately fifty, and a woman can reasonably now expect to live well into her eighties or even beyond, then this span can easily represent more than a third, even up to half, her life. The implications for the individual, her family, and society at large are vast. If the individual is fortunate enough to be free of major debilitating disease and keeps herself properly nourished and mentally, physically and socially active, and finds the work she may be doing to be rewarding, her opportunities for a long and fulfilling life lie before her.

Resolution of the Clinical Vignette

This autonomous, independent woman with intact faculties in her mid-nineties represents a growing cohort of the older old. She is traveling to a place that she knows well, where competent medical care is available if needed: **Bon Voyage!**

References

1. Long Life: A Survival Strategy: Prolonging the Productive, Fulfilling Lives of Women: Ronald M Caplan, MD. Morgan James Publishing. 2008. Pages 183-227.
2. ACOG Practice Bulletin: Cervical Cancer Screening and Prevention: Number 168, October 2016 (reaffirmed 2018)
3. ACOG Practice Bulletin: Breast Cancer Risk Assessment and Screening in Average-Risk Women: Number 179, July 2017 (Reaffirmed 2019)
4. ACOG Practice Bulletin: Management of Menopausal Symptoms: Number 141, January 2014 (Corrected January 2016, March 2018)
5. Bone Density Exam /Testing https://www.nof.org/patients/diagnosis-information/
6. https://www.health.harvard.edu/heart-health/ask_the_doctor_is_bundle_branch_block_serious (Published January 2009, updated April 3, 2019)
7. https://www.nih.gov/news-events/nih-research-matters/genes-linked-abnormal-bone-density-fracture (Published January 15, 2019)

8. Comparison of Denosumab and Bisphosphonates in Patients with Osteoporosis. Lyu,H; Jundi,B et al: J Clin Endocrinol Metab. 2019; 104(5): 1753-1765

9. An atlas of genetic influences on osteoporosis in humans and mice: Nature Genetics 51, 258-266 (2019): John A. Morris, John P. Kemp, J. Brent Richards et al

10. Kannell, WB; Hortland, MC et al: Menopause and Risk of Cardovascular Disease: The Framingham Study. Ann Intern Med Oct 1, 1976; 85 (4): 447-452

11. US Cardiology. Volume 5 Issue 1; 2008:5(1):12-14

12. https://www.uscjournal.com/articles/Menopause-cholesterol-cardiovascular-disease

13. Menopause and the Cardiovascular System: Ouyang, Pamela MD: https://www.hopkinsmedicine.org/heart_vascular_institute/clinical_services/centers_excellence/womens_cardiovascular_health_center/patient_information/health_topics/menopause_cardiovascular_system.ht

14. https://en.wikipedia.org/wiki/RANKL

15. https://www.nature.com/articles/s41413-018-0040-9

16. Perelman, Michael: Sex Coaching for Non-Sexologist Physicians: How to Use the Sexual Tipping Point Model: J Sex Med 2018;15:1667-16672

17. https://www.fda.gov/news-events/press-announcements/fda-approves-new-treatment-hypoactive-sexual-desire-disorder-premenstrual-women

18. http://www.addyi.com

SKIN CARE OF THE OLDER PERSON: THE SKIN AND ITS ASSOCIATED CHANGES

Aziz Khan, MD, Assistant Professor, Department of Internal Medicine, University of Connecticut Health Centre

Hao Feng, MD, MHS, Assistant Professor, Director of Laser Surgery and Cosmetic Dermatology,Department of Dermatology, University of Connecticut Health Centre

Case Scenario:

Mr. X, an 80 year-old male, was referred from the primary care physician's office for evaluation of a growth on the scalp. He was otherwise healthy with no significant past medical or surgical history. He took over the counter multivitamin and vitamin-D tablets. He had noticed multiple growths on the face, scalp, and hands. One of the lesions that had been slowly growing in size over the prior six months was particularly concerning for him and his physician. He had significant sun exposure in the past, including blistering sunburns. On physical examination, he had a firm hyperkeratotic, indurated papulonodule with ulceration. In addition, there were multiple rough, scaly papules on the scalp, ears, face, and hands.

What is the likely diagnosis?

How should you proceed further?

Aging skin:

The skin is the largest organ in the body and acts as a barrier between the body and the external world. As a barrier, the skin protects the body against harmful environmental stimuli, including physical, chemical, and infectious agents. Also, the skin is a dynamic, complex organ with a variety of other functions beyond barrier function and a sensory organ. These functions include temperature, fluid and electrolyte regulation, as well as biosynthesis and metabolism of different substances.

The skin additionally functions as a social organ and is in constant communication with the outside world. In the current society that we are living in, aesthetic appearance is given high importance. Throughout history, people have often been judged based on their appearance and the color of their skin. The visible signs of aging (i.e., wrinkling, grey hair, age spots) mostly involve the skin. The cosmetic industry has invested heavily in improving this aesthetic problem and prevention of signs of aging. However, of late focus has been shifting towards dermatological issues associated with advancing age.

Skin aging involves two processes. Intrinsic aging is genetically encoded and is an inevitable part of the normal aging process. The epidermis becomes thinner, resulting in skin atrophy and increased fragility. Other changes include decreased elasticity, impaired wound healing, loss of thermoregulation, and impaired metabolic functions. Changes in the skin appendages result in other visible signs of aging, including hair loss and grey hair. Extrinsic aging, also known as photo-aging, is skin damage caused by external harmful agents, mainly ultraviolet (UV) radiations from sun exposure. It is often challenging to differentiate changes associated with intrinsic aging from extrinsic aging. Some of the characteristic changes associated with photo-aging include a more pronounced wrinkling, telangiectasia, variation in skin pigmentation, and cellular atypia/dysplasia. Skin growths like actinic keratosis and skin cancers are usually features of sun-damaged skin as UV exposure is a major risk factor for their development.

Common benign skin conditions in the elderly:

Pruritus and Eczematous dermatoses:

Pruritus, or itch, is a common dermatological complaint in the elderly and can be caused by both primarily dermatological and systemic conditions. Dermatological conditions often cause pruritus with associated rash, while systemic diseases can cause pruritus without rash. Common dermatological conditions associated with pruritus in the elderly include skin dryness (xerosis), seborrheic dermatitis, incontinence associated dermatitis, venous stasis dermatitis, allergic contact dermatitis, lichen simplex chronicus, and urticaria.

Xerosis is one of the common conditions associated with aging skin. Decreased production of lipids and sebum contributes to diminished natural skin moisturizing. Xerosis is the most common cause of pruritus in the elderly. Xerosis typically causes pruritus without a rash. However, in severe cases, it can lead to an eczematous reaction, called asteatotic dermatitis. Extremities are the most commonly involved sites in asteatotic dermatitis. Aggravating factors for xerosis include low humidity (cold, dry weather, central heating), frequent bathing, and exposure to harsh detergents or irritants.

A variety of systemic conditions can also cause pruritus without rash in the elderly. These conditions include renal disease, liver disease, iron deficiency anemia, thyroid disease, and malignancy. Drug eruptions cause pruritus with associated rash, depending on the type of drug eruption.

Depression and anxiety can further contribute to pruritus. Chronic pruritus in itself can lead to insomnia and depression. A psychological evaluation should be considered in patients with chronic pruritus, and underlying depression/anxiety should be treated accordingly as appropriate.

Treatment of pruritus involves both topical and systemic agents. Work up for underlying systemic disease, review of medications, and assessment of skin should be performed before initiating therapy. Nutritional status should be assessed as malnutrition can worsen xerosis. Aggravating factors should be avoided. Topical moisturizers (emollients) should be used liberally every day and should be continued to prevent recurrence after treatment. Topical anti-pruritic agents like menthol can be added to the emollients to decrease pruritus in the short term. Other agents for short term relief of pruritus include topical steroids, systemic steroids, and systemic antihistamines.

Seborrheic dermatitis is another common pruritic skin condition affecting the elderly. Dandruff is a mild form of seborrheic dermatitis characterized by scales with minimal inflammation. Seborrheic dermatitis characterized by erythematous patches with overlying scales, distributed mainly in areas with a high density of sebaceous glands (nasolabial folds, eyebrows, retro-auricular folds, etc.) is more common and severe in patients with HIV infection and neurological disease (particularly Parkinson's disease). Treatment options include topical antifungal and/or topical anti-inflammatory agents.

Contact dermatitis is also a frequently seen inflammatory dermatosis in the elderly. Contact dermatitis can be divided into allergic contact dermatitis (a delayed-type hypersensitivity response to a particular substance) and irritant contact dermatitis (direct damage to the skin from a specific material). Irritant contact dermatitis is more common. Treatment involves avoidance of the causative agents and the use of topical anti-inflammatory agents.

Stasis dermatitis is a common inflammatory skin condition in the elderly. Stasis dermatitis mainly involves the lower extremities and is associated with chronic venous insufficiency. Risk factors for chronic venous insufficiency include old age, family history, obesity, standing occupation, deep venous thrombosis, diabetes mellitus, hypertension, certain medications, and heart failure. Stasis dermatitis presents as an ill-defined erythematous patch or plaque in chronically edematous legs. Ulceration may occur in severe cases. Chronic changes include thickening of the skin and hyperpigmentation. Management of stasis dermatitis includes treatment of under-lying venous insufficiency, frequent emollients use, and topical anti-inflammatory agents for pruritus. Bacterial superinfection is common and should be treated with systematic antibiotics when indicated.

Pressure-induced skin and soft tissue injury:

Pressure-induced skin and soft tissue injuries, commonly known as pressure ulcers or bedsores, are common in the elderly. These are caused by sustained, unrelieved pressure resulting in ischemia and tissue damage. Immobility, sensory impairment, reduced perfusion, and malnutrition are major risk factors. Pressure ulcers commonly develop in areas of bony prominence. The deeper tissue is more susceptible to damage than superficial skin. Hence, a small external ulcer may turn out to be a more signifi-cant, extensive ulcer after debridement. Pressure ulcers are classified according to the extent of skin/tissue injury. Management of pressure ulcers requires multidisciplinary care and coordination. Relief of pressure, local wound care, adequate nutrition, pain control, and treatment of underlying medical conditions are the primary treatment measures. Bacterial superinfection is common. Common local signs and symptoms of infection include tenderness, erythema, purulent discharge, and foul odor. However, these are not universally present, and impaired wound healing may be the only sign of infection. Daily monitoring and documentation are essential for wound healing and to prevent a recurrence.

Skin infections:

Common skin infections in the elderly include fungal, bacterial, and viral infections.

Superficial fungal infections (dermatomycoses) are common in the elderly and may go unnoticed for a prolonged period due to their benign nature. Dermatophyte infections can affect any part of the body and are classified according to anatomic involvement. Tinea pedis (infection of feet) and tinea unguium (infection of nails, also known as Onychomycosis) are the most common dermatophyte infections in the elderly. Cutaneous candidiasis often develops in body folds like groins. Obesity and immobility are major risk factors. Diagnosis is usually made from the clinical appearance and can be confirmed with direct microscopy. Topical antifungal therapy is often sufficient; however, in severe or refractory cases, oral antifungals can be used.

Bacterial infections include cellulitis, folliculitis, erysipelas, impetigo, skin abscesses, and erythrasma. Cellulitis often involves the lower extremities. Interdigital fungal infection of the feet is a major risk factor. Cellulitis should be differentiated from stasis dermatitis and contact dermatitis. Deep venous thrombosis should be considered if there is a unilateral swelling with other risk factors for venous thrombosis, including immobility. These conditions can be treated with appropriate topical or systemic antibiotics.

Herpes zoster/shingles is a painful, viral skin infection affecting the elderly. Immune suppression and old age are the major risk factors for the development of shingles. Treatment involves the systemic administration of anti-viral agents and pain medications use. Other viral infections in the elderly include viral warts and molluscum contagiosum.

Scabies is another pruritic skin infection which should be considered in nursing home residents. Scabies mostly involves inter-digital spaces. Visualization of the organism on direct microscopy from skin scraping of burrows confirms the diagnosis. Treatment options include topical permethrin or oral ivermectin.

Benign skin tumors:

Benign skin growths and neoplasms are common in the elderly. Acrochordons (also known as skin tags) are outgrowths of healthy skin. Skin tags are more common in the elderly and are frequently seen in patients with obesity and diabetes mellitus. They appear as pedunculated lesions and commonly occur on the neck and intertriginous areas. They are diagnosed clinically, and treatment options include removal with forceps and fine-grade scissors, cryotherapy, or electrodesiccation.

Seborrheic keratosis is the most common epidermal tumor in the elderly, with a prevalence of up to 60%. Genetic predisposition, old age, and sun exposure are major risk factors. They appear as well-demarcated, round to oval, pigmented papules or plaques with stuck-on appearance. Face, trunk, and upper extremities are the most commonly affected sites. They are diagnosed clinically, and treatment options, if desired, include cryotherapy, curettage/shave excision, or electrodesiccation.

Cherry angiomas are mature capillary proliferations commonly seen in the elderly. They manifest as bright red, blanchable, dome-shaped papules on the trunk. These are asymptomatic but may bleed profusely with traumatic rupture. Treatment options, if desired for cosmetic regions, include electro-cauterization, laser therapy, or cryotherapy.

Solar lentigo, also known as "old age," "liver" spots, occur as a result of the proliferation of normal melanocytes due to chronic sun exposure. These manifest as uniformly pigmented, macules in areas of actinic skin damage. These are asymptomatic. However, lesions with a change in color, border irregularity, or raised lesions should be biopsied to rule out lentigo maligna or melanoma.

Other common benign skin growths in the elderly include lipomas, venous lake, calluses, cutaneous horns, benign nevi, and dermatofibromas.

Pre-malignant growths:

Actinic Keratoses (AKs) occur as a result of the proliferation of atypical keratinocytes in sun-exposed areas. AKs have the potential to progress to squamous cell carcinoma (SCC) of the skin. They manifest as an erythematous, gritty, scaly papules which are more easily felt than seen. Chronic sun exposure is the leading risk factor. Diagnosis is often made clinically; however, a biopsy should be obtained if there is a concern for underlying SCC. Treatment options for AKs include cryotherapy, topical therapies (5-fluorouracil (5-FU) 5% cream, Imiquimod 5% cream), and photodynamic therapy. Protection from the sun is important for prevention. Patients with AKs require ongoing monitoring for lesion recurrence and progression to SCC.

Common malignant tumors in the elderly:

Epidemiology of skin cancer:

Skin cancer is the most common cancer in the United States. It is estimated that one in five Americans will develop skin cancer in their lifetime. The worldwide incidence of skin cancer has increased considerably over the two decades, reaching an "epidemic" proportion. This is attributed mainly to increased cumulative sun-exposure in a progressively aging population. However, skin cancer is preventable in most cases.

Skin cancer greatly affects the quality of life, contributes to the overall burden of skin conditions in the elderly, and can be fatal if not diagnosed early.

There are two main types of skin cancers, cutaneous melanoma (CM), and non-melanoma skin cancers (NMSC). Basal cell carcinoma (BCC) and cutaneous squamous cell carcinomas (SCC) are the two most commons forms of NMSC. NMSC accounts for the majority of skin cancers (80%), the most common being BCC (70%). The majority of the deaths from skin cancer are attributed to CM. BCC and SCCs are highly curable if diagnosed early and treated appropriately.

Exposure to ultraviolet (UV) light is the major risk factor for all types of skin cancer. Cumulative UV light exposure during one's lifetime is associated with an increased risk of CM and NMSCs. Hence, the incidence of skin cancers increases with age. One blistering sunburn in childhood can nearly double the risk of developing melanoma. Skin cancers arise mostly in areas of chronic actinic skin damage. Other risk factors for the development of all types of skin cancers include exposure to tanning beds, skin that burns easily, blond or red hair, immunocompromised conditions (including immunosuppressive medication use), and a history of skin cancer. The presence of multiple moles (more than 50), atypical moles, large moles, family, or personal history of CM increases the risk of developing CM. Patients with a history of melanoma are nine times more likely to develop a second melanoma as compared to the general population.

Caucasians are at increased risk of developing skin cancer; however, skin cancer can develop in anyone, regardless of skin color. In individuals with darker skin types, skin cancer is often diagnosed at a later stage and develops in areas that are not commonly exposed to the sun. Patients with a skin of color are less likely to survive melanoma as compared to Caucasians.

Clinical features:

Cutaneous Melanoma:

There are four main types of invasive cutaneous melanoma. These include superficial spreading melanoma, lentigo maligna melanoma, nodular melanoma, and acral lentiginous melanoma. Superficial spreading melanoma is the most common form of melanoma (accounting for 70% of cases) and presents as a slowly enlarging macule/patch with variable pigmentation. Nodular melanoma is the second most common form and presents as a rapidly enlarging pigmented papule or nodule. Lentigo malgina melanoma (LM) and Acral lentiginous melanoma are less common. Acral lentiginous melanoma is not related to sun exposure and occurs on the palms, soles, and beneath the nails.

The "ABCDEs" rule and the "Ugly Duckling" sign helps clinicians in identifying skin lesions concerning for melanoma. ABCDE is an acronym which stands for A: asymmetry, B: border irregularity, C: color variation, D: diameter > 6 mm, and E: evolving or changing with time. Ugly Duckling refers to a skin lesion/mole, which looks different from the rest and sticks out. Most normal moles on one's skin should look similar. In contrast, a lesion concerning for melanoma stands out like an "ugly duckling." These signs help in the identification of potential melanoma, however, these are not specific for melanoma, and not all melanomas will display these characteristics.

Non-melanoma skin cancers:

Both BCC and SCC develop in areas of chronic actinic damage. The most common variants of BCC include the nodular, superficial, morpheaform subtypes. Nodular BCC typically presents as a pearly, pink, or flesh-colored papule or nodule on the sun-exposed areas of the head and neck. Superficial BCC usually presents as a shiny, erythematous macule, patch, or thin plaque on the trunk. Morpheaform BCC might resemble a scar.

The presentation of invasive SCC varies with the degree of tumor differentiation. Well-differentiated tumors present as firm hyperkeratotic, indurated papules or plaques while poorly differentiated tumors present as flesh-colored papules/nodules with frequent ulceration and bleeding.

Revisiting the case:

Mr. X was evaluated in the dermatology clinic and underwent a full-body skin examination with dermatoscopy. He was found to have multiple actinic keratoses (AKs) on the scalp, ears, nose, and dorsum of hands. Biopsy of the scalp lesion showed a moderately differentiated squamous cell carcinoma with positive margins on biopsy. He was scheduled for Mohs micrographic surgery for definitive removal of the tumor. For the AKs, he was given the option of freezing with liquid nitrogen therapy vs. application of 5-fluorouracil (5-FU) 5% cream. Due to an increased number of lesions, the patient opted for 5-FU therapy.

Management options:

The prognosis of melanoma depends on the stage at the time of diagnosis. The thickness of the tumor (measured on millimeters) is most strongly associated with the probability of metastasis. Patients with stage 0 (in situ melanoma) and stage 1 (localized invasive) have a better prognosis and are curable with surgical treatment. Those with more advanced disease (stage 2-4) are likely to develop metastatic disease. Surgical excision remains the mainstay of treatment. Surgical management of CM is complex and is beyond the scope of this writing. However, wide local excision with regional lymph node sampling is the preferred surgical option. Resection margins depend on the stage of the disease. Immunotherapy can be used as an adjunct to surgery and as primary therapy for metastatic disease.

BCC generally carries a very favorable prognosis, and a complete cure can be achieved with timely intervention. SCC has a higher potential to metastasize as compared to BCC; however, a complete cure can be achieved with early recognition and treatment. Treatment selections depend on patient demographics and patient preference. Mohs micrographic surgery (MMS) provides the best long-term cure rates and cosmetic outcomes. It is the first-line therapy for high-risk BCCs and SCCs. Also, in low-risk patients, MMS can be used as an alternative therapy if the patient desires an improved cosmetic outcome. Standard excision can be used for lower-risk tumors. Non-surgical treatment options including cryosurgery, topical therapies (5-fluorouracil (5-FU) 5% cream, Imiquimod 5% cream), are reserved for patients with BCC who refuse surgery, are poor surgical candidates, and those with multiple superficial BCCs. Topical therapies, however, are not approved by the Food and Drug Administration (FDA) for the treatment of SCCs.

Revisiting the case:
Mr. X successfully underwent MMS. On follow up visit, the wound was healing well with no evidence of local recurrence. There was no regional lymphadenopathy. He was counseled that he will need regular follow-up every 3-6 months for 2 years, followed by every 6-12 months for 3 years, and then annually for life. He was also counseled about skin cancer preventive measures.

Prevention of skin cancer:
Chronic sun exposure is the most important and preventable risk factor for the development of both melanoma and non-melanoma skin cancers. Regular sunscreen use has been associated with a decreased CM risk. Increased incidence of CM in men might be partly due to reduced rates of sun protection. Protection from the sun

(sunscreen use, avoidance of sun, protective cloths) is the most critical defense against the development of skin cancers.

Sun-protection is recommended for all age groups as damaging effects of sun exposure are cumulative over time. A broad-spectrum sunscreen with a Sun Protection Factor (SPF) of at least 30 should be liberally used while out in the sun. Reapplication every two hours is recommended, even on cloudy days. The shade should be sought when possible, especially between 10 am and 4 pm, when UV radiation is the strongest. Shade decreases the amount of UV radiation by 50 to 90%. In contrast, snow, water, metallic surfaces, concrete can reflect up to 90% of the UV rays. In addition to the above, sun-protective clothing, including hats and sunglasses, provide adequate protection against UV radiation. Tanning beds should be avoided. Strict sun avoidance may increase the risk of vitamin-D deficiency; however, oral vitamin-D supplementation is an effective, safe, and well-tolerated alternative for achieving adequate vitamin-D levels.

References:

1. Apalla Z, Nashan D, Weller RB, Castellsagué X. Skin Cancer: Epidemiology, Disease Burden, Pathophysiology, Diagnosis, and Therapeutic Approaches. Vol. 7, Dermatology and Therapy. Springer Healthcare; 2017. p. 5–19.

2. Garcovich S, Colloca G, Sollena P, Bellieni A, Balducci L, Cho WC, et al. Skin cancer epidemics in the elderly as an emerging issue in geriatric oncology. Vol. 8, Aging and Disease. International Society on Aging and Disease; 2017. p. 643–61.

3. Norman RA. Geriatric dermatology. Dermatol Ther [Internet]. 2003 Sep [cited 2020 Jun 28];16(3):260–8. Available from: http://doi.wiley.com/10.1046/j.1529-8019.2003.01636.x

4. Wey SJ, Chen DY. Common cutaneous disorders in the elderly. Vol. 1, Journal of Clinical Gerontology and Geriatrics. Elsevier B.V.; 2010. p. 36–41.

5. Blume-Peytavi U, Kottner J, Sterry W, et al. Age-Associated Skin Conditions and Diseases: Current Perspectives and Future Options. *Gerontologist*. 2016;56 Suppl 2:S230-S242. doi:10.1093/geront/gnw003

ELDER ABUSE

Mark J. Yaffe, MDCM, MCISc, CCFP, FCFP
Professor, Department of Family Medicine
McGill University and St. Mary's Hospital Center

Clinical Vignette

Mrs. L is an eighty-eight year old widow with stable ischemic heart disease and diet-controlled Type 2 diabetes mellitus. She has shown gradual deterioration in short term memory and in judgment. She downplays deficits suggested by her MMSE score of 24, and is angry at her family doctor for notifying the license bureau about concerns about her ability to drive safely. Mrs. L. lives alone, with the exception of a housekeeper who comes to her apartment three half days per week to prepare some meals, do laundry, and to assist with bathing / hygiene. Mrs. L. downplays the need for the latter. The housekeeper had tried a number of times to attend to these issues, but in response to Mrs L.'s lack of cooperation the housekeeper became physically rough with the bathing. As well she has gradually ignored skin sores on the upper legs and buttocks.

Social contact with friends decreased over the preceding few years, aggravated by hearing loss. Following audiology testing Mrs. L. was advised that she would benefit from a particular hearing aid that would be easily useable, despite severe osteoarthritis in her hands. Mrs. L. stated that she could not afford the co-payment cost of the apparatus. The housekeeper frequently yells at her that she is too tight with her money, but Mrs. L. gives into frequent pleas from the housekeeper for extra money to help with troubled members of her family.

The family doctor has suggested a home visit by a community nurse or social worker, but this has been turned down by Mrs. L. She does, however, reluctantly give the physician permission to telephone her only child, a daughter who lives 2000 miles away. The latter is hard to reach and voice messages that are left are not returned. When contact is eventually made, the daughter indicates that she talks to her mother about once every three to four weeks, and that, while her mother might be a little eccentric, she was a "normal 88 year old who requires no new interventions. " The family physician learns that the daughter has power of attorney for mother's affairs, that she hasn't made much attempt to keep track of her mother's finances, and that she was unaware of money regularly being given to the homemaker independent of her usual pay.

What is elder abuse?

Elder abuse encompasses mistreatment and neglect of an older adult (in some communities the use of the word "elder" would be inappropriate as it might be a designation for a community leader of any age). Elder abuse represents single or multiple acts of commission or omission inflicted on an older adult (commonly viewed as aged 60 or 65, or older) within a relationship where there is an expectation of trust. (1) While mistreatment may occur as a result of ignorance, it is usually considered non-accidental or intentional, though intent to harm may in some cases be difficult to substantiate.

Elder abuse is important to detect and respond to not only to address the overt and sometimes covert sequelae of the mistreatment, but also to prolong the lives of the victims: Seniors who have been abused have a significantly higher mortality rate (independent of the abuse) when compared to seniors who have not been abused. (2)

Health care professionals may encounter older adults with signs and / or symptoms of abuse in varied settings: during home visits, in office settings, in emergency rooms, on acute care hospital wards, and in long term care institutions. Within the latter a distinction is encouraged between acts that are uniquely aimed at an individual (elder abuse) and those that may be due to institutional or systemic failure. Both are important to address, but solutions may rest at different levels of care.

As described below elder abuse is commonly divided into four categories: physical, psychological / verbal, financial / material, and neglect (3) :

Physical abuse

Acts associated with physical abuse include:

- Individuals who are hit, slapped, kicked, tied, shaken, choked, grabbed, pushed , shoved, punched, slammed against a wall, pinched, scratched, bit, burned, scalded

- Twisted limbs
- Rough transfers
- Unexplained or poorly explained falls and injuries
- Multiple visits to emergency departments
- Use of a weapon
- Improper use of physical or chemical restraint
- Sexual Abuse: Unwanted sexual contact, touching, or rubbing; Masturbation that is forced, tricked, coerced, manipulated; use of physical threats (hitting, holding down, use of weapon) to give or receive oral, genital, or anal sex

Manifestations of physical abuse: Unexplained or unusual
- Bruises (especially those that are finger or knuckle shaped)
- Need for new dental work
- Lacerations, abrasions, scars
- Sprains, fractures, multiple trauma
- Genital inflammation, pain, tenderness
- Signs of anxiety, depression, withdrawal, low eye contact

Psychological/verbal abuse
Acts associated with psychological abuse include
- Lying
- Humiliating or infantilizing
- Demeaning talk or jokes
- Coercion
- Inappropriate shouting / yelling
- Controlling verbal or physical contact with family or friends
- Threatening to hit or throw something
- Disrespect for privacy
- Insulting, swearing, name calling, putting down
- Threats with weapons, deprivation, punishment, guardianship, abandonment, institutionalization
- Sexual: Verbal threats to give or receive oral, genital, or anal sex; individuals forced to view or participate in pornographic or sexually explicit pictures or videos; offensive sexual talk

Manifestations of psychological abuse: Unexplained or unusual

- Apprehensiveness
- Physical avoidance
- Reduced eye contact or continual eye darting
- Quietness, passivity, withdrawal
- Depression, anger
- Weight loss
- Missed appointments
- Caregivers who try to answer in place of the senior

Financial or material abuse

Acts associated with financial / material abuse include

- Disrespect for property, including taking, misuse, concealment of resources, property, or assets, with or without coercion, enticement, intimidation, or deception
- Misappropriation of funds, bank accounts, or credit/ debit cards against the will of a senior or without his/her knowledge
- Forced to give power of attorney,
- Forged signature
- Use of power attorney or employment of service people by others for personal gain

Manifestations of financial / material abuse: Unexplained or unusual

- Anxiety, apprehensiveness, avoidance
- Social withdrawal
- Depression, tearfulness, weight loss
- Clothes not appropriate to the weather
- Under-medicated

Neglect

Acts associated with neglect include

- Inappropriately left alone or unsupervised
- Withholding of necessary aides: walker, wheelchair, glasses, hearing aid, telephone
- Living environment too hot or too cold

- Clothing inappropriate to weather
- Unsanitary living conditions, bed linens or incontinence products not changed
- Medications not or irregularly supervised
- Inappropriate or poor food supplied
- Delays in seeking treatment
- Inconsistent treatment
- Frequent change of physicians

Manifestations of neglect:
- Poor mobility
- Cachexia
- Decubitus ulcers, pressure sores, bed sores
- Poor hygiene, body odor
- Frequent infections
- Unexplained medical problems
- Fearfulness, anxiety, depression

Systemic or Institutional Failure

Acts associated with institutional or systemic failure include
- Inadequate custodial care or supervision
- Low or unpredictable nursing/nursing aide care
- Delays in response time to seniors' calls for help
- Inadequate nutrition
- Overcrowded or unsanitary living conditions
- Poor staff communication skills
- Limited staff language competency
- Recurrent inappropriate staff- resident interactions
- Misuse of physical or chemical restraints

Detection of elder abuse

Risk Factors
Since physicians of varied backgrounds and experience may be the first or enduring point of contact for an abused senior, a knowledge of elder abuse is promoted despite

sometimes vague signs and symptoms. Guidelines are neither for or against whether physicians should routinely screen for elder abuse. Research into risk factors has generated some of this uncertainty because of a lack of clarity about their impact. Nonetheless it is useful to be aware of such factors and the roles they may play in relation to elder abuse when considered from the perspectives of caregivers (CG) and care receivers (CR) (4):

Weak association	Moderate association	Strong association
Social isolation (CR)	Females (CR)	Poor physical health (CR)
Dementia (CR)	Blacks (CR)	Childhood violence (CG)
Mental illness (CG)	Passive/dependent (CR)	Stress (CG)
Hostility (CG)	CG dependent on CR	CR dependent on CG
Drugs / alcohol (CG)	CG related to CR	Institutional care (CG)

Detection instruments

There are a small number of validated detection tools for use by clinicians. (5) The Elder Abuse Suspicion Index (EASI) © is a practical one because its six questions take only 2-5 minutes to complete. (6) The self-administered version, the EASI-sa, is comprised of 5 questions and is completed in a similar brief time frame. (7) These tools use words understandable by, and acceptable to, older adults (7), and is available in ten languages. (8) A nine question tool derived from the EASI has been specifically designed for use in the long term care setting (EASI-ltc), and is pending formal testing. (9) Copies of the Elder Abuse Suspicion Index tools and practical aspects of their application are found on a website devoted to it: http://www.mcgill.ca/familymed/research/projects/elder

Outcome of suspected abuse

Since a positive response on the EASI can be a false positive arising from cognitive impairment (delirium, dementia), a MMSE (or equivalent tool) should be performed as part of a mental capacity assessment, the EASI being validated for cognition scores of ≥ 24 on the MMSE. If the senior is found by this process to be inapt, then a declaration of such should be made according to the reporting protocol of the jurisdiction in which one is practicing.

Does identification of elder abuse by a cognitively intact senior legally bind a physician to report the mistreatment? It depends on the geographical jurisdiction in which one is practicing. Some do not impose mandatory reporting; some require it for abuse that occurs within a public institution that cares for seniors; and others require reporting irrespective of where the abuse has occurred. A dilemma for practitioners is that some cognitively intact victims do not want the abuse disclosed. There may be reluctance to see the abuser punished; they may be embarrassed, humiliated, or shamed that a family member was abusive; they may fear retaliation from the abuser; or they may realistically worry that removing the abuser may leave their global living situations worse than it was with the abuse.

Such situations are legally and ethically challenging. It would therefore be advisable for clinicians to seek the advice and collaboration of regionally designated resources for elder abuse: Adult Protective Services, social services, or police officers. What can health professionals expect from these experts? Where feasible, social workers will do a complete evaluation of the psychosocial needs of the older person and the caregiver. If indicated, along with a doctor's help, they will begin procedures to have the person declared under a protective regime (public, private curatorship, or homologation of a mandate). They will access homecare services, respite programs, caregiver support groups and placement, if necessary. If the senior is competent, they will respect the right of self- determination, but support the person to have a life without abuse. If indicated, they will involve the police or get a Human Right's Commission (or equivalent) involved.

Clinical vignette continued

The case history described self-neglect; self-neglect, however, does not appear in the cited descriptors of elder abuse. It is considered a different problem, with causes and possible solutions that require a unique approach. The vignette does however suggest neglect on the part of the homemaker and the out-of-town daughter. It does provide evidence of verbal as well as physical abuse by the homemaker. Both daughter and homemaker appear to be abusing the trust mother had in them as far as her finances were concerned.

In the vignette the family physician has not directly used a detection tool to gather data; however he has taken advantage of his knowledge of the content of the EASI to ask Mrs. L. and her daughter relevant questions. As a result he feels more urgency in the situation and in a need to get help for Mrs. L. He reminds her that over his 22 years of care for her that he had tried to respect her best interests. Responding positively to this reminder she agrees to have a visit from a social worker, but reserves the right to keep open whatever options may be available to her.

References

1. World Health Organization. *The Toronto declaration on the global prevention of elder abuse.* Geneva, Switzerland: World Health Organization; 2002.

2. Lachs MS, Williams CS, O'Brien S, Pillemer KA, Chartlson ME. *The mortality of elder mistreatment.* JAMA 1998; 280 (5)428-32.

3. Yaffe MJ, Tazkarji B. *Understanding elder abuse in family practice.* Canadian Family Physician 2012; 58: 1336-40.

4. Yaffe MJ. *Elder Abuse.* Chapter in Calhoun K, Eibling DE, Wax MK, Kost K. Geriatric Otolaryngology. Taylor and Francis, New York, 2006. P 639.

5. McMullen T, Schwartz K, Yaffe M, Beach S. *Elder Abuse and Its Prevention: Screening and detection,* IOM (Institute of Medicine) and NRC (National Research Council: Elder Abuse and Its Prevention: Workshop Summary, pp: 88-93, The National Academies Press Washington, DC, April 2014.

6. Yaffe MJ, Wolfson C, Weiss D, Lithwick M. *Development and validation of a tool to assist physicians' identification of elder abuse: The Elder Abuse Suspicion Index (EASI ©).* Journal of Elder Abuse and Neglect, 2008; 20 (3): 276-300.

7. Yaffe MJ, Weiss D, Lithwick M. *Seniors' Self-Administration of the Elder Abuse Suspicion Index (EASI): A Feasibility Study. Journal of Elder Abuse and Neglect* 2012; 24 (2) 277-292.

8. http://www.mcgill.ca/familymed/research/projects/elder

9. Ballard SA, Yaffe MJ, August L, Cetin-Sahin D, Wilchesky M. Adapting the Elder Abuse Suspicion Index © for use in long-term care: A mixd methods approach. Journal of Applied Gerontology. In press, June 2017.

LATE-LIFE ANXIETY

Jess Friedland, MD, FRCPC,
Geriatric Psychiatrist, Douglas Mental Health University Institute, Program Director,
Geriatric Psychiatry Sub-Specialty Residency Program, McGill University,

Paulina Bajsarowicz, MD, FRCPC,
Geriatric Psychiatrist, Douglas Mental Health University Institute, Assistant Professor McGill University,

Philippe Desmarais, MD, FRCPC, MHSc,
Assistant Clinical Professor, Faculty of Medicine, Universite de Montreal

Clinical vignette

A 75 year-old female presents to her family doctor complaining of increased fatigue and worry. She lives alone, has been widowed for five years and has a son who was a strong source of support after her husband's death and with whom she has a close relationship. After her spouse passed away, she was treated for a first major depressive episode and diagnosed with mild generalized anxiety disorder. She still takes her SSRI antidepressant. Her past medical history includes mild iron-deficiency anemia (untreated), hypertension and dyslipidemia.

For the past six weeks she has been increasingly concerned about her son, who recently became unemployed and is having financial difficulties; she often has insomnia. Two weeks ago, while going to the bathroom, she tripped over the carpet and fell on her right knee; she has fallen several times in the past few months. The pain from this most recent fall has been unrelenting and she has been taking an over-the-counter NSAID regularly.

She has been feeling dizzy, weak, fatigued, feels her heart is racing and is short of breath. She has been taking previously prescribed benzodiazepines for the past week.

Her medications include: Lorazepam 0.5mg PO BID PRN (which she takes regularly), Sertraline 75mg PO QD, Ibuprofen 200mg PO QID, Atorvastatin 20mg PO QHS, and Valsartan 40mg PO QD.

Clinical significance

Anxiety is a universal and potentially useful human emotion, with deep evolutionary roots. It is a complex neurobiological experience, encompassing mind and body and involving the prefrontal cortex, the limbic and autonomic systems. Its primary manifestations are:

- <u>Cognitive:</u> fear, worry, irritability, distress
- <u>Physical:</u> fatigue, muscle tension, insomnia, autonomic hyperreactivity
- <u>Behavioral:</u> avoidance and other safety behaviours

When anxiety's utility is consistently outweighed by associated distress and dysfunction, anxiety is considered disordered. Older adults are typically less prone to anxiety disorders, depression and other negative emotional states than younger adults, and it is relatively rare to have a new onset of an anxiety disorder in late life. However, the potential consequences of anxiety disorders and even subthreshold anxiety are important; they correlate with loneliness and lower life satisfaction, decreased physical and psychosocial functioning, increased risk of depression, heart disease, and dementia, increased use of health services and lower satisfaction with care received.

Epidemiology

A number of large epidemiological studies have investigated the prevalence of late-life anxiety, including notably the National Comorbidity Study Replication (NCS-R) and the Longitudinal Aging Study Amsterdam (LASA). Findings of these and other studies are quite variable, perhaps because older adults tend to under-endorse anxious feelings and excessive worry and rather present more somatic symptoms such as fatigue and pain. For example, the 12-month prevalence of generalized anxiety disorder (GAD) is reported as 0.8-1.8% in the NCS-R, whereas the 6-month prevalence per LASA is reported as 6.9-11.5%. The results converge somewhat when looking at the prevalence of having any anxiety disorder in late life, with the NCS-R finding 6.0-8.9% and LASA finding 10.4-13.9% of people over age 65 to have any anxiety disorder.

Older people living in institutional settings have not been as well described, but small studies indicate that the prevalence of anxiety in these settings is higher than in the community.

For people with neurocognitive disorders, anxiety is a common symptom, occurring in up to one third of patients with mild neurocognitive disorder (mild cognitive impairment) and up to two thirds of patients with major neurocognitive disorder (dementia).

What is clear from epidemiologic studies is that anxiety is common in late life, usually has its onset in childhood to middle age and has a decreasing prevalence with age. GAD, specific phobias and social anxiety disorder remain common throughout the lifespan, while panic disorder, post-traumatic stress disorder (PTSD) and obsessive-compulsive disorder (OCD) become relatively rare in later life.

In terms of course and prognosis, anxiety disorders are typically chronic illnesses with a waxing and waning course. Six-year follow-up of 112 anxiety disorder patients in the LASA study showed persistence of the disorder in about a quarter, subclinical anxiety in about half, high use of benzodiazepines (43%) and low use of antidepressants (7%).

Risk and Protective Factors

A number of risk factors for the development of anxiety disorders have been elucidated:

- Demographic: female sex, being divorced/separated/widowed/never married and/or childless
- Personality: neurotic personality (tendency to have negative reactions to events) and poor coping skills
- Clinical conditions: fear of falling, urinary incontinence, sensory impairment, hypertension, poor sleep, chronic medical condition, functional limitations
- External stressors: early life stress, chronic disability in self or spouse, war experiences

Other potential <u>predisposing factors</u> include new stressors such as losses and the degeneration of adaptation-associated brain regions such as the dorsolateral prefrontal cortex.

To explain the decrease in prevalence of anxiety disorders with age, a number of potential <u>protective factors</u> have been observed or hypothesized. These include the decline in propensity for negative affect over time (though it rises again starting in the mid-70s), increased exposure to stressors over the lifespan ("stress inoculation"), opportunity to practice emotion regulation, degeneration of anxiety-associated brain regions such as the locus coeruleus, and social support, religiosity, physical activity, and cognitive stimulation.

Diagnosis of Anxiety Disorders

Recognition and diagnosis of anxiety disorders in late life can be complicated by under-reporting of anxious feelings and excessive worry by older adults, accumulation of medical and cognitive co-morbidities and the psychosocial losses and transitions that are more common in older adults. The Diagnostic and Statistical Manual of Mental Disorders, 5th Edition, 2013 (DSM-5) provides diagnostic criteria for numerous distinct anxiety disorders along with several other psychiatric disorders, categorized as obsessive-compulsive, stressor-related, somatic or adjustment disorders, that involve significant anxiety components:

- **Specific phobia**; in which immediate and disproportionate fear or anxiety provoked by a specific object or situation leads to persistent avoidance or endurance with intense distress, e.g. fear of falling.
- **Social anxiety disorder**; also known as social phobia, in which the phobic stimulus is a social situation where the individual feels exposed to possible scrutiny by others, about e.g. tremor or forgetfulness.
- **Panic disorder**; involving recurrent, unexpected panic attacks that lead to fear of further panic attacks and maladaptive avoidance of panicogenic situations.
- **Agoraphobia**; involving avoidance of various public situations due to fear of difficulty escaping or getting help in the event of panic or other incapacitating symptoms, e.g. incontinence.
- **GAD (Generalized anxiety disorder)**; in which the individual experiences excessive and difficult-to-control anxiety and worry about everyday, routine

life circumstances, e.g. well-being of family or physical health or safety. The worry leads to cognitive and/or somatic symptoms.

- **Substance/Medication-Induced anxiety disorder**; in which anxiety symptoms are clearly temporally and etiologically linked to medication exposure or to substance intoxication or withdrawal (see examples below).
- **Anxiety disorder due to another medical condition**; in which clinically significant anxiety is demonstrated through history, physical exam or lab findings to be the direct pathophysiological effect of another medical condition (see examples below).
- **Illness anxiety disorder**; previously known as hypochondriasis, in which the anxious preoccupation relates to having or acquiring a serious illness, clearly disproportionate to the individual's absent or mild somatic symptoms and other findings.
- **OCD (Obsessive-compulsive disorder)**; involving obsessions and/or compulsions that are time-consuming or cause significant distress or dysfunction.
- **Hoarding disorder**; whose central feature is a persistent difficulty discarding possessions, leading to accumulation of clutter that compromises living areas.
- **PTSD (Posttraumatic stress disorder)**; in which a number of characteristic symptoms - nightmares, flashbacks and other intrusive phenomena, avoidant behaviours, negative thinking patterns and mood, and hyperarousal - arise following exposure to one or more traumatic events.
- **Acute stress disorder**; similar to PTSD but lasting from three days to one month after the exposure.
- **Adjustment disorder with anxiety**; in which disproportionate anxiety develops in response to an identifiable stressor and resolves within six months of the resolution of the stressor.

In older adults, fear of falling and anxiety in the context of delirium or dementia are also important clinical entities.

Principles of evaluation include ruling out other primary causes, including medication side effects (e.g. prednisone), medical conditions (e.g. chronic obstructive pulmonary disease), and dementia. A thorough physical examination is essential given the many medical conditions that can cause anxiety. The Canadian Network for Mood and Anxiety Treatments (CANMAT) also recommends laboratory work-up including CBC, fasting glucose and lipids, electrolytes, liver enzymes, serum bilirubin, serum creatinine, urine toxicology and TSH. Depending on clinical suspicion, consider urinalysis, vitamin B12 level and ECG. Co-morbidity with depression and substance use are common and must be evaluated. Dangerosity, including suicide risk and pathological avoidance behaviours, must be assessed.

Medical conditions known to have anxiety as a symptom include:

- Endocrine: hypo- and hyperthyroidism, pheochromocytoma, hyperadrenocorticism and hypoglycemia
- Cardiovascular: congestive heart failure, pulmonary embolus, arrhythmia, mitral valve prolapse and coronary artery disease
- Gastrointestinal: ulcerative colitis, diverticulitis, irritable bowel syndrome
- Respiratory: COPD, pneumonia, hyperventilation
- Hematologic: vitamin B12 deficiency and anemia
- Neurologic: Parkinson's disease, neoplasms, vestibular dysfunction, encephalitis and neurodegenerative neurocognitive disorders
- Other: Postural disturbance, dizziness and falls

Medications known to have anxiety as a side effect include anticholinergics, cholinesterase inhibitors, inhaled beta-agonists, insulin, levodopa, montelukast, phenytoin, psychostimulants, steroids, SSRIs, thyroid medications

Substances that can cause anxiety through either intoxication or withdrawal include alcohol withdrawal, amphetamine/cocaine intoxication, benzodiazepine withdrawal, caffeine use/intoxication, cannabis use and nicotine use.

Scales

Validated rating scales for anxiety symptoms can be useful for quantifying symptoms and following response to interventions. Some scales are specific to older people and others are for the general population. Among the numerous anxiety symptoms scales, the following self-rated scales have been sufficiently validated in the older population: seven-item Generalized Anxiety Disorder Scale (GAD-7); Beck Anxiety Inventory (BAI); Geriatric Anxiety Inventory (GAI); Penn State Worry Questionnaire; and Worry Scale.

For people with dementia, for whom caregiver observations need to be taken into account, there is a multimodal anxiety-specific scale and other scales that include an item or set of items on anxiety or anxiety-like symptoms: Reliable Anxiety Scale In Dementia (RAID); Neuropsychiatric Inventory (NPI); and Cohen-Mansfield Agitation Scale.

Key co-morbidities: depression and cognitive disorders

Depression: Clinical pearls to help distinguish pure anxiety from anxious depression include: content of anxiety is more present/future-oriented in pure anxiety vs. related to the past in depression, early morning awakening with worse morning anxiety is more indicative of depression, and anxiety in the context of depression is generally more debilitating than in pure anxiety. About half of older persons with major depressive disorder (MDD) had a comorbid anxiety disorder with severe anxiety symptoms, while about a quarter of older persons with anxiety disorders had MDD. Comorbidity correlates with delayed or diminished response to antidepressants, greater somatic symptoms and greater suicidal ideation and risk of suicide.

Cognitive disorders: A recent systematic review and meta-analysis of the interplay between anxiety and cognition (Gulpers et al. Am J Geriatr Psychiatry 2016) showed incident cognitive impairment in community samples with RR (Relative Risk) 1.77 and incident dementia in community samples RR 1.57 (1.23 for people under age 80 and 2.51 for people over age 80). However, anxiety as a risk factor for conversion to dementia in memory clinic samples was not significant and it is not clear whether anxiety is prodromal or causal. In patients with established dementia, subjective reports of anxiety symptoms in dementia patients were similar in vascular and Alzheimer's dementia (29%) – subjective anxiety and physical tension were the most common complaints. NPI (Neuropsychiatric Inventory) ratings by caregivers showed higher rates of anxiety in vascular (46%) and frontotemporal (39%) dementias vs. Alzheimer's (30%). 5% of patients with Alzheimer's have GAD; psychiatric history is a predictor of this comorbidity.

Treatments

Psychotherapy: Research has focused on GAD and mixed anxiety symptoms. The best evidence is for cognitive-behavior therapy (CBT) for GAD, relaxation training, and mindfulness therapies such as Mindfulness-based Stress Reduction. There is some evidence for supportive therapy. A number of helpful adaptations of CBT in late life have been established, and these adaptations could also be considered for other psychotherapies. The adaptations include: Simplified/less abstract treatment rationale and therapeutic interventions, slower pace with increased repetition and review of previous sessions, audiotaping sessions for patient to review, between-session reminder phone calls, at-home assignments, more focus on behavioural change and health concerns, engagement of the family in the treatment and integration of religion. Some evidence supports the use of telephone or internet-based psychotherapy, and this may help to address access issues.

Pharmacotherapy: The pharmacological treatment of late-life anxiety disorders can be effective based on clinical observations, but is complicated by limited evidence and safety issues. CANMAT recommends that pharmacological choices be guided by the evidence along with prior treatment response, the nature of the targeted symptoms, medication interactions and other safety issues and side effect profiles of the medications. Combination treatment with psychotherapy is recommended.

The available evidence demonstrates efficacy and tolerability for:

- Selective serotonin reuptake inhibitors (SSRIs), including citalopram, escitalopram and sertraline
- Serotonin-norepinephrine reuptake inhibitors (SNRIs), including venlafaxine and duloxetine
- Pregabalin

SSRIs and SNRIs, while generally safe, do increase the QTc (QT interval corrected for heart rate) interval (especially citalopram, which should be limited to a maximum dose of 20 mg QD), the risk of falls and fractures, and the risk of upper GI bleeding.

Although there is no geriatric-specific evidence to guide their use, the tolerability of mirtazapine and buspirone make them reasonable treatment options. Furthermore, our clinical experience and the favourable side effects of quickly improved sleep and appetite support the use of mirtazapine.

Cholinesterase inhibitors may improve anxiety in the context of dementia, though they can in some cases increase anxiety.

Because of issues with their safety profiles, the following medications are not first-line options, and should be used only with caution:

- Benzodiazepines have demonstrated effectiveness for late-life anxiety. However, their safety profile, including sedation, fall and fracture risk, cognitive impairment and link with dementia risk, argues against their regular long-term use. They could be used with great caution in the initial phase of treatment with SSRIs or SNRIs, since those medications can initially increase agitation and insomnia and take several weeks to effectively decrease anxiety.

- Older antidepressants such as tricyclic antidepressants (TCAs) can be effective but are not first-line choices given their significant anticholinergic and cardiac effects. Among the TCAs, nortriptyline is favoured for use in the elderly because it is relatively less anticholinergic.

- Low-dose atypical antipsychotics, particularly quetiapine, olanzapine and aripiprazole, can be effective as augmenting agents in severe mixed anxio-depressive states. Since they have black-box warnings for use in geriatric populations due to a small but significant risk of increased mortality, these should be used only after a well-documented discussion of their pros and cons.

Resolution of the Clinical Vignette

1. How would you approach this patient's problems?
   - High index of suspicion for anxiety disorder given that older adults are less likely to report anxiety and worry.
   - Although anxiety in this patient is multifactorial, a medical cause or exacerbating factor for her symptoms needs to be investigated. She is already known for mild anemia and has been taking NSAID medication regularly and this may be a source of bleeding. Her physical complaints may be primarily somatic symptoms of her anxiety, but an underlying general medical condition needs to be ruled out. Furthermore, pain can exacerbate anxiety and insomnia.
   - After you have investigated the patient, she is found to have a bleeding peptic ulcer which exacerbated her anemia. X-ray showed moderate osteoarthritis. Throughout the assessment, she perseverates about her concerns for her son's financial situation and how she cannot stop thinking about it as she has no means to help him. She tells you she is constantly feeling on edge and keyed up, she cannot concentrate or sleep.

2. How would you address the anxiety?

- The symptoms of her generalized anxiety disorder have worsened due to the stressor of her son's unemployment. If not for the ulcer, we would titrate sertraline to 200 mg as tolerated. However, since her ulcer is a relative contraindication to an SSRI, we can consider a cross taper to mirtazapine which could also help with her insomnia. Supportive therapy, CBT and sleep hygiene instructions can be offered to the patient for both anxiety and insomnia.

3. What else to consider?

- Falls may be due to the weakness from the anemia, but also due to benzodiazepine use. A slow taper may be warranted. Furthermore, since she has been tripping in her apartment a thorough home safety evaluation can be requested. Adequate pain control should be implemented.
- Orthopedic consultation in view of the unrelenting right knee pain

Suggestions for further reading

Alvadaro C and Modesto-Lowe V: Psychotherapeutic Treatment Approaches of Anxiety Disorders in the Elderly. Current Treatment Options in Psychiatry. 2017; 4:47-54.

American Psychiatric Publishing: Diagnostic and Statistical Manual of Mental Disorders, 5th Edition (DSM-5). 2013.

Crocco EA et al: Pharmacological Management of Anxiety Disorders in the Elderly. Current Treatment Options in Psychiatry. 2017; 4:33-46.

Therrien and Hunsley: Assessment of Anxiety in Older Adults: A Reliability Generalization Meta-Analysis of Commonly Used Measures. Clinical Gerontologist. 2013; 36:171-194.

Wolitzky-Taylor KB et al: Anxiety disorders in older adults: a comprehensive review. Depression & Anxiety. 2010; 27:190-211.

AN OVERVIEW OF LATE-LIFE DEPRESSION

Artin Mahdanian, MD, MSc

Silvia Monti De Flores, MD, FRCPC, DFAPA
Department of Psychiatry, McGill University

Clinical vignette

Mr. D is a 73-year-old divorced man who was brought to the emergency room by his daughter for suicidal ideation and depression. He described a few months' history of continuous excessive worry about his future, panic attacks and loss of interest in life. He self-isolated and avoided seeing family and friends. He had gradually stopped all of the physical exercise activities (swimming, jogging and yoga) that he used to do, because he did not have the physical energy and mental joy. He had difficulty sleeping, decreased appetite and had lost about 10 pounds in the past few months. Recently, he had been feeling very guilty about how he had treated his ex-wife who died of suicide by hanging 20 years ago, 10 years after their divorce. He thought he deserved to die and started to think about ending his life. He denied any delusions or hallucinations. He did not have any anxiety or other psychiatric symptoms prior to this episode except for few months of "psychotherapy" with a psychologist 30 years ago after his divorce.

His symptoms started a few months ago when his company went bankrupt following a few months of struggling with a tax audit and numerous financial problems. Then, he decided to retire. He used to be a very successful and high-achieving accountant who ran the company with his brother for more than 40 years. He suffers from diabetes mellitus type II, gout and a frozen shoulder. His medication list includes

Vitamin B12, Metformin-Sitagliptin 1000mg+50mg, Valsartan-HCTZ 160mg+25mg, and Allopurinol. The only important family history was chronic treatment-resistant depression in his mother.

What is depression?

Depression is a general term which is used for Major Depressive Disorder (MDD). Diagnosis is always a clinical one and it is based on meeting the diagnostic criteria for either DSM-5 or ICD-10. For the diagnosis of MDD based on DSM-5, there must be 5 symptoms; one of them should be either depressed mood or lack of interest (anhedonia) and 4 other symptoms out of psychomotor slowness, decreased/increased appetite, weight changes, sleep disturbances, suicidal ideation, decreased energy, decreased concentration, or feeling guilty. The symptoms must be persistent and present most of the time for a period of at least two weeks. Moreover, there should be a decline in baseline functioning of the patient.

Why is depression an important clinical problem in the elderly?

MDD is one of the most common causes of disability worldwide. It is a highly prevalent disorder characterized by episodes of persistent depressed mood or loss of interest/pleasure (affective symptoms) plus other vegetative and cognitive symptoms as described above.

Late-life depression (LLD), with an estimated prevalence of about 15%, is a common psychiatric disorder in people >65y. LLD is associated with increased morbidity and mortality. It is associated with increased healthcare cost. LLD has also been shown to be highly recurrent with research reports varying between 30% and 65% over 3 to 20 years follow-up. The consequences of untreated LLD include poor quality of life as well as worse outcome and exacerbation of other chronic illnesses, and most importantly, suicide.

Predictors of poorer outcome may include adverse childhood events, age of onset, limited education, and the number of previous recurrences and length of untreated episodes. Additionally, personality disorder diagnosis (avoidant, obsessive compulsive, and introvert personality traits) may predict a further episode, while somatoform disorders may predict time to recurrence. Due to the atypical presentation, the diagnosis of LLD is often missed by primary care physicians, which leads to under-treatment of the disease. However, a timely diagnosis can be life-saving and, when treated, it has a good prognosis; up to 70% of treated older patients achieve full remission.

What are the challenges in diagnosis of depression in the elderly?

In the geriatric population, depressive symptoms may be masked by unexplained physical complaints (e.g., fatigue, diffuse pain or back pain, headache, chest pain, etc.) and, subsequently, the classical DSM 5 criteria may sometimes seem to fail in terms of diagnosing depression. Furthermore, the conditions mentioned below can exist concomitantly.

Therefore, the differential diagnosis of LLD in the elderly is broad including, but not limited to, Central Nervous System disorders (dementia, Parkinson disease, and neoplastic lesions), other psychiatric disorders (dysthymia, bipolar, and anxiety disorders), endocrine disorders (hypo- hyperthyroidism, and hyperparathyroidism), medication side effects (e.g., β-blockers, centrally active antihypertensive medications, steroids, H2-blockers, sedatives, certain chemotherapy agents), vitamin deficiency (vitamin B12, vitamin D, and folic acid), life circumstances (e.g., grief, bereavement, financial or autonomy losses), substance use, infectious and inflammatory diseases (e.g., HIV encephalopathy, systemic lupus erythematosus) and sleep disorders (in particular, obstructive sleep apnea).

A complete physical examination, cognitive screening, laboratory tests and/or imaging are the first steps in ruling out these differential diagnoses and in assessing for common comorbidities in the elderly. A physician who has good understanding of the patient's personality can identify nonverbal cues and changes in behavior indicating mood problems. In addition, information from family members and caregivers on the patient's mood and behavior is vital for assessing the older person with depression.

What are the risk factors for depression?

As in all other aspects of depression, the risk factors for LLD are also better described in a biopsychosocial model. The main biological risk factors are old age and female sex. In addition, genetic vulnerability also plays an important role, making people with family history of mood disorders more susceptible to LLD than others. Patients with poor physical health (e.g. multiple comorbidities, sleeping disorders, etc.) and more medication use may also be predisposed to LLD. The notion of frailty affects several domains of functioning, leading to a deterioration in the resilience and capacity for dealing with stressors. Frailty can be defined by the Fried criteria: weight loss, decreased handgrip strength, slowness, exhaustion, and low physical activity. Poor nutritional status is also associated with frailty and LLD; therefore, nutritional supplements (vitamins D, B12, folate and protein) could benefit the depressed frail patient. Neurodegenerative disease (e.g., Parkinson or Alzheimer) and mild cognitive impairment (MCI) are also considered possible risk factors for LLD. We know that LLD and dementia frequently co-occur, and depression can be the first sign of dementia. The vascular hypothesis holds that cerebrovascular disease may cause or predispose to LLD and can be explained by reduced cerebral perfusion, altered brain connectivity, and chronic low-grade inflammation.

Psychological factors such as loss of purpose in life or human relationships seem to be associated with LLD. Moreover, lower level of education, being a widower or single, loneliness, lack of social supports, stressful life events and poverty are all valid risk factors for LLD. Decrease or loss of functional status, visual or hearing impairment, poor lifestyle habits, smoking and alcohol use also increase the risk of developing LLD. In addition, the use of sleep medication such as benzodiazepines and sleep disturbance in general are also correlated with increased risk of LLD.

Useful tools for the diagnosis of depression?

Use of validated scales/tools in screening, diagnosis, and follow-up response to therapy in depression is an important part of providing appropriate care. They can improve diagnostic accuracy, save time, provide more consistent patient care, and monitor a patient's complex emotional and behavioral responses to therapy. Two quick questions from Primary Care Evaluation of Mental Disorders can provide us with a highly sensitive (94%) but not very specific (35%) screening test for depression: 1. Have you been bothered by little interest or pleasure in doing things? 2. Have you been feeling down, depressed, or hopeless in the last month?

If a patient responds positively to either of these two questions, we can screen with the other symptom criteria. Other useful Self- or physician-rated screening tools are also available. The Hamilton Depression Rating Scale (HAM-D), the oldest, most widely used and validated instrument, has numerous versions, both clinician-rated and self-reported, as well as a computer administered version. Many clinicians prefer to use a patient rated scale such as the Beck Depression Inventory (BDI). The BDI has high sensitivity and specificity and is valid and reliable in assessing the severity of depressive symptoms. The Geriatric Depression Scale (GDS) is also a self-report measure designed to minimize the impact of somatic symptoms associated with aging and illness. It has good sensitivity and positive predictive values for diagnosis of major depression. The PHQ-9 also offers a severity score for symptoms, and can also be used to follow outcome. If a clinician is concerned about cognitive impairment, the Mini Mental State Exam (MMSE) and/or Montreal Cognitive Assessment (MoCA) are useful additions.

How is the diagnosis of depression conveyed to the patient?

There is no gold standard for discussing depression diagnosis with elderly patients. It is dependent on the physician's method since research on the topic is lacking. It is helpful to engage the patient with the use of the bio-psychosocial model: inform the patient that the illness is an interaction between physiological (e.g. neurotransmitters hypothesis like serotonin), psychological, and social factors. Creating a good therapeutic alliance and trust is pivotal for a good outcome.

What are the treatment options for depression?

The very first step in the treatment of depression is to treat the modifiable risk factors including nutritional deficiencies (vitamin B12, D, and folic acid), cardiovascular diseases, and any endocrine and electrolyte abnormalities. Risk factors can also be improved by lifestyle changes, physical exercise, healthy diet, sufficient sleep, smoking cessation, discontinuation of alcohol intake as well as optimal treatment for hypertension, hypercholesterolemia, hyperglycemia, and any other comorbid medical condition.

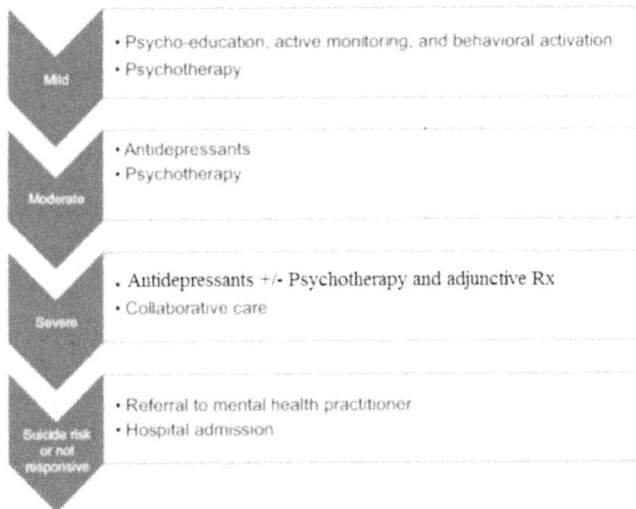

Mild
• Psycho-education, active monitoring, and behavioral activation
• Psychotherapy

Moderate
• Antidepressants
• Psychotherapy

Severe
• Antidepressants +/- Psychotherapy and adjunctive Rx
• Collaborative care

Suicide risk or not responsive
• Referral to mental health practitioner
• Hospital admission

Figure 1. Stepped care approach to late-life depression, based on the severity of depression and patient preference

The treatment options of MDD are based on the biopsychosocial model and the administered choice is according to the severity of the illness and patient preference (figure 1). The severity of the illness is defined based on rating scales, functional impairment and clinical impression. Biological treatments include pharmacotherapy with antidepressants, second generation antipsychotics, neuro-modulation approaches like Repetitive Transcranial Magnetic Stimulation (rTMS), electroconvulsive therapy (ECT), light therapy and supplements (Omega 3, Vit B12). Psychotherapeutic approaches with significant evidence for efficacy include: Supportive Psychotherapy, Cognitive Behavioural Therapy (CBT), Interpersonal Therapy (IPT), Mindfulness-Based Cognitive Therapy (MBCT), Life Review Therapy, Problem-solving Therapy (PST), Bibliotherapy (mostly based on CBT models), Dynamic Therapy, and Existential Therapy. Finally, Social interventions play an important role in treatment of depression in the elderly since losses, loneliness, social isolation, and a limited support network are very common in this population.

Psycho-education: The physician's role is to help patient understand depression, to explain therapeutic options, discuss the bio-psychosocial model of etiology and treatment, to recognize warning signs, and to inform and support the family. Moreover, it is important to try to provide a structure in the patient's life and activate the patient through structured and fun activities.

Behavioral activation: Structured physical activity is recommended for older people with mild or moderate depression who are physically capable.

Psychotherapy: Psychotherapies are the most important type of non-pharmacological treatment and are not inferior to pharmacological treatments in mild to moderate depression. Evidence-based psychotherapeutic treatments of depression in older adults include CBT, IPT, PST, and life review therapy.

Pharmacological treatment: Geriatric patients have different pharmacodynamics and pharmacokinetics due to age-related physiological changes. Therefore, despite the fact that treatment options and algorithms are the same as for other adults, the medications must be administered at lower doses and slowly titrated while actively monitoring the patient. Increased caution is necessary for drug interactions and polypharmacy. In addition, when choosing a psychotropic drug, keep track of the drug's safety profile since some adverse reactions like falls can lead to increased morbidity and mortality. Selective serotonin reuptake inhibitors (SSRIs), Serotonin–norepinephrine reuptake inhibitors (SNRIs), tricyclic antidepressants (TCAs), and atypical antidepressants are the main pharmacological treatments of choice. Existing evidence unanimously suggests that no one class of antidepressant drugs has been found to be more effective than another in the treatment of LLD. However, newer antidepressants are better tolerated and safer. When choosing an SSRI, slight preference goes to an SSRI with the least known drug interactions such as sertraline. TCAs are as effective as SSRIs for LLD, but are less often used because of side effects. TCAs with lesser anticholinergic side effects, such as nortriptyline, are more recommended. SNRIs are not only effective against depression but also effective in the treatment of peripheral neuropathic pain.

An atypical antidepressant that can be used as an alternative for SSRIs is mirtazapine. The sedative side effects of mirtazapine are used as a treatment for insomnia. In addition, mirtazapine increases the appetite and can be used for the symptom of anorexia. Other atypical antidepressants which are commonly used are Bupropion, Vortioxetine and Trazodone.

How Do You Manage Inadequate Response to an Antidepressant?

If a patient has partial or no response to the initial treatment, clinicians should ensure the dose of the medication is optimized to the therapeutic level as much as tolerated (6-8 weeks). There is extensive evidence that shows many patients receive sub-therapeutic doses and/or inadequate duration of treatment.

Evidence shows that switching non-responders to another antidepressant in the same class or another class results in good response and remission rates. However, patients with partial response to the initial antidepressant might benefit from increasing the dose and then the addition of a second medication; i.e. adjunctive treatment which means either combination (adding a second antidepressant to the first) or augmentation (adding another medication that is not an antidepressant, e.g., second generation antipsychotics, mood stabilizers like lithium, triiodothyronine).

Resolution of the clinical vignette

Having confirmed the diagnosis of MDD by a comprehensive history and physical exam, a full blood work up was done that turned out to be negative for other causes or comorbid conditions with MDD as indicated above. Mr. D was then started on

Venlafaxine XR 37.5mg daily. In addition to providing him with psycho-education and support, it was suggested that he restart his physical exercise routine and socialize as much as possible. In the first follow-up visit after 1 week his response to medication and absence of side effects was assessed. His blood pressure and heart rate were monitored and found to to be normal. The dose of the medication was increased to 75mg daily. Mr. D returned in 2 weeks with some response to medication but still far from his baseline. The dose of the medication was slowly increased to 150mg daily. After about 6 weeks on the therapeutic dose of Venlafaxine, Mr. D still complained of some residual depressed mood, decreased energy and sleep disturbances despite some further improvement. At that point the treatment was augmented by adding Quetiapine 50mg at night and the dose very slowly increased to 100mg. When Mr. D was reassessed a few weeks later, he reported that he was completely back to his baseline in terms of mood and interest. He registered in the local community center for Yoga classes twice weekly, went swimming with his friends every other day, and travelled to visit his daughter for one week. He was advised to continue the treatment for 9-12 months as this was the first episode of depression and to taper down the treatment under supervision of a physician to avoid withdrawal symptoms and decrease the risk of relapse.

References

1. Physical exercise for late-life depression: Effects on symptom dimensions and time course. Murri MB, Ekkekakis P, Menchetti M, Neviani F, Trevisani F, Tedeschi S, Latessa PM, Nerozzi E, Ermini G, Zocchi D, Squatrito S, Toni G, Cabassi A, Neri M, Zanetidou S, Amore M. J Affect Disord. 2018 Apr 1;230:65-70. doi: 10.1016/j.jad.2018.01.004

2. Advances in Pharmacotherapy of Late-Life Depression. Beyer JL, Johnson KG. Curr Psychiatry Rep. 2018 Apr 7;20(5):34. doi: 10.1007/s11920-018-0899-6. Review.

3. Late-life depression: issues for the general practitioner. Van Damme A, Declercq T, Lemey L, Tandt H, Petrovic M. Int J Gen Med. 2018 Mar 29;11:113-120.

4. Treatment-resistant Late-life Depression: Challenges and Perspectives. Knöchel C, Alves G, Friedrichs B, Schneider B, Schmidt-Rechau A,

Wenzler S, Schneider A, Prvulovic D, Carvalho AF, Oertel-Knöchel V. Curr Neuropharmacol. 2015;13(5):577-91.

5. Canadian Network for Mood and Anxiety Treatments (CANMAT) 2016 Clinical Guidelines for the Management of Adults with Major Depressive Disorder: Section 3. Pharmacological Treatments. Kennedy SH, Lam RW, McIntyre RS, Tourjman SV, Bhat V, Blier P, Hasnain M, Jollant F, Levitt AJ, MacQueen GM, McInerney SJ, McIntosh D, Milev RV, Müller DJ, Parikh SV, Pearson NL, Ravindran AV, Uher R; CANMAT Depression Work Group. Can J Psychiatry. 2016 Sep;61(9):540-60.

ASSESSMENT OF DECISION-MAKING CAPACITY

Catherine Ferrier, MD
Assistant Professor, Department of Family Medicine,
Faculty of Medicine, McGill University

Vignette

Don is an 83-year-old retired engineer who presents with a one year history of cognitive symptoms. He forgets people's names and conversations he has had, and loses his keys. He lives with his wife; their two children live in the U.S. He remains independent for all basic and instrumental activities of daily living. He scores 29/30 on the MMSE and 27/30 on the MoCA. Some chronic ischemia is noted on brain CT. Laboratory tests are normal. A diagnosis of mild cognitive impairment is made.

He returns for follow-up 6 months later. His wife reports new spatial disorientation and difficulty understanding the use of electronic devices. He got lost once, so has stopped driving. The MMSE score is 22 and the MoCA 21. A diagnosis of mixed AD/vascular dementia is made and he is started on treatment with donepezil. You assess his capacity to assign a general power of attorney and a protection mandate.

A protection mandate in Quebec allows an individual to name someone or several people to take care of personal needs and property management upon incapacity. It is similar to an Advance Directive in the United States which is governed through different statutes in each state: see Chapter "How Do I Protect My Patient?" In other parts of Canada, documents analogous to a protection mandate may go by other names such as powers of attorney or representation agreement. It is important to consult with a qualified professional, usually an attorney, in the jurisdiction where the individual lives to ensure that documentation is correctly done.

It would appear that a protection mandate can be appointed by an individual in the event of future incapacity which is then determined by the appropriate health care provider. The protection mandate would become effective when homologated by the Court, specifically when a judgment is obtained regarding incapacity . In the United States, an Advance Directive can generally be put in place in order to avoid a Guardianship proceeding.

Don fully understands the concept and content of both documents. He signs them shortly after seeing you, naming his wife as a mandatary, the person appointed to act under the protection mandate. His cognition continues to decline gradually. Two years after the initial visit, he needs help with basic activities of daily living and is occasionally incontinent. He has home care services at home. His wife has taken over financial management, using the power of attorney. She has to watch him constantly as he falls easily, including falling off chairs and falling when he gets up at night to urinate. She rarely has a decent night's sleep. His MMSE score is 15/30.

Six months later, he is admitted to hospital with delirium. His wife says that she can no longer take care of him, and he is discharged to a nursing home, with his consent. His wife would like to sell the house, which is in his name, and move into a small apartment close to the nursing home.

Shortly after discharge, you receive a call from the patient's sister in Boston. She says that his wife should be caring for him at home and had no business sending him to the nursing home. She says she will go to court if necessary to have him sent home.

You see the patient to assess decision-making capacity. The patient believes that he can still drive and care for himself. He is not sure whether he has moved recently. He does not know what his income or expenses are. After a detailed examination you find him incapable of making personal decisions and managing his assets. His wife obtains a psychosocial assessment from their social worker, and their notary (who has a distinct legal role in Quebec) initiates the process to have the protection mandate homologated.

*****

Sound ethics requires that we not examine or treat any patient without having obtained their informed consent to do so. If a patient lacks the capacity to make an informed decision about treatment, a substitute decision-maker must be sought.

The terms **Competency**, **Decision-making capacity** and **Aptitude** are sometimes used interchangeably to reflect the same notion. We will use the term **Capacity** or **Decision-making capacity**, which is used widely in the medical literature.

Decision-making capacity is a person's ability to make, and act on, his or her own decisions.

Where do we start?

For a long time capacity was decided on the basis of diagnosis. This is sometimes called the **status approach**. A person who had a cognitive or psychiatric disorder was no longer allowed to make decisions. As our collective understanding of brain disorders improved, it became apparent that this black-and-white distinction lacked the necessary subtlety and unjustly categorized people. In the twentieth century, most jurisdictions updated their laws to require individual capacity evaluation before declaring anyone incapable.

It can also be tempting to base our opinion on the reasonableness of the decision being made by the person, typically a refusal of a medical treatment thought necessary: the **outcome approach**. A "**functional approach**" assesses whether a person's knowledge, skills and abilities allow her/him to make a particular decision in a particular context. Now we commonly use an **integrated approach**, in which a patient's **status** (diagnosis) or foreseen **outcome** (decision-making that is seen as harmful) triggers a **functional** decision-making capacity assessment.

Criteria

There is a widely accepted consensus on four criteria to be used to decide whether a patient is capable of decision-making.[1] They could be summarized as follows:

- Ability to **understand** information relevant to decision-making;
- Ability to **appreciate** the significance of that information for one's own situation;
- Ability to **reason** with relevant information so as to engage in a logical process of weighing options;
- Ability to **express a choice.**

Someone who can **understand**, **appreciate**, **reason** and **express a choice** is capable of decision-making. Someone who lacks all these abilities is not. Of course they all admit of degrees, and a person may have lost some abilities but not others, whence the need to look at each pertinent decision in detail in order to fairly judge the patient's capacity.

The assessment

The fact that the determination of a person's capacity cannot be based on a diagnosis alone does not excuse us from knowing the diagnosis, either through our own examination or by information received from another physician. The situation might be very different depending on whether the patient has a possibly transient disorder such as delirium, a progressive disorder such as dementia, an intermittent and potentially treatable disorder such as psychosis or severe depression, or a fixed disorder such as a developmental disorder or head injury.

Prior to the assessment, it is important to have precise information on the reasons it is being requested. If such an assessment is not required for the patient's well-being or the safety of their property, it should not be done. We also need objective and detailed information about the decisions that need to be made and the alleged lack of judgment or reasoning ability. This allows us to evaluate the patient with respect to her own life and needs, rather than using abstract theoretical examples. For financial capacity we need objective information on the patient's financial situation.

We begin with brief cognitive testing. The Mini-Mental State Examination[2] is by no means an instrument to determine capacity, but the score can provide useful information. For example, one study[3] showed that incapacity is more likely in patients with a score below 19, and capacity more likely if the score is over 23. Psychiatric examination is also necessary, to determine if the patient has a mood disorder severe enough to affect decision-making (e.g. causing loss of hope, diminished self-worth), or psychosis relevant to the decision (e.g. "my doctor wants to harm me"). We then proceed to assess the patient's ability to **understand**, **appreciate**, **reason** and **express a choice**, as applied to the type of decision being questioned. We do so by "walking through" the decision with the patient.

Capacity to consent to medical treatment

Does the patient understand the nature of the illness, the nature and purpose of the proposed treatment, the benefits and risks of the proposed treatment, and alternative treatment options?

Does the patient appreciate how this information applies to his personal situation? Does he/she acknowledge the presence of the medical condition, and appreciate the expected consequences (**to him or herself**) of the proposed treatment and of the alternatives, including no treatment? Is the patient able to reason, i.e. engage in a rational process of manipulating the relevant information? Can the patient express a choice and reasons for the choice? Does the patient consistently express the same choice? If so, the patient is capable of making the decision.

Several tools have been devised to help clinicians assess capacity to make medical decisions. A very helpful one is the **Aid to Capacity Evaluation**, from the University of Toronto.[4] It is essentially a structured interview to help answer the above questions.

Law courts across Canada frequently use the **Nova Scotia criteria**[5]:

"In determining whether or not a person in a hospital or a psychiatric facility is capable of consenting to treatment, the examining psychiatrist shall consider whether the person understands and appreciates: (a) the condition for which the specific treatment is proposed; (b) the nature and purpose of the specific treatment; (c) the risks and benefits involved in undergoing the specific treatment; and (d) the risks and benefits involved in not undergoing the specific treatment."

Capacity to make personal decisions (living situation)

Other personal decisions for which patients' capacity may be questioned often are related to their living situation: can they make capable decisions regarding the safety of living in their own home, or a possible need for help or supervision, or to move into a more structured environment? We apply the same criteria to the patient's approach to these decisions:

Does she/he **understand** any change of health status or circumstances that might affect the living situation; potential risks related to the living situation; and possible interventions to reduce the risk (get help, move, etc.)? Can he/she **appreciate** the effect of a change of health status or circumstances on his/her own safety or well-being in a given living situation; and the expected consequences of living with the risks, or of intervening? Is the patient able to reason, i.e. engage in a rational process of manipulating the relevant information? Can the patient express a choice and the reasons for the choice? Does the patient consistently express the same choice? If so, the patient is capable of making the decision.

Capacity to manage one's assets and make financial decisions

Managing one's financial affairs requires similar abilities to other decision-making: being able to understand, appreciate, reason and express a choice. It also requires certain skills.

Does the patient understand her/his financial situation; any problems there might be, related to financial management; changes in health or cognition that could make it difficult to manage finances; a possible need for help; and other decisions that need to be made? Can the patient appreciate the expected consequences of continuing as is, having help, having someone take over, of a possibly abusive situation, and of the various alternatives, in the case of other decisions? Is the patient able to reason, i.e. engage in a rational process of manipulating the relevant information? Can the patient express a choice? Express the reasons for the choice? Does the patient consistently express the same choice?

Does the patient possess sufficient functional skills to be able to manage his affairs independently? This might include receiving income and paying bills, banking, and budget management, or more complex skills such as making decisions about investments or other property. Are the patient's memory, ability to calculate and organizational abilities sufficient to continue carrying out these tasks? We should keep in mind how the patient organized these tasks in the past: has a meticulous record-keeper lost the ability to maintain and balance his/her chequebook? Or was his/her style always haphazard but good enough for his/her needs? A patient who can understand, appreciate, reason and express choices about financial issues, and has the necessary skills to carry out the financial management required by his own situation, is capable of continuing to do so.

Decision-making for patients with dementia

A patient with early dementia may retain capacity to make decisions in many spheres. We know, however, that the disease is likely to progress, and that decision-making capacity will be gradually lost. It is thus very important, at the time of diagnosis, to find out whether the patient has made plans for the future, and if not to encourage him/her to do so. This may include making a will, giving a power of attorney or protection mandate, and advance care planning.

When a patient with dementia lives alone, safety hazards may arise, such as fire risk, malnutrition, or the effects of forgetting essential medicines or taking them inappropriately. Many such patients lack insight into the presence of the dementia and assume they have normal cognition. Decisions based on this assumption are not competent decisions, and if the patient refuses interventions to improve his/her safety, steps must be taken to formally assess decision-making capacity and name a substitute decision-maker.

Conversely, some patients with early cognitive symptoms may retain insight and be able to address problems and even to competently accept certain risks in order to maintain their independence, thus entering into conflict with family members who want their safety at all costs.

Even when a person is clearly incapable of decision-making, fundamental respect for the person requires us to continue caring for him in keeping with her/his known values and wishes. This might include food preferences and special diets, maintaining his/her appearance and grooming, religious observance, as well as favourite routines and activities. An elder with dementia remains a full member of the human community and should be treated as such.

Capacity to sign legal documents

Power of attorney:
"You can give someone a power of attorney to represent you when you cannot do something yourself…."[6]

A bank or notary may request a letter from a doctor attesting to an older patient's capacity to give a power of attorney. To be capable, the patient must understand the concept and content of the document and its possible implications, including the approximate value of the assets, the power that is being entrusted, the risk of harm to the assets from poor judgment or dishonesty on the part of the mandatary, and the fact that she/he has the right to revoke the power of attorney at any time.

Protection mandate:

A protection mandate "is a document that lets you name, in advance, one or several people to look after your well-being and manage your property if you become incapable of doing this yourself."[7] It has no effect while the person who signed it remains capable of decision-making.

To be capable of signing a protection mandate, the patient must possess the same capacities as for a power of attorney. In addition, she/he must understand that the power given only takes effect if in the future she/he becomes incapable of decision-making, and that after that time it can no longer be revoked. She/he must understand that it applies not only to management of property but also to personal decisions such as health care or housing.

Testamentary capacity

To be capable of making a will, the patient must understand its nature and effect, and recollect approximately what property he/she has and the persons who might expect to inherit from him/her. He/she must understand the extent of what is being given to each beneficiary, and know if he/she has excluded someone who might have expected to benefit.

Protective supervision

Decision-making capacity only needs to be formally assessed if it is required for the protection of the person or her/his property. Many families continue to care for their loved ones and to manage their affairs without any such assessment. For example, they may continue to manage their assets online or using a power of attorney, and to make personal decisions in consultation with the patient. All adults are presumed capable unless there is evidence to the contrary.

"Under the law, the need for protection exists when an incapacitated person must be assisted or represented in the exercise of their civil rights. This need may arise from the person's isolation, the duration of their incapacity, the nature or state of the person's affairs, etc."[8]

We might need to assess capacity, for example, if there is disagreement among family members regarding the needs of the patient, or if major financial transactions are foreseen, such as the sale of a house. In cases of abuse or neglect, a legal decision-maker may be required to protect the person from harm. Finally, if the person refuses interventions essential for his/her safety, or has delusions regarding those caring for him/her, capacity assessment will be needed.

If a person who has become incapable of decision-making has a protection mandate, the family may proceed to have it homologated.[9] This requires a medical assessment and a psychosocial assessment by a social worker. Through a juridical process, the person is declared incapable and the mandatary named. This is usually undertaken by the family with the help of a notary or lawyer.

If there is no protection mandate, the family or another concerned party may apply for private or public curatorship or tutorship. If the person is only partially incapable a tutor is named, who is responsible for some decisions, while the patient retains control of others, as determined by the court. If totally incapable, a curator is named. Wherever possible, the tutor or curator will be a family member or friend of the patient. If no one is available, this role is taken by the Public Curator.[10]

Back to the case

When you first saw Don, he had early cognitive symptoms but still independent, and was presumed capable of making decisions. On your advice he put measures into place to authorize his wife to make personal and financial decisions in his name should he lose capacity. She was able to care for him for several years without any formal capacity assessment; it became necessary when a major financial transaction was being contemplated and a family member was challenging her authority to make decisions on his behalf. You found that Don lacked the necessary understanding, appreciation and ability to reason and express a choice about his personal and financial needs. Protective supervision was put into place.

1. Applebaum PS, Grisso T. Assessing patients' capacity to consent to treatment. NEJM 1988; 319:1635-1638
2. https://www.ncbi.nlm.nih.gov/pubmed/1202204
3. https://www.ncbi.nlm.nih.gov/pmc/articles/PMC271553/
4. http://www/jcb.utoronto.ca/tools/documents/documents/ace.pdf
5. Nova Scotia Hospitals Act article 52.sA: https://nslegislature.ca/sites/default/files/legc/statutes/hospital.pdf
6. https://www.educaloi.qc.ca/en/capsules/power-attorney
7. https://www.educaloi.qc.ca/en/capsules/protection-mandates-naming-someone-act-you
8. Ibid
9. https://www.educaloi.qc.ca/en/capsules/protection-mandates-naming-someone-act-you
10. http://www.curateur.gouv.qc/cura/en/majeur/inaptitude/role/index.html

HOW DO I PROTECT MY PATIENT?

Randy S. Perskin, Esq., JD,
Elder Law Attorney, New York

VIGNETTE

Mary Smith is a 75 year old woman with early onset dementia diagnosed by her physician. She is otherwise healthy and is able to perform ADLs (activities of daily living) such as toileting and bathing. She is married, lives with her husband, and has two adult children who care for her deeply.

As the dementia progresses Ms. Smith becomes confused and although she speaks clearly she cannot follow conversations or express her concerns. Although mobile, she needs direction for purposes of dressing, bathing, toileting and feeding herself. It is no longer safe for her to perform certain daily tasks unattended such as cooking. She can no longer travel outdoors without company as she will often forget where she is, where she is going or where she lives.

Ms. Smith, when suffering from advanced dementia, is not self directing. She becomes unable to coordinate her care and needs assistance with all activities of daily living to the extent that she needs reminders to take her medications, bathe and pay her bills. Although she is still physically healthy it is no longer safe for her to be left to her own devices.

DISCUSSION

Considerations in the care and treatment of the elder population focus on personal needs, including but not limited to healthcare, living situation, and property management. This latter includes payment of bills and managing finances. Elder adults who suffer from physical disabilities which do not impact on their ability to handle their needs or who do not suffer from any significant incapacity can continue to manage their needs as they always have. The issues facing elder persons who suffer from disabilities which impact their ability to understand their needs and manage them can be effectively dealt with if the proper safeguards are in place.

Advance Directives can protect the elder population if and when they can no longer care for themselves. Agents can be appointed to effectively stand in the place of the elder person to make decisions on their behalf should they be unable to do so. In the United States, the Health Insurance Portability and Accountability Act of 1996 (HIPAA) restricts the ability of health care providers and insurance companies to provide personal health information (PHI) without consent.[11] Although protecting a patient's privacy is of significant importance, concerns arise when an individual requires the support of others for care, management and treatment. Pursuant to Federal Law, a health care provider can discuss relevant health information and billing practices if either the patient gives consent, or with family members involved with the care, treatment and payment if in the provider's professional judgment the patient would consent.[12] That being said the patient can limit the amount of information given to family members. A HIPAA Release can be executed allowing the health care provider to release information to the named individual. The Family Health Care Decisions Act (FHCDA)[13] establishes the authority for health care providers in general hospitals and health care facilities, notably nursing homes, to speak with family members or close friends in order to make health care decisions should the patient become unable to do so. FHCDA can be applied when the elder person is in an institutional setting and healthcare decisions need to be made for a patient no longer able to act on their own behalf. However it does not apply to those individuals in the community who may need the assistance of others in making determinations on their own behalf. A Health Care Proxy can be executed, appointing an agent to act on an individual's behalf for purposes of medical care, including care management, in case of an inability to act.[14] An agent should act in accordance, as much as possible, with the principal's wishes even if they disagree. As such, the principal should have a conversation with their agent as to their wishes and desires regarding health care issues. The Health Care Proxy should indicate that the agent is aware of the principal's wishes in such regard. The preferences can be related orally or in writing. The Health Care Proxy will become effective when it is determined that the principal no longer has the capacity to act for him/herself.

A Living Will is a document that sets forth health care wishes regarding life prolonging procedures and other end of life care. A Living Will can specify the types of treatment desired to prolong life or the measures that the principal wishes to be avoided.

A Do Not Resuscitate Order (DNR), on the other hand, is generally written by doctors in a hospital and specifically instructs health care professionals not to perform CPR or other life sustaining measures when the heart beat or breathing stops.

A Power of Attorney is a legal document which appoints an agent to act with regard to financial and legal matters.[15] It can be as broad or as specific as desired and is often used to protect a party who is unable to act on their own behalf with regard to their financial needs. There are three types of Powers of Attorney: Nondurable, Durable and Springing. A Nondurable Power of Attorney usually applies to a specific transaction such as the sale of a home. A Nondurable Power of Attorney is valid until revoked or the principal becomes incapacitated. A Durable Power of Attorney allows an agent to act on behalf of the principal even after incapacity. A Durable Power of Attorney is often used to avoid unnecessary and expensive Guardianships. A Durable Power of Attorney can be revoked and is valid until the death of the principal. A Springing Power of Attorney becomes effective when a named event, such as the incapacity of the principal, arises or after a specified period of time. Generally for incapacity purposes a letter from a physician testifying to that circumstance will work. Powers of Attorney become effective when signed, except for a Springing Power of Attorney. However it is the intent of the Durable Power of Attorney that the agent will act once the principal becomes unable to do so. Effective September 2009 and further amended in September 2010 changes were made to the statutory short form Power of Attorney to the effect that the Power of Attorney must contain the signatures of both the principal and agent; the agent's authority to make gifts be granted through a separate statutory gifts rider that has the signatures of two witnesses; multiple agents must act together unless otherwise designated; a principal can appoint someone to monitor the actions of the agent: this person has the authority to request records of transactions entered into on behalf of the principal; the principal's rights are stated on the first page in bold faced print; the agent's role, fiduciary obligations and legal limitations are explained; and a signature constitutes acknowledgement. A Power of Attorney in New York can also include language allowing for the release of medical information protected under HIPAA for financial planning purposes, specifically the payment of medical bills. A Power of Attorney drafted prior to 2009, if compliant with the General Obligations Law, can remain in full force and effect. It is possible that a Power of Attorney can be accepted multi jurisdictionally if drafted in accordance with the General Obligations Law or the law of the state where it was executed. A conversation with an attorney well versed in the law in this regard is recommended.

Agents acting under a Power of Attorney are fiduciaries and should act in the best interests of the principal. Proper record keeping is imperative. Interested parties, such as financial institutions and family members, can bring special proceedings questioning the agent's actions. The appointment of an agent to act under a Power of Attorney is a decision which should not be taken lightly. The agent should be someone who the principal trusts and has an understanding of their financial situation and needs.

Practical issues in dealing with Advance Directives include capacity. It is hoped that proper planning is put into effect prior to the occurrence of incapacity. Capacity for purposes of executing the proper Advance Directives means the ability to understand the nature of the document being signed and the authority being granted. An attorney skilled in the preparation of such documents, either in conjunction with estate planning or separately, can effectively determine if such capacity exists. By interviewing the principal, asking questions about their wishes, explaining the documents and relating the issues therein, a reputable and knowledgeable attorney can make a determination as to the capacity for these purposes. Optimally, an attorney well versed in elder care issues is consulted. Essentially, a person with diagnoses that affect mental capacity, such as early onset dementia, may not be precluded from creating advance directives.

Even the most comprehensive Advance Directive will not be properly utilized if its existence is unknown. In this regard copies should be provided to any agents appointed, to medical and healthcare providers where necessary, to financial institutions and in the case of Health Care Proxies and Living Wills kept on hand on the principal's person, as in a wallet. Originals and copies should be kept somewhere safe but not necessarily in a safety deposit box which cannot be accessed by the appropriate parties. Discussions with family members, close personal friends or agents as to the existence of Advance Directives and their locations is important.

Under New York law there are two types of Guardianships that can be established. The Surrogates Court Procedure Act (SCPA) Article 17-A can be used to establish a Guardianship for people who are mentally retarded or developmentally disabled attributable to conditions such as cerebral palsy or neurological imbalances.[16] A Guardianship can be established for elderly persons, trauma victims and, at times, mentally ill or developmentally disabled persons pursuant to Article 81 of the Mental Hygiene Law.[17]

A Guardianship proceeding pursuant to Article 81 of the Mental Hygiene Law (MHL) is commenced by Order to Show Cause and Verified Petition in the county where the Alleged Incapacitated Person (AIP), the person to whom the Guardianship proceeding relates, resides or is physically present. The petitioner can be the AIP, the CEO of a facility in which the AIP is a resident, an adult relative, Adult Protective Services, or any other person concerned with the welfare of the AIP. The Order to Show Cause includes identification information for the AIP, such as name and address, as well as the reasons why a Guardianship is being sought. A Verified Petition is more detailed in that in addition to the information given in the Order to Show Cause it will include financial information, a description of the functional level of the AIP including behavior, understanding and appreciation of the nature and consequences of any inability to manage personal needs or property. Factual allegations of actual occurrences, demonstrating that the AIP will suffer harm due to her/his lack of understanding of the consequences of the inability to provide for personal needs or property management, are tailored to relate to the powers being sought, the duration of the powers being sought, and the approximate value and description of the financial assets of the AIP. It is noted whether the AIP is a recipient of public assistance, the nature of any claim, debt or obligation of the AIP, names addresses and telephone numbers of any presumptive distributes, available resources and an opinion as to the sufficiency of those resources as well as other information which would assist the Court Evaluator in conducting an investigation and writing a report.

There are instances where a Temporary Restraining Order is included in the Order to Show Cause, for example where there is an eviction proceeding pending or where abuse is alleged. Language to the effect that personal medical information may be provided should additionally be included in the Order to Show Cause. An AIP may consent to provide health care information protected by HIPAA, or a Court Evaluator can move to obtain a Court Order to obtain medical records. Additional Orders might be necessary where records from financial institutions are required.

Once the Order to Show Cause is signed by a Judge, a hearing date will be set within 28 days of the date of the Order. The Judge will generally appoint a Court Evaluator who is responsible for explaining the Guardianship proceeding to the AIP, investigating the claims made and writing a report, including recommendations, to be supplied to the Court. The report should also relate any jurisdictional and service issues. The report may also be supplied to the attorney for the AIP and Petitioner with prior Court approval.

The Court Evaluator is an independent individual appointed by the Court to effectively act as the eyes and ears of the Court and does not represent any of the parties in the Guardianship proceeding. The Court Evaluator does not have to be an attorney. An attorney for the AIP can also be appointed for representation in the Guardianship proceeding. The attorney for the AIP acts as an advocate. Personal service of the Order to Show Cause and Petition, as well as the Notice of Proceeding which sets forth the time date and place of the hearing, is required. Service of the Order to Show Cause, Verified Petition and Notice of Proceeding should also be effectuated on the Court Evaluator and attorney for the AIP. Service of the Order to Show Cause and Notice of Proceeding, not the Verified Petition, should additionally be effectuated on other interested parties such as the spouse, adult children, siblings and the person with whom the AIP resides.

The AIP is entitled to be present at the Hearing. The AIP's appearance can be waived if it is determined that they cannot meaningfully participate. Generally, the Court will make every effort to allow for the AIP's participation including adjourning the hearing where necessary or conducting bedside hearings. At the Hearing evidence will be presented via testimony, including that of the Court Evaluator, a psychiatric care provider if a psychological assessment was provided, the AIP, as well as family members and other interested parties if available and relevant. Documentary evidence, such as the Court Evaluator's report is introduced into the record. After listening to the testimony and reviewing the evidence the judge will make a determination as to the Guardianship.

The Court's determination as to the Guardianship will be set forth in an Order and Judgment. The Court, in making its determination, should consider the least restrictive alternative thereby giving the AIP the greatest amount of freedom while considering functional limitations that make it difficult to understand or appreciate the nature or consequences of any inability to provide for personal needs or property management. The desires of the AIP are therefore taken into account. The Guardianship can be tailored to the specific needs of the AIP and be broad or narrow. Primary consideration is given to family members, however independent Guardians are often appointed particularly where there are allegations of abuse or neglect, where there is no family member available or where a particular skill set is required to resolve particular issues.

The AIP may be declared an Incapacitated Person, within the scope of Article 81 of the Mental Hygiene Law. It is significant that incapacity in this regard is a legal, not medical, term and limits an individual's ability to enter into contracts or other legal issues that require capacity. However it is not always the case that a person is adjudged incapacitated for purposes of a Guardianship. There are instances where an individual is designated as a Person in Need of a Guardian (PING) usually for specific issues that need to be addressed by a Guardian.

A Guardian can be appointed for personal needs or property management. A Guardian of the Person can be given powers that relate to personal needs such as determining the living situation, health care and placement of aides. A Guardian of the Property can be given powers relating to property management including marshalling and managing assets, paying bills and applying for and maintaining private and public benefits. A Guardianship can be tailored to the specific needs of the AIP. Therefore a Guardian's powers can be limited to a specific issue, such as dealing with an eviction proceeding and relocations issues, stopping abuse, or Medicaid planning. Additionally a Guardian of the Property may be appointed but not a Guardian of the Person. A Temporary Guardian may be appointed during the pendency of the proceeding in order to assist with specific issues that need immediate attention. A Guardian, once appointed, will have the powers set forth in the Order and Judgment upon obtaining a commission to act. If an expansion of powers is necessary an order can be obtained via motion for such purposes. The Guardianship terminates upon the death of the IP or PING or the completion of the duties set forth in the Order and Judgment.

Guardianships are subject to Court oversight. A Guardian is required to submit an Initial Report within 90 days of appointment detailing the ward's current circumstances, and Annual Accounting thereafter. Annual Accountings will be reviewed by a Court Examiner appointed by the Court and a report and proposed order to judicially settle the account will be presented to the Court. Upon the death of the ward, following notice to the Court, a Final Accounting can be presented which can be reviewed by a Referee to Review for purposes of settling the Final Account and discharge. In instances of Temporary or Limited (Special) Guardianships a Report will generally be submitted describing the actions taken to resolve the issues addressed in the Order and Judgment.

Guardianship fees, to the Court Evaluator, Attorney for the AIP and on occasion to the petitioning attorney can be chargeable to the AIP's estate. Additionally, payment to the appointed Guardian is also generally made from the ward's funds. Where limited funds are available fees are often paid by the Department of Social Services to the Court Evaluator or Temporary Guardian and to the attorney for the AIP.

A Guardianship can be transferred to another state pursuant to the Uniform Adult Guardianship and Protective Proceeding Act (UAGPPJA) when adopted by that state. Such a transfer can alleviate the expense and duplicative work required to establish a new Guardianship in a different state. Discussions with an attorney familiar with the UAGPPJA and the states that have adopted it should be entered into when such a transfer may be necessary.

Practical considerations for the aging population include safe living arrangements and financial management. A Geriatric Care Manager, usually a trained nurse or social worker, can assist in determining the specific needs of the elder client and locate housing and other services that are appropriate for care. Various factors need to be considered in determining whether the elder person should remain at home or consider placement in a nursing home or assisted living facility. In determining whether it is safe for an elder adult to live in the community, the condition of the home should be considered, whether assistance is needed to provide for the activities of daily living and whether the individual lives alone or with someone else who can be responsible for their care. Health aides are an invaluable resource to an elder individual who is no longer totally independent but wishes to reside at home. Assisted living facilities and nursing homes are alternatives to a community residence when an elder individual needs more care than can be safely provided in the home. A nursing home generally follows more of a medical model than assisted living facilities do. Assisted living communities therefore provide more of a home atmosphere. Many assisted living facilities in New York do not accept Medicaid or Medicare so financial concerns can come into play.

Financial planning for the elder population includes determining if they are receiving the benefits they need to survive. Long term care insurance is a private policy that covers the expenses for assistance in the community with the activities of daily living, and health aides. The cost of long term care insurance depends on the age at which it was purchased. Medicare parts A, hospital, and B, medical, is available to any person in any state upon reaching age 65. Medicare Part D, for prescription drug coverage, can be obtained through any Medicare approved insurance carrier.

Supplemental insurance can be used to cover those expenses that Medicare does not, such as copays. Medicaid is a needs based program for low income families. The income and asset levels vary from state to state. In New York, community Medicaid can be used to pay for health aides, in addition to healthcare, and institutional Medicaid can be used to pay for nursing homes. Medicaid rules and qualification issues are complicated and the proper planning should be discussed with an elder law attorney expert in the field. Social security retirement benefits in New York can be collected at age 62. A Representative Payee is an individual who is determined to be qualified to collect social security benefits for the senior individual. Supplemental Security Income, SSI, is a federal income supplement program designed to help aged blind and disabled people who have little or no income and is used to meet basic needs such as food, shelter and clothing. Social Security Disability, SSD, is a federal program designed to supplement the income of people whose physical disabilities limit their ability to work. The Supplemental Nutrition Assistance program, SNAP, is a federal income supplement program designed to assist people in obtaining food, previously recognized as food stamps. The Senior Citizens Rent Increase Exemption, SCRIE, freezes the rent of head of households aged 62 and older who live in rent regulated apartments in New York City. Death benefits from a spouse, either from social security or pensions, should also be explored.

Recognizing the signs of elder abuse in the aged population is a key factor in their care. Elder abuse, which can be physical, financial or psychological, may occur at the hands of a caregiver or other person in a position of trust. See the chapter on Elder Abuse for further information.

Financial exploitation can include the misuse of funds or the taking of property. Financial abuse can be recognized by a financial institution if funds are withdrawn without the consent of the account holder or their representative. Additionally, there have been instances where caretakers take their aged clients to the bank to withdraw cash for them or simply use their bank card. In such instances a financial representative can step in to protect the interests of the elder client. Physical and psychological abuse cannot be as easily identified especially where the elder person has a disability that prevents him from communicating what is happening. Physical injuries can be the result of abuse. If the injury resulted from someone pushing or hitting the senior it qualifies as abuse. If the elder person lives in an assisted living community or nursing home there are often cameras set up in the hallways and public areas thereby giving proof positive of abusive behavior. Additionally, such institutions are highly regulated. An incidence report should be generated detailing the incident and steps that were taken to prevent it from happening again. Abuse can take the form of neglect, even self inflicted in the case of an individual who is not properly feeding themselves or obtaining the proper medical treatment. Such incidences can be reported to Adult Protective Services (APS) who can then step in and evaluate whether protection needs to be implemented and the form it should take. The Attorney General of the State of New York has an elder abuse hotline where instances of abuse can be reported. Complaints are investigated and it is then determined whether the incidence rises to the level of a criminal act. The Elder Abuse Education and Outreach Program provides information and advice to elder abuse victims and their caregivers. Even if an act does not rise to the level of elder abuse it still may be negligent, such as in the case where no care or inappropriate care is given for an injury. In such cases a civil action may be brought and discussions with a personal injury attorney can be useful.

It should be noted that all references herein are made to New York Law unless otherwise indicated as Federal Law of the United States. Advice of counsel in the jurisdiction of residence should be used to navigate the legal ramifications of the needs of an elderly client.

CONCLUSION

Mrs. Smith's son consulted counsel when his mother was originally diagnosed with dementia. He was asked whether she had any Advance Directives in place. As he was uncertain, he was advised to see if his mother had a Will, as often Advance Directives are put in place when estate planning is performed. Fortunately Mrs. Smith was able to remember the name of the attorney who prepared her Will. It was discovered that Advance Directives, including a Power of Attorney and Health Care Proxy, had been executed and were effectively used to assist Mrs. Smith when she became unable to manage her finances and personal needs. It was fortuitous that Mrs. Smith had a loving family that was able to work together to protect her interests.

*Disclaimer: The information contained in this chapter is provided only as general information and not intended as legal advice, nor should it be used as a substitute for complete review of your case by an experienced elder law attorney. All situations differ. By reading this chapter there is no attorney client relation established between you and Randy S. Perskin, Esq.

1. 1. HIPAA; PUBL 104-191, 110 flat 1936.
2. 45 CFR 164.510(b)
3. Public Health Law Articles 29-CC & 29-CCC
4. Public Health law Article 29-C
5. General Obligations Law Section 5-1501
6. Surrogates Court Procedures Act Article 17-A
7. Mental Hygiene Law Article 81

FINANCIAL GUIDANCE FOR SENIORS

Karen C. Altfest, Ph.D., CFP®
Principal Advisor and Executive Vice President,
Altfest Personal Wealth Management

Many seniors are primarily troubled by three financial issues:

1. **Will I have enough to support the lifestyle I desire in retirement?**
2. **How can I address healthcare issues and costs?**
3. **How best can I leave my assets to my family, friends and causes I believe in?**

This chapter will address all these issues as they affect seniors and their caregivers in the United States today. It will also offer some tips for physicians caring for older persons who may be losing the cognitive ability to manage their finances on their own.

According to a recent study, only 25% of Americans believe they have prepared adequately for retirement. Reasons include: (a) lack of access to good strategies; (b) poor understanding of the retirement plans that are in place for them; and (c) believing that planning for retirement is just too complicated. For many people, retirement can last almost as long as their work lives. A 30-year retirement period is not uncommon for those who retire in their 60s and live into their 90s. How, they can wonder, can they be secure when the average American retiree has less than $15,000 in retirement savings and they no longer have a regular paycheck?

Of course, the best time to begin preparing for this long period is as early as possible. Savers who begin in their 20s and 30s can end up with enough money to cover costs for decades to come. Those who begin to save in their 40s and 50s may have a greater challenge. The diagram below shows when most Americans begin to save for retirement.

As you can see, some people do begin saving for retirement in their 20s and 30s, while also repaying their own education debt, and planning for children and their first home.

Later in life, if they face a retirement gap (that is, greater expenses than savings), many people work into their late 60s and even 70s, sometimes part-time.

To the best of your memory, at what age did you start saving for retirement?

Of adults who are saving for retirement

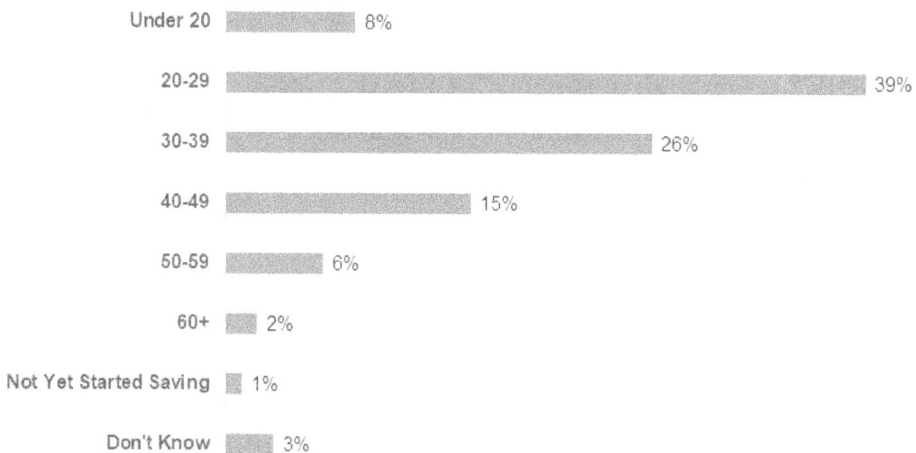

Under 20	8%
20-29	39%
30-39	26%
40-49	15%
50-59	6%
60+	2%
Not Yet Started Saving	1%
Don't Know	3%

Source: Morning Consult, CFP Board Retirement Presentation, April 2019.

The great majority of people living in the United States today would like to continue their current lifestyle after they retire. Few people want to cut back, although their spending may start going for different items, that is, less on travel, but potentially more for healthcare or personal assistance (this can be less true in Canada where medical expenses, shared with the government, are not so great a factor).

A Modern-Day Challenge

Financial literacy is low in the United States for a developed country. The United States places 14th in the world in financial literacy, while Canada lands much higher, in fourth place. Even top universities spend little or no time teaching cash management or providing investing courses to students. People are left to pick up financial wisdom on their own, generally through trial and error, or by way of family example. According to Forbes magazine, two-thirds of Americans cannot pass a basic financial literacy test.

In addition, credit card debt may keep many people from achieving their goals. According to Forbes, the average amount owed on credit cards in the United States is $16,000, which can take 10 years to pay off for those just paying the minimum amount each month.

With that poor showing at financial literacy in mind, here's more on the three most common financial concerns for most older persons.

Will I Have Enough to Support the Lifestyle I Desire in Retirement?

Many people are insecure about calculating how long their money will last. Some want to preserve their capital for the next generation, yet hope for growth in their portfolio; others want to help children and grandchildren now, yet have a substantial estate to divide in the future. Some people, not knowing where to turn for professional help, do their own retirement calculations. They often neglect to factor in inflation, which can have a major effect over an extended retirement period, or to use probability analysis, which can run thousands of scenarios showing what will happen when costs rise while earnings decline, or vice versa. Others neglect to account for lifestyle differences over the decades. They may assume that a stagnant plan, developed on costs while they were still at work can be used as a guide during retirement. But this is not so – a worthwhile retirement plan contains all those elements (such as recognition of inflation and probability analysis results) and more. It should be revisited and updated whenever a person's lifestyle or circumstances change.

Common Sources of Income in Retirement

Most people's income comes from a few of these sources in retirement:

a. Employer-sponsored retirement plans – if a company has a defined contribution plan, such as a 401(k), the worker and the employer can both contribute, and the amount a person ends up with varies, according to savings patterns. Qualified plans are built with pretax dollars, and the money being saved is tax-deferred until withdrawal, which is allowed at age 59½, and currently mandated at age 70½. Defined contribution plans, such as 401(k)s, 403(b) s, and individual retirement accounts (IRAs) are fairly common types of tax-qualified plans. The amount a worker can contribute is decided by federal law, and can be changed.

A Roth 401(k) is a fairly new retirement vehicle, taxed upon contribution to the employer plan, but not later upon withdrawal. In other words, taxes are paid up-front, and then money is allowed to grow in the account. Choosing the most useful retirement savings plan is highly important to that person's ultimate financial health.

a. Social Security – the full retirement age at which workers are eligible for coverage under this government program has risen to age 66 (depending on an applicant's year of birth) and likely will continue to rise as people live longer. By 2050, some estimates project 83.7 million people aged 65 or older living in the United States — nearly twice as many senior citizens as in 2012. In the United States, 10,000 people are turning age 65 every day. Social Security spending on the elderly is greater than income taken out of paychecks to contribute to it for the first time in almost four decades. This should be a reality check for younger generations to take earlier action to protect their own retirement years.

a. Personal savings – this is money that can be kept in a brokerage account or a bank and withdrawn as needed, or left to grow over time. For some people it is their emergency fund--available on very short notice, ready to be put to use for a major and sometimes unexpected need, such as a home repair. There is confidence in knowing that there is a pot of money readily accessible in good times and bad. Simply put, the more a family or individual has saved, the more comfortable they are likely to be in retirement.

How Can a Physician Detect Signs That an Older Person Is Not Financially Prepared for Retirement?

Physicians are often the first to notice signs of stress in the elderly. For example, you may notice that a patient says he or she is fearful of running out of money. Another recurring negative fantasy for some older persons is that they may lose their housing and be homeless. When there is no paycheck coming in, they may worry about how to maintain their current standard of living. They may fear that they could live an overly long life, and worry about how they will support that. The older patient may be afraid to talk to family members about their financial status, worrying that responsibility for financial decisions may be taken away and assumed by an adult child.

One woman whose husband recently died told her doctors she had made plans "to end it all." This brought her to the attention of a psychiatrist, who is now treating her.

What Can Physicians and Caregivers Do to Help Older Patients?

Physicians may spot financial problems with older patients before others do. Here are some ways physicians can help.

Ask relevant questions of the patient and those close to him or her. Determine if the patient is accurately aware of their financial situation, and if they are fiscally responsible. Refer patients, as the physicians in the story above did, to the appropriate specialist or public agency for help. If the case is less extreme, recommend some groups to join or information to read to address their financial misgivings or changes in cognitive ability. Consider having some relevant reading material in your office. Urge patients to communicate with their spouses, children and other loved ones about money questions or fears. Encourage them to use the money they've worked long and hard for to live the life they would like. Check on their mental state, or suggest someone who can. Note when a senior is no longer able to handle his or her finances or to make clear decisions. Ask if there is someone with power of attorney for the older person, or someone the patient can reach out to. Look for signs of abuse or scams against the elderly, and notify the family or the caregivers or government agencies if you suspect this is happening. With people living longer, there are more opportunities both for financial fraud to occur, but also to help steer elderly people toward assistance, perhaps to pro bono elder-care legal counsel or a financial planning organization to address their continuing financial needs.

Check for scams by strangers

Difficult family situations can arise from aging patients' declining money management abilities, so physicians and caregivers can listen for potential scams when a financial situation seems to take an unusual turn. For example, if a patient mentions giving most of his money away to a younger woman he has just met after the woman promised to marry him, that should raise red flags. A son or daughter could be alerted to obtain a court order to gain access to the patient's finances if the situation is thought to be harmful to the older person. This sometimes involves having an attorney start the process to deem the patient mentally incompetent, or bring him into the adult child's home to live.

Listen for stories of abuse

This can include stealing by family or caregivers. These stories may or may not have basis in fact.

Be Alert to Your Older Patients' Signals

Signs of distress may include:

- A sudden change in behavior
- Keeping secrets
- Money missing from accounts
- Personal items gone
- An abrupt rise in expenses
- Sudden new friendships
- A decline in standard of living or quality of care
- Extreme worries about money

Physicians and trained or family caregivers can watch for:

- The illness of a partner
- The death of a spouse
- Significant or long-lasting stress or signs of depression
- Separation from family or friends
- Elder abuse, which is often centered on finances.

Managing Risk

Another aspect of money management to consider is the senior's capacity for, and comfort level with, taking financial risks. There is a saying in financial planning that the most serious risk is one individuals don't know they are taking. Here are some types of risk that financial advisors are aware of and seniors and their caregivers can learn to think about.

Liquidity Risk – An asset may be tied up in an investment and not readily available to the investor, for reasons such as a lockup date, an early withdrawal penalty, a hedge fund redemption date or restrictions arising from private real estate investments. As a result, an investor may only be able to withdraw funds at specified times.

Longevity Risk – A person may live a shorter or longer life than expected. If they die young, they may not have worked long enough to accumulate assets to support their family after they are gone. If they live a very long life, they will need extra assets to cover several years of late-in-life expenses.

Health Risk – In the United States, the possibility of large, unreimbursed medical costs always looms. Healthcare costs have been growing about 4-5% per year in the nation. In 2017, healthcare collectively cost Americans $3.5 trillion, or 17.9% of gross domestic product (GDP). More critically for older persons, medical costs typically more than double between the ages of 70 and 90.

Average Health Spending by Age in the United States

Spending per year based on age group (2016)

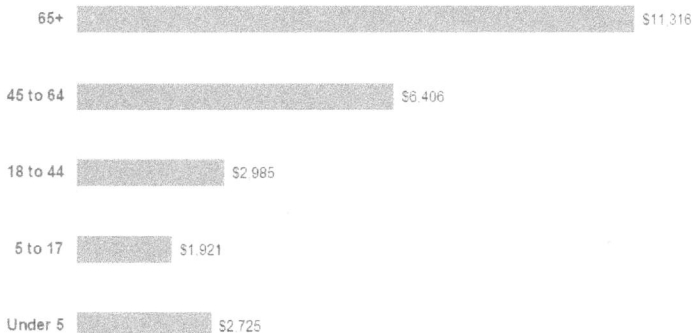

Age group	Spending
65+	$11,316
45 to 64	$6,406
18 to 44	$2,985
5 to 17	$1,921
Under 5	$2,725

Source: The Medical Expenditure Panel Survey (MEPS), The US Department of Health and Human Services, 2016

<u>Investment Risk</u> – Assets placed in financial accounts may not perform as expected, and values can decline.

<u>Withdrawal Risk</u> – This comes from withdrawing money at a disadvantageous time, typically from a portfolio when prices are low, particularly early in the retirement period. At that time more shares of an investment may need to be liquidated, leaving fewer shares to continue to grow and finance future costs.

<u>Inflation Risk</u> – If inflation is not considered when planning for expenses in the future, the individual may be hurt when living costs rise.

How Can I Address Healthcare Costs as a Senior?

In the United States, it is important to make sure that you have appropriate medical insurance coverage in place, either as an individual or through your workplace.

For the elderly, there are usually greater medical or personal needs costs that exceed insurance coverage. Medicare for seniors in the United States, along with supplemental insurance, can fill this gap.

In addition, some people like to have a long-term care insurance policy. This coverage can be costly, but it can defray spiraling costs that may come from the need to live in a care facility in the future or to require assistance at home with basic activities of daily living (ADL). The average age to purchase long-term care insurance in the United States is between 55-64. But seniors cannot wait too long to obtain this coverage because poor health may disqualify them from purchasing a policy or make it prohibitively expensive.

Medicaid is a program for financially needy people who typically have reached the age of 65 that is paid for in part by states and in part by the federal government. The program pays for medical care administered by medical professionals, and also may cover assisted living costs, dental care and continuing-care facility costs, if necessary. To find out more, it is best to check with the applicable state Medicaid office on its eligibility rules or with an elder care attorney who is an expert at guiding seniors in Medicaid planning.

Who Will Take Care of the Older Person?

Many families in the United States are having fewer children and at older ages, and living greater distances from each other around the country. That can mean that there are fewer offspring able to divide the care of the older person. In many families, caregiving becomes the responsibility of one member of the family.

Baby boomers, now between ages 54 and 72, are entering retirement. Gen X, now between ages 38-53, is raising children, concerned about education, coping with the cost of housing, and trying to save for future retirement. They are often in the unenviable and untenable position of having responsibility for two generations other than their own. Millennials are still young, currently ages 22-37, and are newer in the workforce. (Note: all age groups have been recalculated by the Pew Organization, which has recently issued new guidelines.)

People who are concerned about getting proper care for aging parents while simultaneously raising their own children are often referred to as "the sandwich generation," squeezed between the needs of the older person and their own offspring.

As a result of growing longevity, younger elderly people are often caring for parents living into their 90s and beyond. The New York Times in mid-2019 published an article titled "When the Older Care for the Oldest," which gave examples of adult children in their 60s and 70s caring for parents in their 90s. For some of these families, the children sacrifice their own finances to pay for parents' needs, sometimes giving up jobs to care for their elders. Others take parents into their own homes. Sometimes the aging children's health is affected.

Because aging generations are working toward their own retirement, and younger generations may not be available to help, some families choose to hire a caregiver or move an older person into a facility. Caregivers often assist with the ADL (activities of daily living) an older person can no longer handle alone. At times, these caregivers become involved in family and money matters, such as bill-paying. Currently, 43.5 million people in the United States say they have been caregivers. Many say they have given unpaid help, sométimes to children, other times to spouses, and often care to relatives. A major problem, however, is that there is currently a shortage of trained caregivers in the United States. With an aging population, there soon will be many older people without proper care. An equally important challenge to caregiving is high, protracted cost, which can be prohibitive for many families.

Is There a Different Portfolio for Older People?

To arrive at a suitable investment portfolio, first discuss goals with family members, then create a diversified portfolio that makes sense for the older person's needs. Start by dividing the portfolio into two asset classes, stocks and bonds, depending on the amount of risk or volatility that is tolerable in the portfolio. Then divide each of those categories even further. Do some reading or consult a professional financial advisor to determine the best way to do more (see sample diversification diagram below). Basically, the investor's age is just one factor in deciding how much risk to assume in a portfolio. Others have to do with investment growth potential, tolerance level for market declines, and assumed length of the retirement period.

It helps when the older investor is honest about goals, and what they want to happen to the money someday. Are they planning to use it soon, do they have an emergency fund that is not invested in the markets and therefore not subject to fluctuation to see them through unexpected events? Although some older persons wish to take less investment risk as they age, that is a choice, just as it is for all investors. There is no older-investor formula that will suit all people in this age group.

Here is a sample of one way to divide the investment pie:

Investment Management: The Role of Diversification

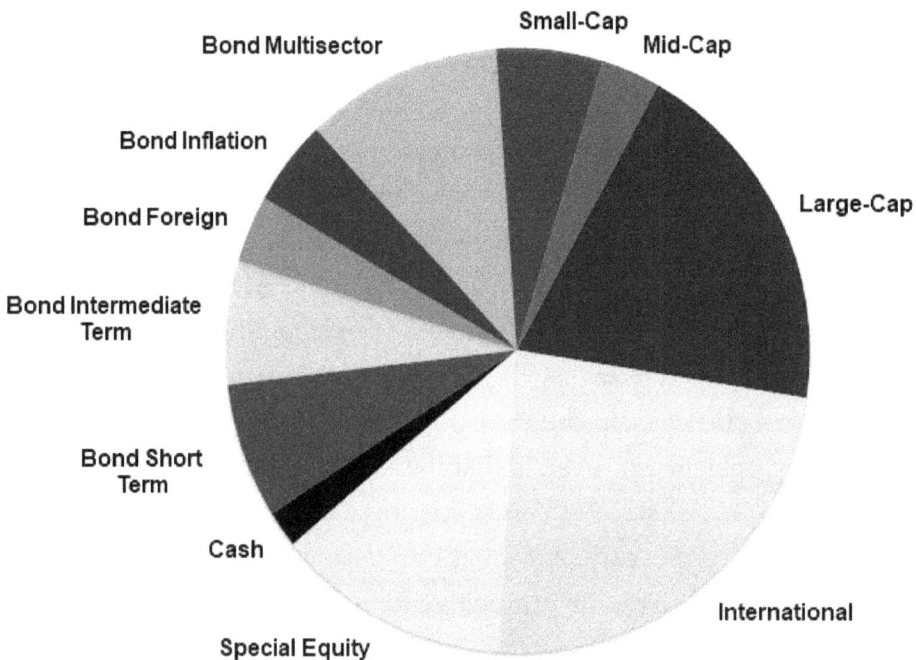

Source: Karen C. Altfest, CFP®, Ph.D. and Lewis J. Altfest, CFA, CFP®, CPA, PFS, Ph.D.

This chart shows one example of how an investor might diversify his or her portfolio. Note the various bond slices on the left, and the stockholdings on the right, beginning with small-capitalization stocks through special equity, generally investments — such as real estate holdings — that do not act the same way as other stocks and bonds in the portfolio.

Of course, an investor might choose a very different asset allocation from the one presented above, depending on goals, appetite for risk, and beliefs about the markets and world events. It is best to have an open discussion with family members and investment professionals when forming a portfolio.

Financial Mistakes the Elderly Commonly Make

1. Cashing out investments in declining markets. People may want a sense of security from knowing their cash is readily available, even at the cost of taking losses or earning very little from certificates of deposit (CDs) or money market accounts.
2. Investing too conservatively. Some people have heard that as they age their appetite for risk should drop. But few people really want their money to be gone at their deaths. They would prefer to pass their assets on to younger generations.
3. Subtracting their age from 100 to find a comfortable asset allocation (stock-to-bond ratio). Because many people today live longer than when that "formula" was popularized, it's likely they would have to raise the 100 by 10-25%, or discard this old saw and invest in a way suitable for their goals.
4. Living beyond their means. This is the hardest behavior to modify. Some seniors do not want to leave the family home they raised their children in, or stop entertaining and buying expensive cars and clothes. People tend to believe that what happened before can happen again, so if they were able to support a lavish lifestyle in the past, they may assume there's no reason to change it now.
5. Forgetting where assets are, how they are titled or even whether they still own an asset. The ability to understand and make clear decisions is key to arriving at good financial choices. If this ability is no longer present, an appropriate person — often an adult child — should assume financial responsibility for the elderly person.

Steps for Seniors or Their Caregivers to Take

To have a successful and comfortable retirement period, it is worthwhile for people to:

1. Decide how much money they will need to support that lifestyle, and work toward it
2. Account for all income and expenses now and in the future
3. Make a plan for when to sell a business, home or other major assets
4. Use realistic aging tables
5. Use probability (known as Monte Carlo) analysis
6. Determine when extra help is indicated
7. Decide where to keep the assets, and let loved ones know how to gain access to them when needed
8. Make sure one's will is up to date; the family and the senior should not do this alone, but with an estate attorney
9. Name beneficiaries for retirement accounts. Be aware of what passes through a will or trust, and what passes outside the will. (In the United States, all retirement accounts should have named beneficiaries – these will transfer outside whatever is stated in a will)
10. Give a trusted relative or friend power of attorney so that designate can make personal and financial decisions on behalf of the senior when necessary while they're still living
11. Leave room for growth in investment portfolios; few people want the assets to "die" when they do, as most people prefer to leave them to the family members. Investor age is a factor but it is not the sole factor in determining asset allocation
12. Identify the best retirement plans for each situation – if you are a small-business owner, this is particularly important

---

How Best Can I Leave My Assets to My Family, Friends and Causes I Believe In?

Many people are reluctant to address their own mortality. But several steps taken now can ease matters at time of death.

It is important for seniors to have an up-to-date will, signed power-of-attorney authorization, a person with healthcare proxy, beneficiaries for retirement accounts, and trusts, if needed.

Meeting with an estate attorney is the best way to accomplish all this preparation. Generally, if a will has gone unchanged for a long period of time, it warrants a fresh look.

Dying intestate (without a will) leaves too much up to others deciding about a person's final wishes.

It helps to have a letter of intent to leave heirs with guidelines for investing or distributing assets after someone is gone.

Conclusion

If physicians and caregivers can help older persons address and seek help with their greatest fears about money (Will I have enough? How can I pay for potentially costly healthcare? How can I best leave my assets when I'm gone?), life in the later years can be much more productive and pleasant. A fee-only financial advisor can offer objective help with these problems. As this chapter has outlined, there are many ways to tackle complex money issues faced by seniors, but often, noticing warning signs, speaking frankly about goals with family and preparing for decline and mortality can be the best prescription for older patients and their finances.

APPENDIX I: References

1. CFP Board. Morning Consult Survey Retirement Presentation, Apr. 15, 2019.

    https://www.cfp.net/docs/default-source/news-events---research-facts-figures/cfp-board-morning-consult-survey-2019.pdf

2. Pascarella, Dani. "4 Stats That Reveal How Badly America Is Failing at Financial Literacy," Forbes. Apr. 3, 2018.
    https://www.forbes.com/sites/danipascarella/2018/04/03/4-stats-that-reveal-how-badly-america-is-failing-at-financial-literacy/#54ce96a62bb7

3. Leatherby, Lauren. "Medical spending among the U.S. elderly," Journalist's Resource, Shorenstein Center on Media, Politics and Public Policy, Harvard Kennedy School. Feb. 22, 2016.
    https://journalistsresource.org/studies/government/health-care/elderly-medical-spending-medicare/

4. Bergman, Adam. "Social Security Feels Pinch as Baby Boomers Clock Out for Good," Forbes. June 21, 2018.

https://www.forbes.com/sites/greatspeculations/2018/06/21/social-security-feels-pinch-as-baby-boomers-clock-out-for-good/

5. Kincaid, Ellie. "The Amount Americans Spend On Healthcare Is Still Growing, But More And More Slowly," Forbes. Dec. 6, 2018. https://www.forbes.com/sites/elliekincaid/2018/12/06/the-amount-americans-spend-on-healthcare-is-still-growing-but-more-and-more-slowly/

6. National Bureau of Economic Research. "Medical Spending of the Elderly" Report Summary, NBER Bulletin on Aging and Health, 2015, No. 2. https://www.nber.org/aginghealth/2015no2/w21270.html

7. Garland, Susan B. "At 75, Taking Care of Mom, 99: 'We Did Not Think She Would Live This Long'," The New York Times, June 27, 2019. https://www.nytimes.com/2019/06/27/business/retirement-parents-aging-living-to-100.html

8. AARP Public Policy Institute and National Alliance for Caregiving. "Caregiving in the U.S. 2015 – Executive Summary, June 2015. https://www.caregiving.org/wp-content/uploads/2015/05/2015_CaregivingintheUS_Executive-Summary-June-4_WEB.pdf

APPENDIX II: Further Reading

1. Altfest, Lewis, Personal Financial Planning 2nd edition (McGraw Hill) July 2007. A comprehensive book on financial planning and investing with case studies

2. Altfest, Karen C., "Personal Finance: Planning Your Future. How to Save, Invest, and Grow Your Assets," Medscape April 25, 2018. An online course for young physicians on all the parts of their financial lives

3. Altfest, Karen C., " Life After a Loss: 6 Smart Steps for Coping With Widowhood," AAII Journal, July 2016. What to do and not to do for widows

4. Kahneman, Daniel, Thinking Fast and Slow, 1st edition (Farrar, Straus and Giroux) April 2013. An introduction to behavioral finance

APPENDIX III: Resource Organizations

AAII (American Association of Independent Investors) provides lectures on investment topics, a journal and speakers in many cities. AAII.com

The Certified Financial Planner™ (CFP®) Board will help you find a financial advisor in many geographic areas.

Letsmakeaplan.org.

NAPFA (the National Association of Personal Financial Advisors) will help you locate a fee-only advisor who works without commissions, on a fee-for-service or investments-under-management basis. Napfa.org/find-an-advisor.

APPENDIX IV: Glossary

Asset

A resource with economic value that an individual, corporation or country owns or controls with the expectation that it will provide future benefit. For personal finances, it's the amount of goods of value, such as your house, and money you've accumulated.

Beneficiary

In the financial world, a beneficiary typically refers to someone who is eligible to receive distributions (payouts) from a trust, will, life insurance policy or a retirement account. Beneficiaries are either named specifically in these documents or have met the stipulations that make them eligible for whatever distribution is specified.

Capital

Capital is a term for financial assets, such as funds held in deposit accounts, as well as for the physical factors of production; that is, manufacturing equipment. Additionally, capital includes facilities, including buildings used to produce and store manufactured goods. Materials used and consumed as part of the manufacturing process do not qualify as capital.

Defined benefit plan

A defined benefit plan, or traditional pension, is an employer-sponsored retirement plan in which employee benefits are computed using a formula that considers several factors, such as length of employment and salary history. The company administers portfolio management and investment risk for the plan. There are also restrictions on when and by what method an employee can withdraw funds without penalties. Benefits paid are typically guaranteed for life and rise slightly to account for increased cost of living.

Diversified portfolio

Diversified portfolios include investments spread across different asset categories, such as fixed-income, often bonds and cash, equities, commodities and sometimes derivatives. Further diversification is possible within each asset category, such as growth and value stocks within equities or domestic and international bonds within fixed income. The asset mix of a portfolio depends on an investor's risk tolerance and financial objectives.

Emergency fund

An emergency fund is an account for funds set aside in case of the event of a personal financial dilemma, such as the loss of a job, a debilitating illness or a major repair to your home. The purpose of the fund is to improve financial security by creating a safety net of funds that can be available to meet emergency expenses.

Financial literacy

Financial literacy is the education on and understanding of various financial areas including topics related to managing personal finance, money and investing. This topic focuses on the ability to manage personal finance matters efficiently, and it includes the knowledge of making appropriate decisions about personal finance such as investing, insurance, real estate, paying for college, budgeting, retirement, estate and tax planning.

Inflation

Inflation is a quantitative measure of the rate at which the average price level of a basket of selected goods and services in an economy increases over a period of time. It is the constant rise in the general level of prices that causes a unit of currency to buy less than it did in prior periods. Often expressed as a percentage, inflation indicates a decrease in the purchasing power of a nation's currency.

IRA

A traditional individual retirement account (IRA) allows individuals to direct pretax income toward investments that can grow taxdeferred; no capital gains or dividend income is taxed until it is withdrawn. Contributions to a traditional IRA may be tax-deductible, depending on the taxpayer's income, tax-filing status and other factors.

Qualified retirement plans

A qualified retirement plan meets the requirements of Internal Revenue Code Section 401(a) of the Internal Revenue Service (IRS) and is therefore eligible to receive certain tax benefits. Such a retirement plan is established by an employer for the benefit of the company's employees. Qualified retirement plans give employers a tax break for the contributions they make for their employees. Qualified plans that allow employees to defer a portion of their salaries into the plan can also reduce employees' present income-tax liability by reducing taxable income.

Real estate

Property comprising land and the buildings on it, as well as the natural resources of the land. It can be grouped into three broad categories based on its use: residential, commercial and industrial.

Roth 401(k)

A Roth 401(k) is an employer-sponsored investment savings account funded with after-tax dollars up to the plan's contribution limit. This type of investment account is well-suited to people who think they will be in a higher tax bracket in retirement than they are in their working years. In contrast, the traditional 401(k) plan is funded with pretax money, which results in a tax on future withdrawals.

Roth IRA

A Roth IRA is a type of qualified individual retirement account (IRA) that accrues gains tax-exempt but uses after-tax money to fund it. This can be contrasted with a traditional IRA, which uses pre-tax funds and then defers that income tax until the time of withdrawal.

Social Security

Social Security is the term used for the Old-Age, Survivors and Disability Insurance (OASDI) program in the United States, run by the federal Social Security Administration (SSA). While best known for retirement benefits, it can also provide disability income and survivor benefits.

Titling of assets

In estate planning, the way one titles his or her property determines which method of distribution is used when the estate is settled upon death. There are several asset-titling options that can help ensure heirs receive the assets according to the owner's wishes. An estate attorney can help with decisions in this area.

THE ROLE OF RELIGIOUS BELIEF IN THE END-OF-LIFE CARE OF OLDER PERSONS

A. Mark Clarfield MD, FRCPC

Medical School for International Health,

Faculty of Health Sciences, Ben-Gurion University of the Negev

Clinical Vignette:

An 88-year-old moderately demented woman with coronary artery disease and atrial fibrillation presents with a massive stroke. For several months, she remains unconscious with complete hemiplegia and difficulty swallowing. Her prognosis is bleak and she has no Advance Directive. The patient's family has strong Jewish religious convictions and requests a permanent feeding tube. While this discussion occurs, she becomes febrile and is diagnosed with pneumonia.

Furthermore, the patient's three children insist that the doctor must under no circumstances tell the patient's elderly husband their mother's bleak prognosis, because "the news will surely kill him". For his part, the husband is cognitively intact and keeps asking about his wife's condition.

Questions:

1. Is it appropriate to insert or refuse to insert a feeding tube in this patient?
2. Should her pneumonia be treated?
3. How should one respond to the husband's queries?

Introduction

Words have meaning. For example, "feeding", "food", "nutrition", "hydration", "hunger", "thirst", "starvation" and "truth" are all terms fraught with meaning, the problem being that they may mean different things to different people, and at different times. Misunderstandings can thus occur. This is especially the case with various ethnic/religious groups, especially when they come into conflict with the majority culture which in Canada and most developed countries today is largely, or at least avowedly, secular. And it behooves us to keep in mind that this has only been the case for a few short decades.

Before we continue, it must be clear that not everyone who is brought up in a particular religious group will necessarily strictly follow their respective credos and rules. For example, while it is clear that for the Jewish (and Muslim) religions, although some people brought up in these traditions will partake, eating pork is clearly forbidden. As well, in these two religions, some forms of birth control (even abortion) will be allowed under somewhat restricted conditions. Yet, according to Catholicism, most forms of birth control and certainly abortion are strictly forbidden, although there are Catholics who do undergo the procedure. That being said, even avowedly secular people are often influenced, consciously or not, by the belief systems in which they have been raised. As such, certain things may appear more or less acceptable (or not) to them by dint of these early and perhaps ongoing influences.

In this chapter, we examine the above scenario and explore the Jewish approach, with some brief comparisons to Islamic and Catholic belief systems. I choose to discuss Judaism because I am a member of this faith group and as such am more familiar with its credos and rules than those of other faiths. That being said, Judaism is used simply as an example. While exact belief systems may differ, in this chapter I will try to bring out the principles of how religious belief can influence end-of-life care, especially for older persons. As well, I offer some general guidelines as to how the members of the treating team might best react, especially if there is a conflict between what the formal caregivers think is in the patient's best interests and the beliefs/wishes of the patient or her family.

Whether religious or not, it behooves doctors to have at least some awareness of how patients' and families' belief systems might affect decisions - either for themselves and/or for their loved ones. This is especially the case when a conflict in management arises. The more the doctor can understand where the patient is "coming from" religiously, the more empathy expressed (but without need of formal agreement or approval), the easier it will be to manage many ethical conflicts. The doctor need not be a religious expert but should be ready to query the patient/family enquiring whether there might be any religious concerns behind a conflicted issue. At times the physician may ask for clarification or even consult with the relevant pastoral authority.

Feeding tube insertion

With respect to the first question relating to the clinical scenario above, for the Jewish religion (and Islam too) "feeding" (food and water) can never, as may be held by the believing Catholic, be considered "extraordinary". In such a Christian consideration, logic suggests that we thus need not apply "extraordinary" measures in every case. However, according to Jewish law, given that feeding is considered an "ordinary" measure, it can almost never be denied the patient, at least in some form. The analogy of access to air is sometimes used.

That being said, according to Jewish law there is no injunction as to how nor how much feeding is to be given, with the understanding that invasive percutaneous endoscopic gastrectomy (PEG) and forced nasal gastric (NG) feeding need not always be utilized, especially if such use causes disproportionate pain and suffering. Spoon feeding (however expensive and time-consuming) would be allowed as long as the patient did not show any signs of distress from aspiration or from hunger and/or thirst and was not associated with other harms such as recurrent aspiration.

However, many elderly Jewish patients (and their children) will frequently have a long historical memory of outrages such as the Holocaust - during which millions of Jews were worked, gassed and often just starved to death. These fraught memories can make the use of feeding (or its withholding) a charged issue. While one need not be an expert on religious Jewish law nor in the dolorous history of the 20th century, a sensitivity as to where the patient and especially family may be coming from will help in the management of such fraught cases. While Muslim patients will not have the same historical pressures, they will however usually insist in the same way on feeding and hydrating an end-stage patient for similar religious reasons. Furthermore, the general practice in countries from which most Muslim immigrants to Canada come will usually push the family in the same direction as their Jewish counterparts.

Use of antibiotics

With respect to the use of antibiotics when faced with suspected infection in a dying patient, again since both Jewish and Islamic law follow a "Choose Life" approach, the usual religious practice would be to agree to (even to insist upon) the use of antibiotics. This would be the case, even if antibiotic use is judged as medically "futile" by the treating team. However, that being said, in both this scenario and that relating to feeding tubes, Jewish religious law will also recognize that if the intervention causes undue suffering with little clinical benefit, it may be scaled back or even forgone.

Although it may seem illogical and perhaps even hypocritical to the treating team, many families will be satisfied by even a partial approach - for example giving antibiotics orally rather than IV to cut down on the use of invasive procedures, especially if venous access is difficult to initiate and/or maintain. When distributive justice is invoked as trumping beneficence (for example, "Using an antibiotic in your mother is not only futile but is likely to cause an increase in antibiotic resistance for others"), this claim will hold less water. Jewish law will tend to put more emphasis on the patient in front of the clinician than on a theoretical population.

Should the spouse be told the truth?

In this vignette, the children demand that their elderly father be shielded from the stress of learning the truth about his wife's dire prognosis. In most cases, however odd this might seem, the family's concern is real and the doctor should treat it as such. According to Jewish law (as is the case with both Islam and Catholicism too), truth telling is always the preferred option in most of life's situations. However, Jewish law does allow for "bending" of the rules but only in the case when the doctor in his/her professional opinion (not the family) is actually convinced that this is indeed the case.

Of interest is the fact that apart from religious law as a specific rationale, there are many cultures around the world which believe that older persons (in an analogy to children) sometimes need to be protected, usually by the family, from hearing the truth. Practice in Japan is a good example. Again, it is important for members of the treating team to see where the patient and their family are coming from – that is, usually from a sincere desire to protect their loved ones from avoidable travail.

It may be easy for many clinicians nowadays to look down on these requests as "primitive" or "illiberal". However, a little cultural humility and some historical perspective are in order. This author easily recalls that during his own training in Toronto just a few decades back, senior physicians would routinely withhold the truth from patients; again, in an attempt to protect them from bad news. Our clinical frankness is a much more recent development.

How to approach this case

Simply recognizing that religious law (or the patient's interpretation of same – even when "incorrect") might be an issue is a good first step. Again, while the physician need not be an expert in these belief systems, even a little knowledge can be helpful. For example, for many years and even up to the present day, many observant Jews incorrectly thought that organ transplantation was forbidden by religious law. In fact, this is actually <u>not</u> the case and being able to explain this theological fact to a patient, or if they are still skeptical suggesting that they ask for a rabbinical opinion, will usually reconcile any disagreement.

Specifically, with respect to feeding, it is worth recognizing early on that not offering such sustenance is against Jewish law and insisting on allowing the patient to "starve" will hold no influence on the family who is insisting on such feeding. However, since there is no injunction as to how or how much a patient must be fed, one can suggest that the family (or a surrogate) take the time to spoon feed the patient, explaining that "like a baby" most patients will take just as much as they want. When they "refuse" to take any more, it is unlikely that they are suffering from hunger or thirst and the episode can be stopped until the next mealtime.

However, if this does not work, either due to the family's refusal or inability to cooperate, there is usually no choice but to insert a PEG. However if this form of tube feeding causes complications and the patient is obviously exposed to pain and suffering or risk to life and health, the physician may well be able to convince the family that on balance the goal must be to minimize suffering. In this way, with careful mouth hygiene and occasional top-ups with fluids, preferably in this case via hypodermoclysis the terminal patient can be left to die in a humane manner and one in which the family can accept. Issues such as feeding should not be considered photographs but rather more like a video, that is they often will gradually evolve. Most families can, with time, patience and empathy be helped to find the right balance - whatever their practices and religious beliefs.

With respect to antibiotic therapy, again this issue can be dealt with via careful explanation and the family's opinion may change over the course of illness. This might especially be the case if repeated fevers ensue. In this case, use of IV antibiotics for a few days switching to p.o. as soon as possible is an option. However, after multiple bouts of fever (source found or as is often the case not), families can often be convinced that repeated attempts to find intravenous access with the resultant patient suffering would tip the balance towards a more conservative approach. Again, the metaphor of a video rather than snapshot is helpful to keep in mind.

To tell, or not

Requests to withhold the truth can be dealt with by explaining that in <u>your</u> clinical experience, telling the truth (even difficult ones) is extremely unlikely to cause harm to those who seek information. In fact, the case can be made that trying to withhold the facts is usually counterproductive. Almost always, the truth does slip out and then the person from whom it was withheld will with justice feel betrayed. Again, this process may not occur in one episode and sometimes it takes people time to be convinced.

It is true and helpful that in many countries, Canada and USA included, the secular law in fact demands that patients and families be responded to honestly when the team is queried. This fact, when explained gently, can help the family cope with any guilty feelings about letting their father know the facts. When the physician explains to those who may object that he/she really has no legal choice, usually the issue is resolved.

That being said, our thoughts on truth telling have evolved over the past few decades. It is now more widely known that giving out facts can, like a medication, be offered in various doses and gradually (cf "start low, go slow"). In this way the physician can answer the patient's and/or family's queries but need not feel the need to tell the "whole truth" especially if it is not asked for. A graded and nuanced practice is probably the best approach over these fraught questions.

Conclusion

Whatever the treating physicians own specific religious upbringing or level of religiosity, it is useful to recognize that religious faiths may play a large role with our patients and their families, especially around the difficult issues surrounding death and dying. The more we know or discover about how their belief systems may be influencing decisions, the better the physician can effectively handle the case. Many people do not realize that it is only a small minority of humankind that have no religious belief. Most people around the globe have some and this can often affect their lives, especially in moments of illness and in the situation of death and dying. The more we physicians can know of and empathize with our patient's health belief models, especially as they relate to religious and spiritual beliefs, the better we can care for them and theirs in the hour of need.

Acknowledgments: I would like to thank Dr. Shimon Glick and Dr. Shabbir Alibhai for their helpful comments on an earlier draft of this manuscript.

References

1. Clarfield AM, Gordon M, Markwell H, Alibhai S. Ethical issues in end-of-life geriatric care. The approach of three monotheistic religions: Judaism, Catholicism and Islam. J Amer Geriatr Soc; 2003; 51:1149-54.

2. Clarfield AM, Monette J, Bergman H, Monette M, Ben-Israel Y , Caine Y, Charles J, Gordon M, Gore B. Enteral feeding in end-stage dementia: a comparison of religious, ethnic and national differences in Canada and Israel. J Gerontol: Med Sci. 2006; 61A(6):621-627.

3. Jotkowitz AB, Clarfield AM, Glick S. The care of patients with dementia: a modern Jewish ethical perspective. J Amer Geriatr Soc 2005; 53:881- 884.

4. Marcus EL, Clarfield AM, Moses AE. Ethical issues relating to the use of antimicrobial therapy in older adults. Clin Infect Dis 2001; 33 (15 Nov): 1697-1705.

5. Goldsand G et al. Jewish medical ethics. CMAJ 2001;164: 219-22

6. Markwell H et al. Catholic medical ethics. CMAJ 2001;165: 189-192

7. Daar AS et al. Islamic medical ethics. CMAJ 2001;164: 60-63

8. Horton R. Offline: Medicine and the Holocaust - it's time to teach. The Lancet 2019: Jul13: 394 (10193):105

9. Baycrest Hospital. Caring for Holocaust Survivors (see http://holocaust-survivors.baycrest.org/)

GLOSSARY: MEDICAL TERMS AND THEIR MEANING

Ronald M. Caplan, MD, CM, FACS, FACOG, FRCS(C)

ABSCOPAL EFFECT: Radiation given to a targeted tumor causes untreated tumors elsewhere in the body to shrink.
https://www.ncbi.nlm.nih.gov/pmc/articles/PMC6775241/

ACCOUNTABLE CARE ORGANIZATION (ACO): Medical provider organization that incentivizes cost and quality control, for example by reducing inpatient utilization and specialist referrals. Includes **Medicare Shared Savings Program (MSSP),** which sets a target cost of care for patients.

ACE INHIBITOR: Drug that inhibits the angiotensin-converting enzyme, stopping the formation of Angiotensin II which constricts blood vessels. Blood pressure is lowered, because blood vessels are opened up, and blood can flow more freely.
http://www.medicinenet.com/ace_inhibitors/article.htm
https://www.webmd.com/heart-disease/guide/medicine-ace-inhibitors#1
https://www.bmj.com/content/363/bmj.k4209

ACETYLCHOLINE: A neurotransmitter.
http://www.ncbi.nlm.nih.gov/books/NBK11143/

ACNE: Chronic skin condition characterized by seborrhea (oily secretion) and blocked follicles (comedomes) including blackheads and whiteheads that may become infected.
https://online.epocrates.com/diseases/10111/Acne-vulgaris/Key-Highlights

ACRYLAMIDE: Chemical that can form during high heat food preparation of high starch foods from the amino acid asparagine in combination with some sugars. Possible carcinogen in high doses.
https://www.cancer.gov/about-cancer/causes-prevention/risk/diet/acrylamide-fact-sheet

ACUTE FLACCID MYELITIS: Post-viral neurologic syndrome sometimes seen following COVID19 infection in young children largely in the three to six year old range https://www.mdlinx.com/news/physicians-issue-warning-about-rare-neurological-condition-expected-to-appear-this-fall/41HVQbOXEV8SDxaEXYnegB?i-post_environment=m3usainc&iqs=9z2z6d5v1f2le52i8k9pvb8c2ksg7hbdc6ovbphn-b90&utm_medium=email&utm_campaign=All%

ADDICTION: Physiologic compulsive need for a substance, use of that substance, inability to abstain, development of tolerance to it, and distinctive withdrawal symptoms and signs. See "**Opioid**".
https://www.cdc.gov/drugoverdose/index.html

ADHESION: Abnormal union of surfaces, or fibrous tissue bands between structures.
https://www.ncbi.nlm.nih.gov/pmc/articles/PMC5295619/

ADOPTIVE CELL TRANSFER (ACT): Use of **Tumor-Infiltrating Lymphocytes (TILs)** to overcome immunosuppressive signals and eradicate cancer cells.
https://www.cancer.gov/about-cancer/treatment/types/immunotherapy

ADVANCE DIRECTIVE: Legal document that ensures one's wishes are followed in the event a person cannot make their own decisions. See: The Care of the Older Person: How do I protect my patient?: Randy S. Perskin. RMC Publishing, LLC www.careoftheolderperson.com
https://ag.ny.gov/sites/default/files/advancedirectives.pdf

AGING: Gradual loss of physiological functions accompanied by increasing risk of mortality and decreasing fertility. The Rate of Aging is the ratio between damage accumulation and compensatory mechanisms. See: The Care of the Older Person: Introduction: Jose Morais. RMC Publishing, LLC www.careoftheolderperson.com
http://journal.frontiersin.org/article/10.3389/fgene.2016.00119/full
https://www.nature.com/articles/s41551-017-0093?WT.mc_id=EMI_NBME_1707_JULYISSUE_PORTFOLIO&spMailingID=54556746&spUserID=MTc-

3MDI4ODk5NQS2&spJobID=1203835636&spReportId=MTIwMzgzNTYzNgS2
https://jamanetwork.com/journals/jama/article-abstract/2703112?utm_
source=silverchair&utm_medium=email&utm_campaign=article_alert-jama&utm_
content=olf&utm_term=091718
https://www.frontiersin.org/articles/10.3389/fimmu.2019.01614/full?utm_
source=F-AAE&utm_medium=EMLF&utm_campaign=MRK_1046250_35_Immu-
no_20190718_arts_A

AGONIST: Exogenous substance that goes to a cell receptor and produces a response.
https://en.wikipedia.org/wiki/Agonist

AIDS: **A**utoimmune **D**eficiency **S**yndrome: Sexually transmitted infection caused
by **H**uman **I**mmunodeficiency **V**iruses HIV-1 and HIV-2 which compromise the
immune system.
https://www.aids.gov/
http://www.thelancet.com/journals/lancet/article/PIIS0140-6736(14)60164-1/fulltext
https://jamanetwork.com/journals/jama/article-abstract/2703112?utm_
source=silverchair&utm_medium=email&utm_campaign=article_alert-
jama&utm_content=olf&utm_term=091718
https://jamanetwork.com/journals/jama/article-abstract/2678246?utmsource=
silverchair&utmmedium=email&utmcampaign=articlealert-jama&utmcontent=

AKATHISIA: A movement disorder with restlessness that may be a drug side effect.
See: The Care of the Older Person: Psycho oncology: Living with the Fear of Death:
Norman Straker. RMC Publishing, LLC 2018, 2019 www.careoftheolderperson.com
https://www.ncbi.nlm.nih.gov/pmc/articles/PMC1123446/

ALBUMIN: Water soluble single chain protein synthesized in liver. Present in egg
white and blood serum.
http://albumin.org/properties-of-human-serum-albumin-and-albumin-atomic-
coordinates/

ALDOSTERONE: Mineralocorticoid hormone from adrenal cortex. Increases
blood pressure. Implication in alopecia.
https://en.wikipedia.org/wiki/Aldosterone

ALGORITHM: Set of instructions to perform a specific task. **DATA-DRIVEN
AlGORITHM: Machine Learning** utilized to design algorithm, with data to learn

from, and ongoing data collection.
https://www.techopedia.com/definition/3739/algorithm https://ieeexplore.
ieee.org/stamp/stamp.jsp?arnumber=8290925

ALKALINE PHOSPHATASE: Immune protein enzymes that catalyze the
hydrolysis of phosphate groups, freeing inorganic phosphate.
http://journal.frontiersin.org/article/10.3389/fimmu.2017.00897/full?utm_
source=F-AAE&utm_medium=EMLF&utm_campaign=MRK_352999_35_
Immuno_20170808_arts_A

ALLELE: One of the two forms of a gene, derived from either the mother or the
father. Genes are carried on chromosomes. Chromosomes are paired, with one
chromosome in each pair coming from the father, and one coming from the mother.
http://mcat-review.org/genetics.php

ALLOGRAFT: Transplant from human donor to genetically nonidentical human
recipient.
http://ndt.oxfordjournals.org/content/early/2013/04/25/ndt.gft087.full.pdf

ALOPECIA: Baldness
https://www.ncbi.nlm.nih.gov/pmc/articles/PMC3149477/

ALZHEIMER'S DISEASE: AD. Common form of dementia. One characteristic is
amyloid plaque deposition in the brain. See: The Care of the Older Person: Update
On Alzheimer's Disease Diagnosis and Management: Serge Gauthier: Doctor, My
Wife Is Getting Forgetful: Serge Gauthier: Why Does My Patient Have Gait And Balance Disorders ?: Olivier Beauchet; Incontinence In Older Adults: Samer Shamout,
Lysanne Campeau, RMC Publishing, LLC www.careoftheolderperson.com
http://www.thelancet.com/journals/laneur/article/PIIS1474-4422(16)00062-4/abstract
http://www.ncbi.nlm.nih.gov/pubmed/24028956
http://www.nature.com/nature/journal/v537/n7618/full/537036a.html?WT.
feed_name=subjects_neuroscience
http://www.jwatch.org/na42506/2016/10/06/new-biologic-treatment-dramati-
cally-shrinks-plaques
https://www.ncbi.nlm.nih.gov/pubmed/27025652
http://www.nature.com/neuro/multimedia/alzheimers/index.html?WT.mc_
id=BAN_NN_1612_Alzheimers
www.nature.com/neuro/multimedia/alzheimers/index.html?WT.mc_id=TOC_

NN_1216_Alzheimers&spMailingID=54002625&spUserID=MTc2NTUxNjM-5NAS2&spJobID=1160

https://pubs.acs.org/doi/10.1021/acschemneuro.8b00160

https://www.nature.com/articles/s41593-018-0101-9?utm_source=Springer_Nature_website&utm_medium=Website_links&utm_content=AngWan-SN-OD-Neuroscience-Global&utm_campaign=SNOR_USG_SFN18

https://www.alzheimersanddementia.com/article/S1552-5260(18)30068-2/fulltext?rss=yes

https://www.ncbi.nlm.nih.gov/pmc/articles/PMC6194148/

https://alzres.biomedcentral.com/articles/10.1186/s13195-018-0441-4

https://www.nature.com/articles/s41591-018-0311-4?WT.ec_id=NM-201901&sap-outbound-id=D7CBD8E437538AF66B-20183215057C627E43F6DB

https://jamanetwork.com/journals/jamaneurology/fullarticle/2722842?guestAccessKey=94b79aa8-7c1d-45f8-9e0b-545a2484647a&utm_source=silverchair&utm_campaign=jama_network&utm_content=weekly_highlights&cmp=1&utm_medium=email

https://www.nature.com/articles/d41586-019-00879-3?WT.ec_id=NATURE-20190321&utm_source=nature_etoc&utm_medium=email&utm_campaign=20190321&sap-outbound-id=01A2C014D0D47D9CED5

https://academic.oup.com/brain/advance-article/doi/10.1093/brain/awz099/5481202

AMINO ACIDS: The building blocks of protein. Some amino acids can be synthesized in the human body. Essential amino acids must be supplied in the diet, as they cannot be synthesized in the human body.
http://www.biology.arizona.edu/biochemistry/problem_sets/aa/aa.html

AMNIOTIC FLUID: The fluid surrounding the developing fetus, contained in the amniotic sac. The thin amniotic membrane is closely applied to the inner walls of the uterus.
http://iaimjournal.com/wp-content/uploads/2014/11/9-Amniotic-fluid-derived-stem-cells.pdf

AMYLOID: Beta amyloid. Protein fragments that can clump in amorphous plaques in degenerative disease.

https://www.nia.nih.gov/alzheimers/publication/part-2-what-happens-brain-ad/hallmarks-ad

http://www.nature.com/nature/journal/v537/n7618/full/nature19323.html

AMYOTROPHIC LATERAL SCLEROSIS: Motor Neuron Disease. Characterized by degeneration of both upper and lower motor neurons leading to muscle weakness and paralysis.

https://www.nature.com/articles/550S105a

https://www.ncbi.nlm.nih.gov/pubmed/17023659

https://jamanetwork.com/journals/jama/fullarticle/2724169?guestAccess Key=cefbe6c9-c210-49d6-aca6-9ebca2eaaf86&utm_source=silverchair&utm_medium=email&utm_campaign=article_alert-jama&utm

ANASTOMOSIS: Relinking of a tubular structure so that the lumen is patent.
http://plasticsurgery.stanford.edu/education/microsurgery/intraoperative.html

ANDROGEN: The "male" sex hormones. Present in women in different amounts than in males. In men, the testicles are the main source of androgens. In women, androgens are mainly derived from the adrenal glands that sit atop the kidneys, and from the ovaries.

https://www.britannica.com/science/androgen

https://www.frontiersin.org/articles/10.3389/fimmu.2018.00794/full?utmsource=F-AAE&utmmedium=EMLF&utmcampaign=MRK63294735Immuno20180508artsA

ANDROGEN RECEPTOR ANTAGONISTS: Drugs that competitively inhibit testosterone from binding to prostate cancer cells.

http://www.nejm.org/doi/full/10.1056/NEJMra1701695?query=main_nav_lg

http://www.nejm.org/doi/full/10.1056/NEJMoa1715546?query=main_nav_lg

ANDROSTENEDIONE: A form of androgen.
https://pubchem.ncbi.nlm.nih.gov/compound/androstenedione#section=Top

ANEMIA: Deficiency of red blood cells or hemoglobin.
https://www.jwatch.org/na45561/2017/11/29/anemia-elderly-review?query=etoc_jwgenmed&jwd=000012066693&jspc=OBG

ANEURYSM: Weakening in a blood vessel wall, leading to a bulge.
http://stroke.ahajournals.org/content/44/12/3613

https://journals.lww.com/cardiologyinreview/Abstract/2016/
03000/Abdominal_Aortic_Aneurysms_and_Risk_Factors_for.5.aspx
https://www.jwatch.org/na47426/2018/09/11/natural-history-small-ascending-
aortic-aneurysms?query=etoc_jwcard&jwd=000012066693&jspc=OBG

ANGINA (PECTORIS): Chest pain caused by inadequate oxygenation (ischemia) of, and circulation to heart muscle, secondary to arteriosclerotic disease in the coronary arteries which supply the heart.
https://emedicine.medscape.com/article/150215-overview

ANGIOGENESIS: New blood vessel formation.
http://www.nature.com/nrd/journal/v3/n5/full/nrd1381.html

ANGIOGRAPHY: Radiologic visualization of blood vessels after injecting them with radiopaque dye.
https://emedicine.medscape.com/article/1603072-overview

ANGIOPLASTY: The opening of a narrowed blood vessel by balloon inflation, along with stent placement to preserve patency.
http://www.ncbi.nlm.nih.gov/pubmedhealth/PMH0021296/

ANGIOTENSIN: A vasoconstricting hormone. Stimulates aldosterone release from the adrenal cortex.
http://www.ncbi.nlm.nih.gov/pubmed/8583476

ANGIOTENSIN RECEPTOR BLOCKER: ARB. Drug that blocks the angiotensin receptor.
http://www.ncbi.nlm.nih.gov/pmc/artichttps://www.bmj.com/content/363/
bmj.k4209les/PMC4395832/

ANHEDONIA: Loss of the capacity to experience pleasure. See: The Care of the Older Person: Psycho oncology: Living with the Fear of Death: Norman Straker. RMC Publishing LLC www.careoftheolderperson.com
https://www.medicinenet.com/script/main/art.asp?articlekey=17900

ANOREXIA: Eating disorder with self starvation and marked weight loss. The Care of the Older Person: Could My Patient Be Malnourished ?: Jose Morais. RMC Publishing, LLC www.careoftheolderperson.com
https://jeatdisord.biomedcentral.com/articles/10.1186/s40337-015-0040-8

ANOSMIA: Loss of the sense of smell. Can be a feature of COVID19
https://www.ncbi.nlm.nih.gov/pmc/articles/PMC7265845/#:~:text=Anosmia%20
is%20a%20prominent%20sign,also%20be%20presented%20%5B26%5D.

ANTHRAX: Serious bacterial infection caused by Bacillus Anthracis. Can be
acquired cutaneously, and via the respiratory and gastrointestinal tracts.
https://www.cdc.gov/anthrax/specificgroups/health-care-providers/index.html

ANTIBIOTIC: A drug that kills or inactivates bacteria. Often works by binding
and disrupting bacterial ribosomes (see "Ribosome")
http://www.nature.com/nrmicro/journal/v13/n1/full/nrmicro3380.html
http://www.nature.com/ja/journal/v67/n1/full/ja201349a.html
https://en.wikipedia.org/wiki/List_of_antibiotics
http://mdlinx.pdr.net/pharma-news/news-article.cfm/6885214/antibiotic-
resistant-bacteria-star-shaped-peptide

ANTIBODY: A substance that reacts with a foreign invader (antigen) inactivating it.
https://www.ncbi.nlm.nih.gov/pmc/articles/PMC4284445/
http://www.nature.com/milestones/mileantibodies/timeline/index.html

ANTIBODY-DRUG CONJUGATES: Antibodies linked to a toxic substance, such
as radioactive material, bacterial product, or chemical.
https://www.ncbi.nlm.nih.gov/pubmed/27299281
https://www.ncbi.nlm.nih.gov/pubmed/26589413
https://www.ncbi.nlm.nih.gov/pubmed/24423619

ANTIGEN: Foreign invader of the body.
http://www.annualreviews.org/doi/abs/10.1146/annurev-
immunol-032712-095910

ANTIMETABOLITE: Substance that interferes with cell metabolism by inhibiting
or replacing a normal metabolite. Used as chemotherapeutic agents in cancer.
http://www.ncbi.nlm.nih.gov/pubmed/23361267
http://www.slideshare.net/OribaDanLangoya/antimetabolites-in-cancer-
chemotherapy-23606975

ANTIMULLERIAN HORMONE: Produced by ovarian granulosa cells. Prevents
the depletion of follicles in the ovary.
http://www.ncbi.nlm.nih.gov/pubmed/22646322

ANTIOXIDANT: Substance that prevents the chemical combination of oxygen with various other substances, such as fats.
http://dspace.uni.lodz.pl:8080/xmlui/bitstream/handle/11089/17754/bartosz2.pdf?sequence=1&isAllowed=y

ANTISENSE TECHNOLOGY: Turning off genes by introducing pieces of the genetic code.
http://smart-therapeutics.com/Technology/RNAi-Antisense-Technologyb

ANXIETY: Feeling of unease that can rise to the level of panic attacks.   See: The Care of the Older Person: Late-Life Anxiety: Jess Friedland, Paulina Bajsarowicz, Philippe Desmarais. RMC Publishing, LLC www.careoftheolderperson.com
http://www.ajgponline.org/article/S1064-7481(16)30147-6/abstract

AORTA: The main artery from the heart to other parts of the body.
http://teachmeanatomy.info/abdomen/vasculature/arteries/aorta/

APHERESIS: Removing blood from the body for the purpose of eliminating a specific component, then reintroducing the blood into the body.
https://health.ucsd.edu/specialties/apheresis/Documents/2011%20
Conventional-apheresis-therapies.pdf

APOLIPOPROTEIN E (ApoE): Protein involved in fat metabolism. A variant is a disease risk factor.
http://www.ncbi.nlm.nih.gov/pubmed/11882522
http://www.ncbi.nlm.nih.gov/pubmed/16432152

APOPTOSIS: Programmed cell death
http://www.ncbi.nlm.nih.gov/pmc/articles/PMC2117903/
https://www.ncbi.nlm.nih.gov/books/NBK26873/
http://journal.frontiersin.org/article/10.3389/fimmu.2017.00961/full?utm_source=F-AAE&utm_medium=EMLF&utm_campaign=MRK_368025_35_Immuno_20170822_arts_A
https://www.frontiersin.org/articles/10.3389/fimmu.2018.00241/full?utm_source=F-AAE&utm_medium=EMLF&utm_campaign=MRK_571163_35_I
https://www.frontiersin.org/articles/10.3389/fimmu.2018.02379/full?utm_source=F-AAE&utm_medium=EMLF&utm_campaign=MRK_812127_35_Immuno_20181030_arts_A

APPENDICITIS: Inflammation of the appendix. Can be treated by minimally invasive surgery. Incidence has possibly been lowered with antibiotic use.
http://www.bmj.com/content/357/bmj.j1703.full

APTAMER: Single stranded DNA or RNA molecule that can bind to preselected targets.
http://www.basepairbio.com/research-and-publications/what-is-an-aptamer-2/

AROMATASE INHIBITORS: The enzyme aromatase catalyzes conversion of testosterone to estradiol. Aromatase inhibitors are drugs that prevent this type of estradiol formation.
http://www.nature.com/nrc/journal/v15/n5/abs/nrc3920.html
http://erc.endocrinology-journals.org/content/20/4/R183.full

ARRHYTHMIA: (Cardiac) Abnormal beating of the heart. Includes tachycardia (abnormally fast heartbeat), bradycardia (abnormally slow heartbeat) and irregular heartbeats.
http://www.clevelandclinicmeded.com/medicalpubs/diseasemanagement/cardiology/cardiac-arrhythmias/

ART: **A**dvanced **A**ssisted **R**eproductive **T**echnology. Techniques that enhance the ability to conceive children, including ovum and sperm retrieval, and ICSI.
http://www.cdc.gov/reproductivehealth/infertility/
http://www.hfea.gov.uk/ICSI.html

ARTERIOSCLEROSIS: Literal meaning is hardening of the arteries. In **atherosclerosis**, a common type, calcified fat deposits build up in the lining of arteries, narrowing and obstructing them.
http://www.ncbi.nlm.nih.gov/pubmed/11001066
http://bmcmedicine.biomedcentral.com/articles/10.1186/1741-7015-11-117

ARTERY: A blood vessel that usually carries oxygenated blood from the heart to other areas of the body. Exceptions are the pulmonary artery, which carries blood from the heart to the lungs for oxygenation, and the umbilical arteries in the fetus, which carry blood from the fetus to the placenta for oxygenation.
https://training.seer.cancer.gov/anatomy/cardiovascular/blood/classification.html

ARTHRITIS: A group of conditions of varying etiology characterized by inflammation in the joints.

http://www.rheumatology.org/Practice-Quality/Clinical-Support/Criteria/ACR-Endorsed-Criteria

ARTHROSCOPY: Direct visualization into the joints by minimally invasive technique.
http://www.arthroscopytechniques.org/
http://www.bmj.com/content/357/bmj.j1982

ARTIFICIAL HEART: Mechanical device that replaces the heart. **Mechanical Cardiac Support** refers to devices that assist the failing heart.
https://www.nature.com/articles/d41586-018-07197-0?WT.mc_id=EMX_NJOBS_1103_NATUREJOBSNEWSLETTER_A&WT.ec_id=EXTERNAL&spMailingID=57708268&spUserID=NjYxMzYyNDIyMjIS1&spJobID=1520347411&spReportId=MTUyMDM0NzQxMQS2
http://www.jhltonline.org/article/S1053-2498(14)00976-0/abstract

ARTIFICIAL INTELLIGENCE: Computer systems able to perform tasks normally attributable to human intelligence. These include visual perception, speech recognition, decision-making and language translation. Ideally, the computer systems would think and act humanly and rationally. Utilizes **Machine Learning** in which data is fed to a computer and statistical techniques are used to help the computer get better at a task without specifically programming it for that. **Deep Learning** is a type of machine learning that runs data inputs through multiple layers of biologically inspired neural network architecture. See **DEEP LEARNING, MACHINE LEARNING**
https://www.lexico.com/definition/artificial_intelligence
https://builtin.com/artificial-intelligence

ASBESTOS: A mined mineral formerly used for insulation and fireproofing. Fibers can be released into the air which can be responsible for asbestosis, a serious lung disease.
http://www.ncbi.nlm.nih.gov/pubmed/25444537

ASTROCYTES: Cells in the brain between neurons.
https://www.nature.com/articles/d41586-018-07197-0?WT.

ATHEROSCLEROSIS: See "Arteriosclerosis"
http://www.atherosclerosis-journal.com/

ATP: **A**denosine **T**ri**p**hosphate: A nucleotide involved in intracellular energy transfer.
https://pubchem.ncbi.nlm.nih.gov/compound/Adenosine_triphosphate

ATROPHY: Wasting of body tissue. **SARCOPENIA** is the loss of skeletal muscle mass and function. **CACHEXIA,** which incorporates sarcopenia, is a complex metabolic wasting syndrome associated with underlying disease, characterized by unwanted weight loss, muscle atrophy, fatigue, weakness, and loss of appetite.
https://www.ncbi.nlm.nih.gov/pubmed/22773188
https://www.ncbi.nlm.nih.gov/pmc/articles/PMC3940510/
https://www.ncbi.nlm.nih.gov/pubmed/20886766
https://www.ncbi.nlm.nih.gov/pmc/articles/PMC4269139/
https://www.ncbi.nlm.nih.gov/pmc/articles/PMC3117995/

AURA: A perceptual disturbance.
http://www.medicinenet.com/script/main/art.asp?articlekey=2395

AUTOANTIBODY: Immune protein (mainly IgM) produced by the immune system that is directed against (targets) an individual's own proteins, tissues, or organs
https://www.ncbi.nlm.nih.gov/pmc/articles/PMC2703183/
http://journal.frontiersin.org/article/10.3389/fimmu.2017.00603/full?utm_source=F-AAE&utm_medium=EMLF&utm_campaign=MRK_294450_35_Immuno_20170608_arts_A

AUTOIMMUNE DISEASES: Diseases in which the immune response is inappropriately triggered and attacks the individual's own tissues and organs. Includes systemic lupus erythematosus, rheumatoid arthritis, multiple sclerosis and Sjogren's syndrome.
http://www.nature.com/nm/journal/v21/n7/full/nm.3897.html
http://journal.frontiersin.org/article/10.3389/fimmu.2016.00587/full?utm_source=newsletter&utm_medium=email&utm_campaign=Immunology-w52-2016
http://www.clevelandclinicmeded.com/medicalpubs/diseasemanagement/rheumatology/laboratory-evaluation-rheumatic-diseases/
https://www.ncbi.nlm.nih.gov/pmc/articles/PMC4122257/

AUTOPHAGY: Intracellular degradation delivering cytoplasmic constituents to the lysosome. May have implications in anti-aging and starvation adaptation.
http://genesdev.cshlp.org/content/21/22/2861.long

http://journal.frontiersin.org/article/10.3389/fimmu.2016.00657/full?utm_
source=newsletter&utm_medium=email&utm_campaign=Immunology-w1-2017

BABY SHAKING SYNDROME: Abusive head trauma. Brain tissue injury, as well
as hemorrhage and edema, may result.
https://emedicine.medscape.com/article/1176849-overview

BACTERIUM: (Pleural: Bacteria) An old name for a microscopic organism that can
be present in, or invade, humans. A pathogenic bacterium , or microorganism is
one that causes disease.
http://www.bode-science-center.com/center/relevant-pathogens-from-a-z.html

BARIATRIC (METABOLIC) SURGERY: Weight loss surgery for selected Type
2 Diabetics and obese patients. Includes gastric binding, stomach stapling, gastric
bypass, and stomach shortening sleeve gastrectomy.
https://asmbs.org/patients/bariatric-surgery-procedures

BASAL GANGLIA: Region at the base of the brain with clusters of neurons
including the caudate nucleus, putamen, and globus pallidus.
http://webspace.ship.edu/cgboer/basalganglia.html
https://nba.uth.tmc.edu/neuroscience/m/s3/chapter04.html

BASE PAIR: Two (out of four) **nucleic acid bases** on a rung of the spiral ladder of
DNA. The four nucleic acids involved are adenine (**A**), cytosine (**C**), guanine (**G**),
and thymine (**T**). They code the sequences of amino acids that, in turn, make up
the proteins.
http://www.dictionary.com/browse/base-pair

BETA BLOCKER: A drug that lowers blood pressure by taking up the receptor
sites that control blood pressure.
http://www.medicinenet.com/beta_blockers/article.htm

BETA CAROTENE: An antioxidant. Precursor of Vitamin A.
http://www.medicalnewstoday.com/articles/252758.php

BILE ACID SEQUESTRANT: Drug that binds bile acids in the intestine, so that
they are excreted.
http://www.medicinenet.com/bile_acid_sequestrants/article.htm

BIOENGINEERING: Rearranging DNA. Manufacturing recombinant DNA.
http://www.mdpi.com/journal/bioengineering

BIOFEEDBACK: Training to acquire voluntary control of a body function, such as heart rate.
http://www.ncbi.nlm.nih.gov/pubmedhealth/PMH0070200/

BIORHYTHM: Cyclic pattern of activity; recurring biologic process. See **Circadian Rhythm**

BIOSIMILAR: Product that is highly similar to an approved biologic product
http://www.fda.gov/Drugs/DevelopmentApprovalProcess/
HowDrugsareDevelopedandApproved/ApprovalApplications/
TherapeuticBiologicApplications/Biosimilars/default.htm
http://jamanetwork.com/journals/jama/fullarticle/2590051
http://jamanetwork.com/journals/jama/article-abstract/2590049

BISPHOSPHONATES: Class of drugs that prevent loss of bone mass by inhibiting bone resorption by blocking osteoclasts.
http://www.bmj.com/content/351/bmj.h3783

BLEPHAROPLASTY: Cosmetic eyelid surgery.
https://www.ncbi.nlm.nih.gov/pmc/articles/PMC2840922/

BLOCKCHAIN TECHNOLOGY in HEALTHCARE: Interoperable platform that memorializes every event or step ("Block") in a data stream, or chain. Implications in personalized medicine, research, and appropriate healthcare data sharing with enhanced security.
http://bulletin.facs.org/2017/12/blockchain-technology-in-health-care-a-primer-for-surgeons/#.WlezLK6nHX4

BODY MASS INDEX: BMI. A calculation of body fat. Weight (kilograms) divided by height (meters squared). The Care of the Older Person: Could My Patient Be Malnourished?: Jose Morais . RMC Publishing, LLC www.careoftheolderperson.com

BONE DENSITY: Measurement of Calcium and other minerals in bone.
http://www.ncbi.nlm.nih.gov/pmc/articles/PMC2685234/

BONE DENSITY SCAN: Low exposure Xray to measure bone density.
https://www.bones.nih.gov/health-info/bone/bone-health/bone-mass-
measurement-what-numbers-mean

BONE SCAN: NUCLEAR: Imaging bone after radiotracer uptake to identify
tumors, usually metastatic.
https://www.ncbi.nlm.nih.gov/pmc/articles/PMC4553252/

BOTOX: Botulinum **tox**in type A. Inhibits acetylcholine release.
http://www.ncbi.nlm.nih.gov/pmc/articles/PMC2856357/

BRCA GENES: Breast **Ca**ncer Genes 1 and 2. Inherited mutations that predispose to
breast and ovarian cancer. BRCA1 may increase risk of endometrial cancer as well.
http://oncology.jamanetwork.com/article.aspx?articleid=2531470
https://www.sgo.org/wp-content/uploads/2016/10/2016-SGO-Genetics-
Toolkit3.pdf https://jamanetwork.com/journals/jama/fullarticle/2748515?guestA
ccessKey=99eb27c0-0cd5-45e6-870f-b8251b23d4be&utm_source=silverchair&utm_
medium=email&utm_campaign=article_alert&utm_content=etoc&utm_
term=082019

BREAST CANCER: Malignant tumor in breast tissue.
http://www.jwatch.org/na44519/2017/07/06/asco-2017-report-breast-
cancer?query=topic_breastcan&jwd=000012066693&jspc=OBG
https://www.acog.org/-/media/Practice-Bulletins/Committee-on-Practice-
Bulletins--Gynecology/Public/pb179.pdf?dmc=1&ts=20170710T0228314803
https://tools.bcsc-scc.org/BC5yearRisk/intro.htm
https://insights.ovid.com/crossref?an=00006250-201709000-00035 https://
www.partnershipagainstcancer.ca/wp-content/uploads/2019/05/Breast-
Cancer-Surgery-Standards-EN-April-2019.pdf http://hormonebalance.org/
images/documents/Shyamala%2099%20Progesterone%20differentiation%20
Mammary%20gland%20JMGB&N_1311167749.pdf

BRONCHITIS: Inflammation of the bronchial passages.
https://www.ncbi.nlm.nih.gov/pubmed/23204254

BULEMIA: Eating disorder. Food consumption followed by self-induced vomiting.
https://www.ncbi.nlm.nih.gov/pmc/articles/PMC2927890/

BUNDLE BRANCH BLOCK: Delay in the pathway of electrical impulses to the left or right ventricle of the heart, resulting in a delay of contraction of that ventricle. http://www.acc.org/latest-in-cardiology/journal-scans/2016/08/05/11/45/effect-of-the-antihypertensive-and-lipid-lowering-treatment?w_nav=LC

CANCER: Malignant tumor (growth). The hallmark of cancer is its ability to invade normal tissue. Cancer can often metastasize, spreading to distant areas in the body. It is likely to recur even though it has been removed or destroyed at its initial (primary) site. The Care of the Older Person: Cancer in Older Adults: Doreen Wan-Chow-Wah, Cancer Screening in the Older Adult: Catalina Hernandez-Torres, Tina Hsu. RMC Publishing, LLC
www.careoftheolderperson.com
http://www.cell.com/cell/fulltext/S0092-8674(18)3032-7
http://www.cell.com/pb-assets/consortium/pancanceratlas/pancan/index.html
https://www.cancer.gov/about-cancer/treatment/types/targeted-therapies/targeted-therapies-fact-sheet
https://cancerstaging.org/About/news/Pages/-Cancer-Staging-Manual,-Eighth-Edition,-Just-Released-by-American-Joint-Committee-on-Cancer-(AJCC).aspx
http://www.jcso-ejournal.com/jcso/november_2016?pg=34#pg34
http://journal.frontiersin.org/article/10.3389/fimmu.2017.00374/full?utm_source=F-AAE&utm_medium=EMLF&utm_campaign=MRK_243180_20170411_arts
https://www.nature.com/articles/s41551-017-0067?WT.mc_id=EMI_NBME_1704_APRILISSUE_PORTFOLIO&spMailingID=53957850&spUserID=MTc3MDI4ODk5NQ
http://stm.sciencemag.org/content/9/400/eaan2966
http://science.sciencemag.org/content/early/2018/01/17/science.aar3247
https://www.empr.com/home/news/fda-approves-tumor-agnostic-oral-cancer-therapy-vitrakvi/
https://www.nature.com/articles/d41586-018-07602-8?utm_source=briefing-
https://www.nature.com/articles/d41586-018-07602-8?utm_source=briefing-dy&utm_medium=email&utm_campaign=briefing&utm_content=20181206dy&utm_medium=email&utm_campaign=briefing&utm_content=20181206
https://www.frontiersin.org/articles/10.3389/fimmu.2019.00467/full?utm_source=F-AAE&utm_medium=EMLF&utm_campaign=MRK_943967_35_Immuno_20190326_arts_A

https://www.frontiersin.org/articles/10.3389/fimmu.2019.00467/full?utm_
source=F-AAE&utm_medium=EMLF&utm_campaign=MRK_943967_35_
Immuno_20190326_arts_A

CANCER MARKER: Substances produced by tumor cells or by other cells in
response to a tumor. See: Tumor Specific Antigen (TSA).
https://www.nature.com/articles/s41551-017-
0065?WT.mc_id=EMI_NBME_1704_APRILISSUE_
PORTFOLIO&spMailingID=53957850&spUserID=MTc3MDI4ODk5NQS

CANNABIS: Plant from which cannabinoids are obtained. Tetrahydrocannabinol
(THC) is the principal psychoactive compound.
https://medicalmarijuana.procon.org/view.resource.php?resourceID=000141
https://www.ncbi.nlm.nih.gov/pubmed/16463612
https://www.frontiersin.org/articles/10.3389/fimmu.2018.02009/full?utm_
source=F-AAE&utm_medium=EMLF&utm_campaign=MRK_779779_35_
Immuno_20180927_arts_A
https://www.empr.com/drugs-in-the-pipeline/cannabidiol-cbd-ischemia-
reperfusion-injury-organ-transplantation-revive-therapeutics-orphan-drug/
article/813111/?utm_source=newsletter&utm_medium=email&utm_
campaign=mpr-dailydose-cp-20181109&cpn=obg
https://pubchem.ncbi.nlm.nih.gov/compound/cannabidiol#section=Substances-
by-Category
https://jamanetwork.com/journals/jamanetworkopen/fullarticle/2716990?utm_
source=silverchair&utm_medium=email&utm_campaign=article_alert-
jamanetworkopen&utm_content=olf&utm_term=113018
https://www.empr.com/features/medical-marijuana-clinical-practice-
geriatric-pain-insomnia-elderly/article/815102/?utm_source=newsletter&utm_
medium=email&utm_campaign=mpr-dailydose-cp-201812

CANNABIS WITHDRAWAL SYNDROME: Can include irritability, hostility,
nervousness, anxiety, sleeplessness, restlessness, appetite loss, depression,
shakiness, tremors, sweating, fever, headaches.
https://www.mailman.columbia.edu/public-health-now/news/more-one-ten-
heavy-cannabis-users-experience-withdrawal-after-quitting-cannabis

CARBOHYDRATE: Simple and complex sugars that are the energy source for the body. Excess carbohydrate can be converted to fat for storage.
http://www.fao.org/docrep/w8079e/w8079e0h.htm

CARCINOGEN: Substance or radiation that predisposes to cancer.
http://mdlinx.pdr.net/internal-medicine/news-article.cfm/6931990/?utm_
source=in-house&utm_medium=message&utm_campaign=mh-im-nov16
https://en.wikipedia.org/wiki/Carcinogen

CARPAL TUNNEL SYNDROME: CTS: Restriction of the median nerve by the transverse carpal ligament at the wrist resulting in compression neuropathy.
https://www.ncbi.nlm.nih.gov/pmc/articles/PMC3314870/

CAR-T: Chimeric **A**ntigen **R**eceptor **T**-Cell therapy: T-cells genetically modified to enhance tumor destruction.
https://www.cancer.gov/about-cancer/treatment/research/car-t-cells
http://www.nejm.org/doi/full/10.1056/nejmoa1407222#t=article
https://jhoonline.biomedcentral.com/articles/10.1186/s13045-017-0423-1
www.empr.com/news/first-gene-therapy-antigen-receptor-t-cell-acute-
lymphoblastic-leukemia/article/685222/?DCMP=EMC-MPR_DailyDose_
cp_20170830&cpn=obgyn_all
https://jamanetwork.com/journals/jama/fullarticle/2664338?utm_
source=silverchair&utm_medium=email&utm_campaign=article_alert-jama&utm_
content=olf&utm_term
The Promise and Challenges of CAR-T Gene Therapy | Genetics and Genomics | JAMA | The JAMA Network

CAT SCAN: Computerized Axial Tomography. An advanced, computerized imaging technique that very quickly takes serial Xrays through the body in thin "slices", so that very small abnormalities can be found. With a helical (spiral) three dimensional CAT scan the Xray tube revolves around the patient. A four dimensional CAT scan takes multiple images during phases of the breathing cycle, particularly useful in cases of lung tumors that have to be precisely localized and that move with respiration. The fourth dimension is Time.
https://radiopaedia.org/articles/computed-tomography
http://www.jwatch.org/na43480/2017/03/16/radiation-exposure-and-cancer-risk-
low-dose-ct-lung-cancer?query=etoc_jwgenmed&jwd=000012066693&jspc=OBG

CATALYST: A substance that facilitates a chemical reaction without being changed by that reaction.

CATARACT: Clouding, loss of transparency, of the lens of the eye.
http://www.webmd.com/eye-health/cataracts/extracapsular-surgery-for-cataracts

CAUTERY: (**Electrocautery**) Surgical destruction of tissue by direct current heating. **Electrosurgery** utilizes radio frequency (RF) alternating current to heat tissue.
https://en.wikipedia.org/wiki/Electrosurgery

CELL: The basic living microscopic structure in the human body. Each cell is surrounded by a cell membrane. Cells generally have a center, the nucleus, which is itself surrounded by a membrane. The nucleus contains the chromosomes, on which rest the genes.
https://en.wikipedia.org/wiki/Cell_(biology)

CEREBROVASCULAR ACCIDENT: See "**Stroke**"

CERVICAL CANCER: Cancer of the uterine cervix. Most often caused by specific Types of sexually transmitted Human Papilloma Virus (**HPV**), which can also cause **carcinoma of the penis**. Largely preventable by **vaccines**.
https://www.ncbi.nlm.nih.gov/pubmed/12120445
https://www.cancer.gov/about-cancer/causes-prevention/risk/infectious-agents/hpv-vaccine-fact-sheet
https://emedicine.medscape.com/article/2006486-overview

CERVIX: The mouth, or neck, of the uterus, projecting through the vaginal vault. Its opening is the cervical os.
http://www.obgyn.net/gynecological-oncology/identifying-squamous-cancer-colposcopy

CHECKPOINT: T-lymphocyte locus that can shut off T-cell and suppress the immune response. (See T-lymphocyte)
http://www.cgen.com/focus-areas/immuno-oncology/immune-checkpoints
http://journal.frontiersin.org/article/10.3389/fimmu.2017.00692/full?utm_source=F-AAE&utm_medium=EMLF&utm_campaign=MRK_307979_35_Immuno_20170622_arts_A

CHECKPOINT INHIBITOR:(Immune Checkpoint Inhibitor, ICI) Drug that blocks a checkpoint, allowing T-lymphocyte to respond to malignant cell. Ref: Pardoll, Drew: Nature Reviews Cancer 12, 252-264 (April 2012)
http://blog.dana-farber.org/insight/2015/09/what-is-a-checkpoint-inhibitor/
http://ascopubs.org/doi/full/10.1200/JCO.2017.74.6065
http://jamanetwork.com/journals/jama/fullarticle/2653953?amp;utm_source=JAMAPublishAheadofPrint&utm_campaign=08-09-2017
http://ard.bmj.com/content/76/10/1747

CHIMERA: A single organism composed of cells from different zygotes. A **chimeric gene** combines portions of different coding sequences to produce a new gene.
https://en.wikipedia.org/wiki/Chimeric_gene

CHIP: **C**lonal **H**ematopoiesis of **I**ndeterminate **P**otential: Acquired mutations in hematopoietic stem cells that accumulate in bone marrow, associated with an increased risk of heart attack and stroke.
https://www.ncbi.nlm.nih.gov/pmc/articles/PMC4961884/
http://www.nejm.org/doi/full/10.1056/NEJMoa1701719

CHOLESTEROL: Normally occurring lipoproteins in the body. If cholesterol levels, and levels of low density lipoprotein (LDL) are too high, atherosclerosis can result.
http://emedicine.medscape.com/article/121187-overview https://www.ahajournals.org/doi/pdf/10.1161/CIR.0000000000000625 https://www.ahajournals.org/doi/10.1161/CIR.0000000000000625

CHOLESTEROL INHIBITOR: Drug that inhibits the intestine from absorbing cholesterol.
http://www.health.harvard.edu/blog/pcsk9-inhibitors-a-major-advance-in-cholesterol-lowering-drug-therapy-201503157801

CHORIONIC VILLI: Microscopic projections from the placenta in which fetal blood circulates.
https://en.wikipedia.org/wiki/Chorionic_villus_sampling

CHROMATIN: The protein (**histone**)/DNA complex in the cell nucleus that forms the chromosome.
https://en.wikipedia.org/wiki/Chromatin

http://www.nature.com/news/plot-a-course-through-the-genome-1.22553?WT.
ec_id=NATURE-20170907&spMailingID=54864391&spUserID=MjA1NjIyNjc4OAS
2&spJobID=1244089361&spReportId=MTI0NDA4OTM2MQS2

CHROMOSOME: An elongated, stringlike structure in the nucleus of the cell that
carries the genes. There are forty six chromosomes in each cell, arranged in twenty
three pairs. One of each pair is originally derived from the mother, and one from
the father.
https://www.genome.gov/26524120/chromosomes-fact-sheet/

CILIA: Tiny hairlike projections on cells.

CIRCADIAN RHYTHM: Biologic process that exhibits endogenous circadian (24
hour, diurnal) cycle. Can be influenced by external factors.
https://www.ncbi.nlm.nih.gov/pmc/articles/PMC4353305/
https://en.wikipedia.org/wiki/Circadian_rhythm

CIRRHOSIS: Chronic degeneration of liver cells accompanied by fibrous scarring
of the liver.
https://www.niddk.nih.gov/health-information/health-topics/liver-disease/
cirrhosis/Pages/facts.aspx

CLAUDICATION: Pain in the legs, or arms, after exercising, usually a symptom of
peripheral arterial disease. See: **peripheral artery disease**.
https://www.mayoclinic.org/diseases-conditions/claudication/symptoms-
causes/syc-20370952

CLITORIS: The erectile organ above the urethral orifice at the entrance to the vagina.
https://www.ncbi.nlm.nih.gov/pubmed/23169570

CLONE: An exact genetic copy. An identical twin is a clone because the fertilized
egg splits in two. A fraternal twin is not a clone because two different eggs,
fertilized by two different sperm develop in the uterus at the same time.
https://www.genome.gov/25020028/cloning-fact-sheet/
http://www.cell.com/cell/fulltext/S0092-8674(18)30057-6

COCHLEAR IMPLANT: Medical device that replaces the function of the inner ear,
sends signals to the brain via the auditory nerve.
https://www.nidcd.nih.gov/health/cochlear-implants

CODON (TRIPLET): Sequence of three consecutive nucleotides. Part of the genetic code. There are sixty-four codons. Sixty-one code for specific amino acids. The other three codons are stop signals. See: **Nucleotide** https://www.genome.gov/genetics-glossary/Codon?id=36

COGNITION: Conscious mental activities of thinking, learning, understanding and remembering.
https://www.sciencedaily.com/releases/2016/09/160909095045.htm
http://psychcentral.com/lib/in-depth-cognitive-behavioral-therapy/
https://www.mdlinx.com/family-medicine/medical-news-article/2016/12/13/coffee-chlorogenic-acid-vascular-phenolics-flow-mediated-dilatation-fmd-/6965864/?category=last-month&page_id=1
http://journal.frontiersin.org/article/10.3389/fimmu.2017.01101/full?utm_source=F-AAE&utm_medium=EMLF&utm_campaign=MRK_398354_35_Immuno_20170921_arts_A

COGNITIVE IMPAIRMENT: Mild Cognitive Impairment (**MCI**) is a dysfunction of conscious mental activities with minimal impairment of the instrumental activities of daily life (IADL). In Amnestic MCI memory dysfunction predominates. There can be progression to **Dementia.** The Care of the Older Person: "Doctor, my wife is getting forgetful": Serge Gauthier ; Management of older patients in the Emergency Department: Cyrille Launay ; Assessment of decision-making capacity: Catherine Ferrier. RMC Publishing, LLC www.careoftheolderperson.com
http://n.neurology.org/content/90/3/126
http://n.neurology.org/content/90/13/e1158
https://academic.oup.com/brain/article/141/3/877/4818093

COLON, COLORECTAL CANCER: Cancer of the large intestine and rectum. Detectable at precancerous and early stage by colonoscopy and biopsy. Cancer markers can be used in screening.
https://www.ncbi.nlm.nih.gov/pubmed/26151224
https://emedicine.medscape.com/article/1948929-overview
https://cancerstaging.org/references-tools/quickreferences/Documents/ColonMedium.pdf
https://www.cancer.org/cancer/colon-rectal-cancer/detection-diagnosis-staging/how-diagnosed.html
https://gi.org/guideline/colorectal-cancer-screening-recommendations-for-

physicians-and-patients-from-the-u-s-multi-society-task-force-on-colorectal-cancer/

https://annals.org/aim/article-abstract/2726664/performance-characteristics-fecal-immunochemical-tests-colorectal-cancer-advanced-adenomatous-polyps

https://www.asco.org/practice-guidelines/quality-guidelines/guidelines/resource-stratified#/3494

https://www.asco.org/practice-guidelines/quality-guidelines/guidelines/resource-stratified#/34946

COLONOSCOPY: Direct inspection of the entire large intestine with a flexible fiberoptic instrument called a colonoscope.
http://www.asge.org/assets/0/71328/9cf71f1d-ef18-4a34-9259-31f487a6213c.pdf

COLOR FLOW DOPPLER: Ultrasound with color coding of blood flow velocity and direction. Doppler effect refers to the measurable difference in sound as it moves away.
https://123sonography.com/content/1821-principles-color-doppler

COMA: Deep, unarousable unconsciousness
https://www.medicinenet.com/script/main/art.asp?articlekey=2803
https://www.ncbi.nlm.nih.gov/pubmed/19001840

CONCUSSION: Traumatic injury to the brain.
https://www.cdc.gov/headsup/basics/concussion_whatis.html
https://www.cdc.gov/traumaticbraininjury/severe.html
https://www.fda.gov/NewsEvents/Newsroom/PressAnnouncements/ucm596531.htm

CONSCIOUSNESS: Awareness.
https://bmcneurosci.biomedcentral.com/articles/10.1186/1471-2202-5-42

https://plato.stanford.edu/entries/consciousness-neuroscience/

CORD BLOOD: Fetal blood in the umbilical cord. Can be banked in order to retrieve stem cells.
http://www.acog.org/Resources-And-Publications/Committee-Opinions/Committee-on-Genetics/Umbilical-Cord-Blood-Banking

COVID19: Corona Viral Disease caused by SARS-CoV-2 virus: Causative RNA virus of global pandemic that emanated from Wuhan, China in 2019. Affects multiple organ systems. Elders, and people with coexisting medical conditions, especially older persons in nursing homes and similar facilities, markedly vulnerable to severe sequelae and death.

https://www.nejm.org/doi/full/10.1056/NEJMoa2008457 https://www.cdc.gov/coronavirus/2019-ncov/lab/grows-virus-cell-culture.html https://www.uptodate.com/contents/coronaviruses

https://www.niaid.nih.gov/diseases-conditions/covid-19

https://www.frontiersin.org/articles/10.3389/fimmu.2020.01880/full?utm_source=F-AAE&utm_medium=EMLF&utm_campaign=MRK_1417202_35_Immuno_202009

https://pubs.acs.org/doi/10.1021/acsnano.0c06726

COX-1 INHIBITOR: Drugs including aspirin, ibuprofen, and Naprosyn are both COX-1 and COX-2 inhibitors, inhibiting cyclooxygenase-I as well as cyclooxygenase 2.

http://www.ncbi.nlm.nih.gov/pubmed/11566042

COX-2 INHIBITOR: Non-steroidal anti-inflammatory drugs (NSAID's). These drugs target cyclooxygenase-2 (COX-2) enzyme that encourages prostaglandin production, leading to inflammation and pain.

http://journal.frontiersin.org/article/10.3389/fimmu.2016.00375/full?utm_source=newsletter&utm_medium=email&utm_campaign=Immunology-w40-2016

C-REACTIVE PROTEIN: CRP. Plasma protein with increased concentration in the presence of inflammatory disorders. The Care of the Older Person: Could My Patient be Malnourished?: Jose Morais RMC Publishing, LLC 2018, 2019 www.careoftheolderperson.com

https://www.frontiersin.org/articles/10.3389/fimmu.2018.02745/full?utm_source=F-AAE&utm_medium=EMLF&utm_campaign=MRK_838932_35_Immuno_20181129_arts_A.

CRISP R: **C**lustered **R**egularly **I**nterspaced **S**hort **P**alindromic **R**epeats: DNA sequences found in genomes of bacteria. Segments of prokaryocytic DNA containing repetitions of base sequences, followed by segments of spacer DNA. Used in **genome editing**. Useful in detecting viral infection.

https://www.empr.com/news/vitrakvi-larotrectinib-advanced-solid-tumors-ntrk-gene-fusion-approval/article/816725/?utm_source=newsletter&utm_medium=email&utm_campaign=mpr-dailydose-cp-20181129&cpn=obgyn_all,obgyn_md,cambia_august201&hm

https://www.nature.com/articles/d41586-019-00601-3?WT.ec_id=NATURE-20190228&utm_source=nature_etoc&utm_medium=email&utm_campaign=20190228&sap-outbound-id=F3F53CF91C70386022609FDF29CEFA2072F7C0D6

CRISPR-Cas9: Complex of RNA and protein (nucleases): Recognizes sequence of bases in target gene. Cas9 (an enzyme) unwinds double helix. CRISPR RNA sequence binds to target. Cas9 cuts both strands of target DNA. In a modification, DNA sequences are not cut: the Cas9 enzyme carries a molecular switch that turns on target genes.

http://www.ncbi.nlm.nih.gov/pmc/articles/PMC4786927/

http://link.springer.com/article/10.1186/s12977-016-0270-0?view=classic

https://www.nature.com/articles/d41586-019-01824-0?WT.ec_id=NATURE-201906&sap-outbound-id=D57BDD0F2FB94BAE156838EBF274B4C29D863CA1&mkt-key=005056B0331B1ED782E8AD53A869855D

http://www.bloomberg.com/features/2016-how-crispr-will-change-the-world/

http://jamanetwork.com/journals/jama/article-abstract/2600454

https://en.wikipedia.org/wiki/CRISPR

http://journal.frontiersin.org/article/10.3389/fimmu.2016.00375/full?utm_source=newsletter&utm_medium=email&utm_campaign=Immunology-w40-2016

https://www.technologyreview.com/s/608350/first-human-embryos-edited-in-us/

http://jamanetwork.com/journals/jama/fullarticle/2646800?utm_medium=alert&utm_source=JAMAPublishAheadofPrint&utm_campaign=10-08-2017

https://www.nature.com/news/crispr-hacks-enable-pinpoint-repairs-to-genome-1.22884?WT.ec_id=NATURE-20171026&spMailingID=55217903&spUserID=MjA1

https://www.ncbi.nlm.nih.gov/pubmed/27052831

http://www.cell.com/cell/fulltext/S0092-8674(17)31247-3

https://www.extremetech.com/extreme/281232-chinese-scientist-reportedly-creates-genetically-engineered-babies-immune-to-hiv

https://www.technologyreview.com/s/612458/exclusive-chinese-scientists-are-creating-crispr-babies/amp/

CRYOSURGERY: Surgical destruction of tissue by freezing.
http://emedicine.medscape.com/article/1125851-overview

CUL DE SAC: Rectouterine peritoneal pouch between the posterior wall of the uterus and the rectum.
https://en.wikipedia.org/wiki/Recto-uterine_pouch

CYBERNETICS: Control and communication with living tissue, as with a chip implanted in a muscle.
http://www.asc-cybernetics.org/foundations/definitions.htm

CYST: A fluid-filled growth (tumor). May be benign or malignant.
https://www.ncbi.nlm.nih.gov/pubmed/21845969
http://www.pathologyoutlines.com/topic/ovarytumorwhoclassif.html

CYSTOCELE: Bulge of the urinary bladder into the anterior wall of the vagina.
https://www.niddk.nih.gov/health-information/health-topics/urologic-disease/cystocele/Pages/facts.aspx

CYSTOSCOPE: Operating telescope used to visualize the interior of the urinary bladder and the ureteral orifices. P. 237, 238. See : The Care of the Older Person: Incontinence in Older Adults : Samer Shamout, Lysanne Campeau. RMC Publishing, LLC
www.careoftheolderperson.com
https://www.ncbi.nlm.nih.gov/pmc/articles/PMC4457046/
https://en.wikipedia.org/wiki/Cystoscopy

CYTOKINE: Factor released by a cell that has an effect on other cells. Implications in aging.
http://www.ncbi.nlm.nih.gov/pmc/articles/PMC2785020/
http://journal.frontiersin.org/article/10.3389/fimmu.2017.00930/full?utm_source=F-AAE&utm_medium=EMLF&utm_campaign=MRK_352999_35_Immuno_20170808_arts_A
https://www.frontiersin.org/articles/10.3389/fimmu.2018.00422/full?utm_source=F-AAE&utm_medium=EMLF&utm_campaign=MRK_571163_35_I
https://www.frontiersin.org/articles/10.3389/fimmu.2018.00586/full?utm_source=F-AAE&utm_medium=EMLF&utm_campaign=MRK_608868_35_I
https://www.frontiersin.org/articles/10.3389/fimmu.2019.00480/full?utm_

source=F-AAE&utm_medium=EMLF&utm_campaign=MRK_943967_35_
Immuno_20190326_arts_A

CYTOPLASM: The contents of a cell outside the nucleus.
https://en.wikipedia.org/wiki/Cytoplasm

D-DIMER: Fibrin degradation product of blood clot degraded by fibrinolysis
that can be detected in blood after a pulmonary embolus (blood clot in the lung).
Reference values are adjusted for age.
https://www.google.com/search?q=d-dimer+definition+medical&rlz=1C1EJ
FA_enUS783US783&oq=d-dimer+definition+&aqs=chrome.1.69i57j0l5.64272j0j4&s
ourceid=chrome&ie=UTF-8

DEATH: Cessation of life https://jamanetwork.com/journals/jama/fullarti
cle/2769148?guestAccessKey=c234904b-79e4-4fa8-970e-dbac5739205a&utm_
source=silverchair&utm_campaign=jama_network&utm_content=ped_
weekly_highlights&cmp=1&utm_medium=email https://jamanetwork.com/
journals/jama/fullarticle/2769149?guestAccessKey=002dcb34-be0f-4f21-986b-
a78ed29ccb96&utm_source=silverchair&utm_campaign=jama_network&utm_
content=ped_weekly_highlights&cmp=1&utm_medium=email

DEEP LEARNING: Deep neural network model. Machine learning technique
analyzing large amounts of data, enabling prediction of outcomes (prognosis)
when new data is presented. May be used to predict cardiovascular disease risk by
observation of the eye retina, and to help clarify psychiatric diagnosis.
https://arxiv.org/abs/1708.09843
https://en.wikipedia.org/wiki/Deep_learning https://www.nature.com/
articles/s41746-018-0029-1 https://jamanetwork.com/journals/jamapsychiatry/
article-abstract/2664960https://jamanetwork.com/journals/jamapsychiatry/
article-abstract/2664960

DELIRIUM: Confusional state with altered attention and awareness. See: The Care
of the Older Person: How to Diagnose and Manage Delirium: Haibin Yin. RMC
Publishing, LLC 2018, 2019
www.careoftheolderperson.com
https://www.ncbi.nlm.nih.gov/pubmed/25300023
https://www.uptodate.com/contents/diagnosis-of-delirium-and-confusional-states

DELIVERY: The birth of the baby as it exits the birth canal.

DEMENTIA: Loss of cognitive functioning. Frontotemporal Dementia refers to a heterogenous group of conditions. See: The Care of the Older Person: Dementia: "Doctor, My Wife is Getting Forgetful": Serge Gauthier; How do I protect my patient? Randy

S. Perskin. RMC Publishing, LLC 2018, 2019

www.careoftheolderperson.com

http://www.ncbi.nlm.nih.gov/pmc/articles/PMC2211335/

http://www.bmj.com/content/347/bmj.f4827

https://www.jwatch.org/na45523/2017/12/05/healthy-life-healthy-brain-lifestyle-factors-and-dementia?query=etoc_jwneuro&jwd=000012066693&jspc=OBG

http://n.neurology.org/content/90/3/126

http://geropsychiatriceducation.vch.ca/docs/edu-downloads/depression/cornell_scale_depression.pdfhttps://jnnp.bmj.com/content/early/2018/08/26/jnnp-2018-318650

https://www.bmj.com/content/361/bmj.k1315

https://www.jwatch.org/na48784/2019/04/16/revisiting-plasma-total-tau-levels-dementia-biomarker?query=etoc_jwneuro&jwd=000012066693&jspc=OBG

DEMOGRAPHY: The study of groups of people and their environment.
http://www.pewresearch.org/fact-tank/2016/03/31/10-demographic-trends-that-are-shaping-the-u-s-and-the-world/

DEPRESSION: Depressive disorder marked by prolonged sadness, mood alteration, often with feelings of loss, anger and frustration. See: The Care of the Older Person: An Overview of Late-Life Depression: Artin Mahdanian, Silvia Monti De Flores. RMC Publishing, LLC 2018, 2019 www.careoftheolderperson.com
http://www.ncbi.nlm.nih.gov/pmc/articles/PMC2922383/
http://geropsychiatriceducation.vch.ca/docs/edu-downloads/depression/cornell_scale_depression.pdf https://ajp.psychiatryonline.org/doi/10.1176/appi.ajp.2018.17060595

DERMABRASION: Surgical procedure to remove skin imperfections by abrading the skin surface.

https://ajp.psychiatryonline.org/doi/10.1176/appi.ajp.2018.17060595

http://emedicine.medscape.com/article/1297069-treatment

DETRUSOR MUSCLE: Muscular coat of the urinary bladder. See: The Care of the Older Person : Incontinence In Older Adults : Samer Shamout, Lysanne Campeau. RMC Publishing, LLC

www.careoftheolderperson.com

http://emedicine.medscape.com/article/1949017-overview

DHEA: Dehydroepiandrosterone. Androgenic steroid hormone secreted largely by adrenal cortex.

https://en.wikipedia.org/wiki/Dehydroepiandrosterone

DIABETES MELLITUS: Chronic disease characterized by abnormally high blood glucose levels. See: The Care of the Older Person: How to manage type 2 diabetes in frail elderly patients : Young-Sang Kim, Jose Morais; Could My Patient Be Malnourished? : Jose Morais ; Frailty : Sathya Karunananthan, Howard Bergman ; Polypharmacy And Deprescribing In The Elderly : Louise Mallet. RMC Publishing, LLC www.careoftheolderperson.com

http://www.merckmanuals.com/professional/endocrine-and-metabolic-disorders/diabetes-mellitus-and-disorders-of-carbohydrate-metabolism/diabetes-mellitus-dm

http://www.onlinejacc.org/content/early/2018/11/23/j.jacc.2018.09.020

DIASTASIS RECTI: Widening of the linea alba ("white line") with separation of the rectus abdominis ("ABS") muscles

https://www.ncbi.nlm.nih.gov/pmc/articles/PMC5715079/

https://radiopaedia.org/articles/linea-alba

https://www.ncbi.nlm.nih.gov/pmc/articles/PMC3649122/

DIET: Food intake. See: The Care of the Older Person: Could My Patient Be Malnourished?: Jose Morais. RMC Publishing, LLC www.careoftheolderperson.com

http://www.pubfacts.com/detail/27465379/Relation-between-mealtime-distribution-of-protein-intake-and-lean-mass-loss-in-free-living-older-adu

http://jamanetwork.com/journals/jama/fullarticle/2636710

https://www.nature.com/articles/s41398-018-0293-5

DISEASE: Aberrant state of morphology or pathophysiology Boudreau, JD, Cassell, EJ, Fuks, A: Physicianship and the Rebirth of Medical Education. Oxford University Press 2018

DIURETIC: Drug that causes increased passage of fluid by the kidneys. See: The Care of the Older Person: Polypharmacy And Deprescribing In The Elderly: Louise Mallet; Incontinence In Older Adults: Samer Shamout , Louise Campeau. RMC Publishing, LLC www.careoftheolderperson.com
http://emedicine.medscape.com/article/2145340-overview

DNA: Deoxyribonucleic acid. DNA makes up the chromosomes that carry the genes. DNA is arranged in a distinctive double helix, three dimensional pattern. It resembles a tight spiral staircase, with rungs (steps) each of which holds two (out of four) nucleic acid bases, called **base pairs**.
https://www.genome.gov/25520880/deoxyribonucleic-acid-dna-fact-sheet/

DNA MICROARRAY: DNA Biochip. Collection of microscopic DNA spots on a surface. Used to measure gene expression patterns.
https://www.genome.gov/10000533/dna-microarray-technology/

DNA MISMATCH REPAIR: During DNA replication, erroneous insertion, deletion and misincorporation of bases can occur in the daughter DNA strand. Such errors can also occur during DNA recombination. DNA Mismatch Repair involves the recognition and correction of these abnormalities.
https://en.wikipedia.org/wiki/DNA_mismatch_repair
https://jamanetwork.com/journals/jamasurgery/article-abstract/2647248?utm_medium=alert&utm_source=JAMA+SurgLatestIssue&utm_campaign=15-11-2017
https://www.nature.com/scitable/topicpage/dna-is-constantly-changing-through-the-process-6524876

DNA PROBE: A highly specific test to detect the DNA of an individual, or a virus. It is used to detect the human papilloma virus (HPV) that is the usual causative organism of cancer of the cervix. The test is used in the criminal investigation of rape, and in identification. An individual male can be identified by the distinctive DNA in his sperm.
http://www.nature.com/subjects/dna-probesv

DOPAMINE: A neurotransmitter.
http://www.dictionary.com/browse/dopamine

DUODENUM: First part of the small intestine after the stomach.
http://emedicine.medscape.com/article/1948951-overview

DYSGEUSIA: Distorted sense of taste. Can be present in cases of COVID19.
https://www.ncbi.nlm.nih.gov/pmc/articles/PMC7308993/

DYSKINESIA: Abnormality of voluntary movement.
https://en.wikipedia.org/wiki/Dyskinesia

DYSMENORRHEA: Pain with menses.
https://academic.oup.com/epirev/article/36/1/104/566554

DYSPAREUNIA: Painful intercourse. See: The Care of the Older Person: After the Menopause: Ronald M. Caplan RMC Publishing, LLC
https://www.ncbi.nlm.nih.gov/pmc/articles/PMC2671314/

DYSPLASIA: An abnormal, benign, microscopic cell change that can be a precursor of cancer.
http://www.cancer.gov/publications/dictionaries/cancer-terms?cdrid=45675

ECTOPIC PREGNANCY: Pregnancy outside of the normal location in the uterus. Usually in a fallopian tube.
https://academic.oup.com/humupd/article/20/2/250/663951

EDEMA: Swelling by accumulation of fluid in tissues. See: The Care of the Older Person: Could My Patient Be Malnourished?: Jose Morais. RMC Publishing, LLC
www.careoftheolderperson.com
http://www.ncbi.nlm.nih.gov/books/NBK53445/

ELDER ABUSE: The intentional or neglectful causing of harm to an aging person See: The Care of the Older Person: Elder Abuse: Mark J. Yaffe. RMC Publishing, LLC
www.careoftheolderperson.com
https://online.epocrates.com/diseases/69735/Elder-abuse/Differential-Diagnosis
https://jamanetwork.com/journals/jama/fullarticle/2708121?utm_source=
silverchair&utm_medium=email&utm_campaign=article_alert-jama&utm_cont

ELECTROCARDIOGRAM: Noninvasive test that measures the electrical activity of the heart.

https://www.ncbi.nlm.nih.gov/pmc/articles/PMC1614214/

EMBOLIZATION: Therapeutic introduction of a substance into a blood vessel to occlude it. **Transcatheter Arterial Chemoembolization (TACE)** combines the introduction of therapeutic substances into a tumor in conjunction with occlusion of the blood vessels of the tumor.

http://www.hopkinsmedicine.org/liver_tumor_center/treatments/intraarterial_therapies/tace.html

EMBOLUS: Detached thrombus (blood clot) that travels through blood vessels to another site.

http://emedicine.medscape.com/article/300901-overview
http://emedicine.medscape.com/article/1916852-overview

EMBRYO: The developing baby in the uterus during the fourth to eighth weeks of development, to the end of the second month, by which time all major features of the body are recognizable. All the main organ systems in the body have been laid down by the end of the second month.

https://embryology.med.unsw.edu.au/embryology/index.php/Ultrasound
https://www.nature.com/articles/d41586-018-07317-w
https://www.nature.com/articles/d41586-018-07317-w

EMOTION: Affective state of consciousness. Feeling.

https://www.ncbi.nlm.nih.gov/pmc/articles/PMC3950961/

ENDOCRINE GLANDS: Glands that secrete (produce) hormones, including the pituitary gland at the base of the brain, the thyroid gland, the adrenal glands , the ovaries, and the testes.

https://en.wikipedia.org/wiki/Endocrine_gland

ENDOCYTOSIS: Active transport of molecules into the cell in an energy using process

https://www.ncbi.nlm.nih.gov/books/NBK9831/

ENDOMETRIAL BIOPSY: Surgical sampling of the uterine lining.

https://academic.oup.com/humupd/article/23/2/232/2632344

ENDOMETRIAL CANCER: Cancer of the lining of the uterus.
https://www.ncbi.nlm.nih.gov/pmc/articles/PMC5288678/

ENDOMETRIAL HYPERPLASIA: Benign overgrowth condition of the lining of the uterus with crowding of glands. **ATYPICAL (ADENOMATOUS) HYPERPLASIA** of the endometrium is considered to be premalignant.
https://pdfs.semanticscholar.org/3b81/8cfedf864fca863c378a8028f91e0280b299.pdf

ENDOMETRIOSIS: Abnormal deposition of endometrium outside the uterus.
http://www.gponline.com/clinical-review-endometriosis/womens-health/endometriosis-fibroids/article/1150448

ENDOMETRIUM: The lining of the uterus.

ENDORPHINS: Hormones that affect receptors in the brain. May reduce pain by binding to opioid receptors.
http://www.ncbi.nlm.nih.gov/pmc/articles/PMC3104618/

ENDOTHELIN I: A vasoconstrictor.
http://www.ncbi.nlm.nih.gov/pmc/articles/PMC3005421/

ENTEROCELE: True hernia of small bowel covered by peritoneum bulging into the vaginal vault.

ENTROPY: Measurement of molecular disorder or randomness in a system.
https://www.britannica.com/science/entropy-physics

ENZYME: An organic catalyst. Enzymes facilitate chemical reactions within the human body.
https://www.mcat.me/review/bb/enzyme-structure-and-function/

EPF: **Early Pregnancy Factor**. Pregnancy-specific protein that is present in pregnant woman's serum 48 hours after fertilization.
http://www.ncbi.nlm.nih.gov/pubmed/9196793

EPIDEMIC: Increase in the number of cases of a disease in a population.
https://www.cdc.gov/ophss/csels/dsepd/ss1978/lesson1/section11.html
https://www.hhs.gov/opioids/about-the-epidemic/index.html

EPIDIDYMIS: Duct behind the testis that carries sperm to the vas deferens.
http://emedicine.medscape.com/article/1949259-overview

EPIGENETIC CLOCK: Essentially refers to DNA Methylation Age. DNA **methylation**: adding a methyl group (CH3) to one of the bases of DNA: is an epigenetic mechanism involved in gene regulation.
https://www.whatisepigenetics.com/dna-methylation/
http://clinicalepigeneticsjournal.biomedcentral.com/articles/10.1186/s13148-019-0656-7 https://www.ncbi.nlm.nih.gov/pmc/articles/PMC6826138/

EPIGENETICS: Study of the processes that regulate the turning on and off of genes. http://epi.grants.cancer.gov/i/epigen-lg.jpg

EPIGENOME: Description of all the chemical modifications to DNA and DNA-associated proteins in the cell which alter gene expression. Epigenetic changes can drive aging. Much of the epigenome is reset when the genome is passed to offspring.
https://www.genome.gov/27532724/
http://www.nature.com/news/an-epigenetics-gold-rush-new-controls-for-gene-expression-1.21513?WT.ec_id=NATURE-20170223&spMailingID=53480287&spUserID=MjA1NjIyNjc4OA
https://www.nature.com/articles/s41467-020-15847-z

EPIGENOMICS: Analysis of epigenetic changes.
http://anatomyandphysiologyi.com/epithelial-tissue/

EPITHELIUM: A microscopic cellular covering of surfaces, including skin and mucous membranes.
http://anatomyandphysiologyi.com/epithelial-tissue/

EPITOPE: Antigenic determinant. The part of the antigen molecule that is recognized by the antibody, and to which the antibody attaches.
https://www.britannica.com/science/epitope

ERECTILE DYSFUNCTION: ED. Difficulty with achieving or maintaining penile erection. See: The Care of the Older Person: After the Menopause: Ronald M. Caplan RMC Publishing, LLC
http://www.bmj.com/content/348/bmj.g129

ERYTHROPOIETIN: Stimulates the formation of red blood cells. Produced by recombinant DNA technology.
https://en.wikipedia.org/wiki/Erythropoietin

ESTRADIOL: A form of estrogen produced in the ovaries.
https://pubchem.ncbi.nlm.nih.gov/compound/estradiol

ESTROGEN: Female sex hormones, mainly made in the ovary.
https://en.wikipedia.org/wiki/Estrogen
http://journal.frontiersin.org/article/10.3389/fimmu.2017.00108/full?utm_source=newsletter&utm_medium=email&utm_campaign=Immunology-w7-2017

ESTROGEN REPLACEMENT THERAPY: ERT. Treatment of menopausal symptoms, usually in conjunction with progesterone. See: The Care of the Older Person: After the Menopause: Ronald M. Caplan RMC Publishing, LLC www.careoftheolderperson.com
http://emedicine.medscape.com/article/276104-overview

EUKARYOTE: Any organism whose cells contain a nucleus which contains DNA within chromosomes.
http://www.dictionary.com/browse/eukaryote

EXERCISE (AEROBIC): Generally refers to sustained physical activity designed to promote oxygen utilization. The Care of the Older Person: Why Does My Patient Have Gait and Balance Disorders?: Olivier Beauchet. Physical Activity as a Countermeasure to Frailty: Guy Hajj Boutros, Antony Karelis: RMC Publishing, LLC www.careoftheolderperson.com
http://cardiology.jamanetwork.com/article.aspx?articleid=2530563
https://www.frontiersin.org/articles/10.3389/fimmu.2018.02187/full?utm_source=F-AAE&utm_medium=EMLF&utm_campaig
https://jamanetwork.com/journals/jama/fullarticle/2712935?guestAccessKey=c09863bb-66ff-4c16-88c3-06ab0357f57d&utm_source=silverchair&utm_medium=email&utm_campaign=article_alert-jama&utm
https://jamanetwork.com/journals/jamainternalmedicine/fullarticle/2714300?guestAccessKey=55c4f5ef-9957-470d-9691-071330b0644d&utm_source=silverchair&utm_campaign=jama_network&utm_content=weekly_highlights&cmp=1&utm_medium=email
https://jamanetwork.com/journals/jama/fullarticle/2712935?guestAccessKey=2364bbfc-d62a-4d49-9fdb-9d0114d00fc8&utm_source=silverchair&utm_medium=email&utm_campaign=article_alert-jama&utm_content=etoc&utm_term=112018https://n.neurology.org/content/92/9/e905 https://

jamanetwork.com/journals/jamanetworkopen/fullarticle/2724776?utm_source=silverchair&utm_medium=email&utm_campaign=article_alert-jamanetworkopen&utm_content=etoc&utm_term=030119

EXOME: All the **exons** in a **genome. Whole Exome Sequencing:** Identifies variations in the protein-coding region of a gene. Most disease-causing mutations occur in **exons.**
https://ghr.nlm.nih.gov/primer/testing/sequencing
https://jamanetwork.com/journals/jama/fullarticle/2769138?guestAccessKey=e9f01f60-c67f-4a71-8ee7-a0cbd1f876c0&utm_source=silverchair&utm_campaign=jama_network&utm_content=ped_weekly_highlights&cmp=1&utm_medium=email

EXONS: The pieces of DNA that provide instructions for making proteins
https://ghr.nlm.nih.gov/primer/testing/sequencing

EXOSOME: Extracellular vesical involved in cell communication and immune function. Role in cancer cells.
https://www.frontiersin.org/articles/10.3389/fgene.2018.00092/full

EXTRAPYRAMIDAL SYSTEM: Part of the motor system network incorporating the Basal Ganglia, involved with involuntary actions performed at a subconscious level. Distinguished from the tracts of the motor cortex that travel through the pyramids of the Medulla.
https://www.sciencedirect.com/topics/neuroscience/extrapyramidal-system

FABRY'S DISEASE: Alpha-galactosidase-A deficiency: enzyme utilized in lipid metabolism. Rare X-linked lysosomal storage disease.
http://www.ninds.nih.gov/disorders/fabrys/fabrys.htm

FALLOPIAN TUBE: The fine tubular structure arising from each side of the uterus near the fundus, ending in fingerlike projections called fimbria that are close to each ovary, essentially forming the "pickup" mechanism for the egg released at ovulation.

FERTILITY: The ability to conceive children.
http://emedicine.medscape.com/article/274143-overview

FERTILIZATION: The fusion of the ovum (oocyte, egg) and the spermatozoon (sperm).
https://en.wikipedia.org/wiki/Human_fertilization

FETUS: The baby developing in the uterus is known as the fetus from the beginning of the third month until the baby is born. The fetal period is the longest period of intrauterine life.
http://www.nature.com/news/secrets-of-life-in-a-spoonful-of-blood-1.21430?WT.ec_id=NATURE-20170209&spMailingID=53380605&spUserID=MjA1NjIyNjc4OAS2&spJobID=1101425398&spReportId=MTEwMTQyNTM5OAS2 https://www.nature.com/articles/d41586-018-07317-w

FHIT GENE: Fragile **hi**stidine **t**riad. Aberrant transcripts from this gene are found in some cancers, notably esophageal, stomach and colon cancer.
http://www.ncbi.nlm.nih.gov/gene/2272

FIBEROPTICS: Light images sent through fine fibers of glass or plastic.
http://www.laserfocusworld.com/articles/2011/01/medical-applications-of-fiber-optics-optical-fiber-sees-growth-as-medical-sensors.html

FIBRIN: In blood clotting, thrombin causes fibrinogen to polymerize, forming fibrin. Polymerized fibrin and platelets form a hemostatic plug , or clot.
https://www.britannica.com/science/fibrin

FIBROID: A benign solid tumor of the uterus.

FIBROMA: A benign solid tumor that can occur in the breast or ovary.

FISTULA: An abnormal passage from one body cavity to another, or out to the body surface.

FOLLICLE (OVARIAN): The fluid-filled structure surrounding the developing egg (ovum)in the ovary.
http://www.embryology.ch/anglais/cgametogen/oogenese02.html

FOMITE: Inanimate object that can be contaminated and transmit disease, eg countertop. https://www.google.com/search?q=fomite+definition&rlz=1C-1CHBF_enUS821US821&oq=fomite&aqs=chrome.1.69i57j0l7.7262j0j4&sourceid=-chrome&ie=UTF-8

FRAILTY SYNDROME: Weakness, slowness, minimal physical activity, exhaustion and low energy, weight loss. See: The Care of the Older Person: Frailty: Sathya Karunananthan, Howard Bergman; Critical Care of the Older Person: Astrid Pilgrim, Michael R. Pinsky; RMC Publishing,LLC www.

careoftheolderperson.com

https://jamanetwork.com/journals/jamasurgery/article-abstract/2656841

http://www.ncbi.nlm.nih.gov/pubmed/17634320

http://annals.org/aim/article-abstract/2668215/effect-physical-activity-frailty-secondary-analysis-randomized-controlled-trial https://documentcloud.adobe.com/link/track?uri=urn%3Aaaid%3Ascds%3AUS%3Af24df018-1e90-454d-af5f-7a345b6d5190

https://jamanetwork.com/journals/jamanetworkopen/fullarticle/2733174?utm_source=silverchair&utm_medium=email&utm_campaign=article_alert-jama

https://jamanetwork.com/journals/jamanetworkopen/fullarticle/2740784?utm_source=silverchair&utm_medium=email&utm_campaign=article_alert-jamanetworkopen&utm_content=wklyforyou&utm_term=08022019

FREE RADICAL: Short lived uncharged molecule.

https://documentcloud.adobe.com/link/track?uri=u

https://jamanetwork.com/journals/jamanetworkopen/fullarticle/2733174?utm_source=silverchair&utm_medium=email&utm_campaign=article_alert-jaman%3Aaaid%3Ascds%3AUS%3Af24df018-1e90-454d-af5f-7a345b6d5190

http://www.ncbi.nlm.nih.gov/pmc/articles/PMC3249911/

FSH: Follicle stimulating hormone.

http://www.ncbi.nlm.nih.gov/pubmed/9741710

GABA: **G**amma-**a**mino**b**utyric **a**cid. A neurotransmitter.

http://www.webmd.com/vitamins-supplements/ingredientmono-464-gaba%20gamma-aminobutyric%20acid.aspx?activeingredientid=464&

GALACTOGRAPHY: Mammography with injection of contrast to image milk ducts.

GAMETE: A germ (sex) cell: the female ovum, or the male spermatozoon.
https://www.khanacademy.org/science/biology/cellular-molecular-biology/meiosis/a/phases-of-meiosis

GENE: The determinant of human characteristics and behavior from a cellular level on upwards. Each gene is a section on a DNA molecule and usually resides at a specific point (locus) on a chromosome. Each gene has a counterpart on the other

chromosome that makes up the pair. The genes elaborate proteins.
http://www.ncbi.nlm.nih.gov/genbank/

GENE EDITING (**Genome Editing**): A form of **Genetic Engineering.** Insertion, deletion or replacement of DNA at a specific site on the genome using engineered nucleases ("molecular scissors") See **CRISP R**
https://www.technologyreview.com/s/608350/first-human-embryos-edited-in-us/
https://www.horizondiscovery.com/gene-editing
http://jamanetwork.com/journals/jama/fullarticle/2646800?utm_medium=alert&utm_source=JAMAPublishAheadofPrint&utm_campaign=10-08-2017
https://www.technologyreview.com/s/612458/exclusive-chinese-scientists-are-creating-crispr-babies/amp/?__twitter_impression=true

GENE EXPRESSION PROFILING: Measurement of activity (expression) of thousands of genes, giving a picture of cellular functioning. In breast cancer for example, identifies distinct molecular entities associated with differential prognoses and response to cytotoxic drugs.
http://www.ncbi.nlm.nih.gov/pubmed/11823860
https://www.mdedge.com/hematology-oncology/clinical-edge/summary/breast-cancer/optimizing-gene-expression-profiling-early?utm_source=ClinEdge_OP_cedge_110816&utm_medium=email&utm_content=Gene%20Profiling%20in%20Early%20BC%20|%20CTC%20Clusters%20and%20MBC%20|%20Impact%20of%20Chemo%20Events%20|%20

GENE SILENCING: Regulation of gene expression. siRNA: **s**mall interfering RNA potentially can inhibit genes in genetic disease (See RNAi)
http://www.ncbi.nlm.nih.gov/probe/docs/applsilencing/ https://jamanetwork.com/journals/jama/fullarticle/2712406?guestAccessKey=22414c3e-162a-4ff0-8b50-5477ff58735b&utm_source=silverchair&utm_campaign=jama_network&utm_content=weekly_highlights&cmp=1&utm medium=email
https://www.ncbi.nlm.nih.gov/pmc/articles/PMC5542916/

GENE THERAPY: Treating a disorder by inserting a gene into cells.
http://www.ama-assn.org/ama/pub/physician-resources/medical-science/genetics-molecular-medicine/current-topics/gene-therapy.page?

https://www.frontiersin.org/articles/10.3389/fimmu.2018.00554/full?utm_
source=F-AAE&utm_medium=EMLF&utm_campaign=MRK_589856_35_
Immuno_20180403_arts_A

GENETIC ENGINEERING: Manipulating the genome.
http://www.fda.gov/AnimalVeterinary/DevelopmentApprovalProcess/
GeneticEngineering/
https://www.frontiersin.org/articles/10.3389/fimmu.2018.00153/full?utm_
source=F-AAE&utm_medium=EMLF&utm_campaign=MRK_536191_35

GENOME: The complete DNA sequence. The human genome project deciphered
the complete DNA sequence of humans. **Whole Genome Sequencing** determines
the order of all the **nucleotides** in a person's **DNA.**
https://ghr.nlm.nih.gov/primer/testing/sequencing
http://www.ncbi.nlm.nih.gov/projects/genome/guide/human/

> **Next Generation Sequencing:** Technologies that sample multiple DNA
> sequences in parallel.
> https://www.cancer.gov/publications/dictionaries/genetics-dictionary/def/
> next-generation-sequencing

GENOTYPE: The individual genes of each person. The expression of the
person's genetic code. **SNP genotyping** refers to variations in Single Nucleotide
Polymorphisms between individuals.
https://www.niehs.nih.gov/news/assets/docs_p_z/snp_genotyping_508.pdf
http://www.nature.com/tpj/journal/v3/n2/full/6500167a.html
https://www.britannica.com/science/genotype

GERD: Gastroesophageal Reflux Disease.
https://gi.org/guideline/diagnosis-and-managemen-of-gastroesophageal-reflux-
disease/

GERIATRICS: Medical specialty that focuses on health care, diseases, and issues
of elderly people, and the aging process. See: The Care of the Older Person:
Introduction: Jose Morais. RMC Publishing, LLC www.careoftheolderperson.com
http://www.merckmanuals.com/professional/geriatrics/provision-of-care-to-
the-elderly/overview-of-geriatric-care

http://bulletin.facs.org/2016/12/improving-quality-in-geriatric-surgery-a-blueprint-from-the-american-college-of-surgeons/

GERONTOLOGY: The multidisciplinary study of aging and its issues in all its aspects http://biomedgerontology.oxfordjournals.org/content/59/1/M24.full

GEROPROTECTOR: Drug that targets the fundamental mechanisms of aging. https://www.nature.com/articles/d41586-018-01668-0?utm_source=briefing-dy&utm_medium=email&utm_campaign=20180215

GEROSCIENCE: The study of the intersection of aging, biology, chronic disease and health.
Covers Epigenetics, Inflammation, Adaptation to stress, Proteostasis, Stem cells and Regeneration, Metabolism, and Macromolecular damage. https://pubmed.ncbi.nlm.nih.gov/25417146/ https://www.nia.nih.gov/research/dab/geroscience-intersection-basic-aging-biology-chronic-disease-and-health

GLAND: Organ that synthesizes and secretes a substance required by the body. http://www.histology.leeds.ac.uk/glandular/exocr_endocr_properties.php

GLAUCOMA: Condition that causes optic nerve damage and vision loss, often by an increase in intraocular pressure.
https://www.ncbi.nlm.nih.gov/pubmed/24825645vg

GLOBULINS: Include **alpha globulins**, beta **globulin**, and **gamma globulin**, including **(Ig)A, (Ig)G: immunoglobulin G, (Ig)M, (Ig)E and (Ig)D** synthesized by B lymphocytes, important in the immune response. Identified by **serum protein electrophoresis**, which separates the proteins.
https://www.aafp.org/afp/2005/0101/p105.html
https://www.ncbi.nlm.nih.gov/pmc/articles/PMC2715434/
https://www.reference.com/science/gamma-globulin-2944770f90b33e6c?aq=Gamma+Globulins&qo=cdpArticles

GLOBUS PALLIDUS: A subcortical structure in the brain. Part of the basal ganglia. http://webspace.ship.edu/cgboer/basalganglia.html

GLOMERULONEPHRITIS: Lesions of kidney glomeruli (capillary networks that filter blood) resulting from deposition or formation of immune complexes. In the acute phase, hematuria (blood in the urine), proteinuria (protein in the urine), and

red blood cell casts in the urine are seen.
http://emedicine.medscape.com/article/239278-overview#a4
http://www.sci.utah.edu/~macleod/bioen/be6000/prevnotes/L18-kidney.pdf

GLP-1R: Glucagon-like peptide 1 receptor agonist. Used in treatment of Type 2 (adult onset) Diabetes.
http://www.diabetesincontrol.com/newly-updated-glp-1-agonist-medications-chart/

GLYCOENGINEERING: Altering a cell surface so that infused tumor-specific immunocytes can enter the tumor parenchyma (functional tissue).
https://www.frontiersin.org/articles/10.3389/fimmu.2018.03084/full?utm_
source=FAAE&utm_medium=EMLF&utm_campaign=MRK_889258_35_
Immuno_20190122_arts_A

GOITER: Enlargement of the thyroid gland.
http://www.uptodate.com/contents/clinical-presentation-and-evaluation-of-goiter-in-adults

GNRH: Gonadotropin releasing hormone from the hypothalamus.
http://emedicine.medscape.com/article/255152-overview

GRAFT: Healthy tissue taken from one part of the body to replace diseased or damaged tissue in another part.

GRANULOSA CELL: A cell in the lining of an ovarian follicle. Granulosa cells manufacture estrogen, and to a lesser extent androgens and progestins. Conversion of androgens to estrogen takes place in granulosa cells.
https://embryology.med.unsw.edu.au/embryology/index.php/Granulosa_cell

GREENHOUSE GASES: Include carbon dioxide, sulfur dioxide, nitrous oxide, methane.
https://www.epa.gov/ghgemissions/overview-greenhouse-gases

GROWTH HORMONE: Somatotropin. Secreted by the pituitary gland.
http://www.ncbi.nlm.nih.gov/pubmed/20020365

HCG: **Human chorionic gonadotropin**. Produced by the placenta.
http://www.fda.gov/Drugs/ResourcesForYou/Consumers/
BuyingUsingMedicineSafely/MedicationHealthFraud/ucm281834.htm

HEART FAILURE: Congestive heart failure. Heart muscle contraction not sufficiently strong to properly circulate blood. Fluid accumulates.
http://heartfailure.onlinejacc.org/article.aspx?articleid=1568320

HEMORRHAGE: Excessive bleeding.

HER-2 GENE: Human Epidermal Growth Factor Receptor-2. Linked to breast cancer.
http://www.cancer.gov/research/progress/discovery/HER2

HEREDITY: Parent to child transmission of traits, by inheritance of genes.
https://ghr.nlm.nih.gov/primer/inheritance/inheritancepatterns

HERNIA: Intraabdominal contents enclosed by peritoneum bulging into a weakened wall.

HEURISTICS: Strategies or mental processes used to quickly form judgments, make decisions, or find a solution to a complex problem by focusing on the most relevant aspects of the problem.
https://en.wikipedia.org/wiki/Heuristics_in_judgment_and_decision-making#:~:text=Heuristics%20are%20simple%20strategies%20or,situation%20to%20formulate%20a%20solution.

HIGH DENSITY LIPOPROTEIN: **HDL**. Complex of lipids and proteins that transports cholesterol in the blood to the liver.
http://www.ncbi.nlm.nih.gov/pmc/articles/PMC3787738/
https://www.jwatch.org/na45882/2018/01/17/continuing-enigma-hdl?query=topic_lipid&jwd=000012066693&jspc=OBG

HIPPOCAMPUS: Area of the brain involved with spatial memory which is important in navigation, and episodic memory (remembering autobiographical events). Located in the medial temporal lobe of the brain. Includes a gray matter ridge on the floor of each lateral ventricle.
https://en.wikipedia.org/wiki/Hippocampus
https://www.nature.com/nature/journal/vaop/ncurrent/full/nature22067.html
https://en.wikipedia.org/wiki/Episodic_memory

HIRSUTISM: Excess hair growth.
http://emedicine.medscape.com/article/121038-overview

HISTOCOMPATIBILITY: Antigenic similarities between tissue donor and recipient so that a transplant is not rejected.
https://www.hindawi.com/journals/jtrans/2012/842141/

HISTONE: Protein in chromosomes that binds to DNA, giving shape to the chromosome. Role in controlling gene activity.
https://www.cancer.gov/publications/dictionaries/cancer-terms/def/histone

HMO: Health maintenance organization. Essentially a health insurance plan.

HOLOGRAPHY: The scattered light from an object is captured, then illuminated by a beam. Multiple two dimensional pictures are assembled into a three dimensional display.
http://holocenter.org/what-is-holography

HOMEOSTASIS: State of balance with constant adjustment among body systems so that body can survive and function correctly. See: The Care of the Older Person: Critical Care of the Older Person: Astrid Pilgrim, Michael R, Pinsky. RMC Publishing, LLC www.careoftheolderperson.com
https://www.cancer.gov/publications/dictionaries/cancer-terms/def/homeostasis#:~:text=homeostasis%20(HOH%2Dmee%2Doh,to%20survive%20and%20function%20correctly.

HOMEOSTENOSIS: Decreased ability to maintain homeostasis under stress; a narrowing (stenosis) of reserve capacity. See: The Care of the Older Person: Critical Care of the Older Person: Astrid Pilgrim, Michael R. Pinsky. RMC Publishing, LLC www.careoftheolderperson.com
https://www.sharecare.com/health/aging-mental-health/what-ishomeostenosis#:~:text=As%20people%20get%20older%20or,homeostasis%20(balance)%20under%20stress.

HOMOCYSTEINE: Amino acid derived from the dietary amino acid methionine. Homologue of the amino acid cysteine.
http://www.ncbi.nlm.nih.gov/pmc/articles/PMC4146172/

HOMOGRAFT: Transplanted tissue from another human individual.
http://bja.oxfordjournals.org/content/108/suppl_1/i29.full

HORMONE: A substance formed in an endocrine gland and carried by the blood stream to other organs which it affects. Such organs are called end organs. For example, follicle stimulating hormone and luteinizing hormone from the pituitary gland act on the ovary, controlling ovarian secretion of estrogen and progesterone. Estrogen and progesterone act on the endometrium lining the uterus.
http://biology.freeoda.com/chemical_composition_of_the_hormones.htm
http://www.news-medical.net/health/Hormone-Interactions-with-Receptors.aspx

HORMONE REPLACEMENT THERAPY: HRT. Treatment of menopausal symptoms with estrogen and progesterone.
http://press.endocrine.org/doi/abs/10.1210/jc.2015-2236

HOT FLASHES: Sudden onset of a feeling of heat and flushing of short duration.
http://theoncologist.alphamedpress.org/content/16/11/1658.long

HUMAN CONNECTOME PROJECT: Mapping the human brain connectivity.
http://www.humanconnectomeproject.org/

HYALURONIC ACID: An anionic nonsulfated glycosaminoglycan. Component of skin.
http://www.ncbi.nlm.nih.gov/pmc/articles/PMC3583886/

HYDROFLUOCARBONS: HFC. Several organic compounds. Decreasingly used as refrigerants.
https://www.britannica.com/science/hydrofluorocarbon

HYPERGLYCEMIA: Abnormally increased blood glucose levels.
https://ccforum.biomedcentral.com/articles/10.1186/cc12514
http://joe.endocrinology-journals.org/content/204/1/1.full.pdf

HYPERPLASIA: Overgrowth of tissue. Increase in cellular reproduction rate.
http://journals.lww.com/jaapa/Fulltext/2016/08000/Benign_prostatic_
hyperplasia   A   clinical_review.2.aspx
http://emedicine.medscape.com/article/269919-overview

HYPERTENSION: High blood pressure. Sometimes defined as 130 mm Hg systolic (pressure during heart muscle contraction), and 80 mm HG diastolic (pressure during relaxation).
http://jaha.ahajournals.org/content/4/12/e002315.full

http://www.jwatch.org/na43262/2017/03/02/pharmacologic-treatment-hypertension-older-adults?query=etoc_jwgenmed&jwd=000012066693&jspc=OBG
http://hyper.ahajournals.org/content/early/2017/11/10/HYP.0000000000000065
https://jamanetwork.com/journals/jama/fullarticle/2664350?utm_source=silverchair&utm_medium=email&utm_campaign=article_alert-jama&utm_content=olf&u
https://jamanetwork.com/journals/jama/fullarticle/2664350?&utm_source=191323&utm_medium=BulletinHealthCare&utm_term=120217&utm_content=Mornin

HYPOTENSION, ORTHOSTATIC: Low blood pressure on standing.
http://www.ncbi.nlm.nih.gov/pubmed/27225359?access_num=27225359&link_type=MED&dopt=Abstract

HYPOTHALAMUS: Part of the brain below the thalamus. Forms the major portion of the ventral region of the diencephalon. Forms part of the wall of the third ventricle.
http://press.endocrine.org/doi/abs/10.1210/jc.2015-2236

HYSTERECTOMY: Surgical removal of the uterus.

HYSTEROSALPINGOGRAM: Injection of radiopaque dye into the uterus via the cervix to radiologically visualize the uterine cavity, the fallopian tubes, and their patency.

HYSTEROSCOPY: A minimally invasive surgical technique in which a fiberoptic telescope (hysteroscope) is introduced through the cervical os into the uterine cavity. The endometrial lining of the uterus and the interior openings of the fallopian tubes can be seen.

ICSI: Intracytoplasmic sperm injection.
http://americanpregnancy.org/infertility/intracytoplasmic-sperm-injection/

IMMUNE SYSTEM: The system that allows the body to ward off invasion by foreign substances, including infectious agents. Cells including T-lymphocytes that go to infected sites are elaborated in bone marrow and other areas. Antibodies (immunoglobulins) that target specific invaders (antigens) circulate in the bloodstream. Infected areas drain through lymphatic channels to the lymph nodes,

where invading organisms are processed.
http://emedicine.medscape.com/article/1948753-overview

IMMUNOCYTE: Leukocyte that induces immune response by antibody production in reaction to an antigen.
http://www.feinsteininstitute.org/programs-researchers/immunology/immunocytes-cytokine-biology/

IMMUNOGLOBULIN: Ig. Proteins that function as antibodies and bind to antigens.
http://www.ebioscience.com/knowledge-center/antigen/immunoglobulin.htm

IMMUNOME (CELLULAR): Immune cell subset phenotype and activation/functional status. Used to predict whether a patient will respond to immunotherapy.
https://www.frontiersin.org/articles/10.3389/fimmu.2019.01767/full?utm_source=F-AAE&utm_medium=EMLF&utm_campaign=MRK_1064098_35_Immuno_20190808_arts_A

IMMUNOSENESCENCE: Age associated immune change, notably with a reduction in peripheral blood naïve cells , and a relative increase of memory cells, along with the inflammatory changes that accompany aging, so-called **inflammaging**
https://www.frontiersin.org/articles/10.3389/fimmu.2019.02247/full?utm_source=F-AAE&utm_medium=EMLF&utm_campaign=MRK_1111535_35_Immuno_20191001_arts_A

IMMUNOSUPPRESSION: Suppression of the immune response.
http://emedicine.medscape.com/article/432316-overview

IMMUNOTHERAPY: Prevention or treatment of disease with substances that stimulate the immune response. Blocking the shut-off of the immune response. Anticancer vaccines.
https://www.mdanderson.org/treatment-options/immunotherapy.html
http://journal.frontiersin.org/article/10.3389/fimmu.2016.00621/full?utm_source=newsletter&utm_medium=email&utm_campaign=Immunology-w1-2017
http://journal.frontiersin.org/article/10.3389/fimmu.2016.00621/full?utm_source=newsletter&utm_medium=email&utm_campaign=Immunology-w1-2017
http://www.mdedge.com/jcso/article/135689/gastroenterology/meeting-potential-immunotherapy-new-targets-provide-rational/pdf?channel=213
http://journal.frontiersin.org/article/10.3389/fimmu.2017.00555/full?utm_

source=F-AAE&utm_medium=EMLF&utm_campaign=MRK_275249_35_
Immuno_20170518_arts_A
https://www.frontiersin.org/articles/10.3389/fimmu.2018.00384/full?utm_
source=F-AAE&utm_medium=EMLF&utm_campaign=MRK_571163_35_

IMPLANTATION: The sperm fertilizes (fuses with) the egg (ovum) in the fallopian tube. The fertilized egg then migrates from the fallopian tube into the uterus at a specific time , when the endometrium is most receptive, and attaches to and burrows into the uterine lining.

IMPRINTING: (Genomic Imprinting) The process by which only the copy of a gene from one parent gets switched on in an offspring.
https://www.genome.gov/27532724/
https://ghr.nlm.nih.gov/primer/inheritance/updimprinting

INDUCED PLURIPOTENT STEM CELLS: IPS. Cells from an adult human that have been reprogrammed into an embryonic-like state.
http://stemcells.nih.gov/info/basics/pages/basics10.aspx
http://www.nature.com/news/japanese-man-is-first-to-receive-reprogrammed-stem-cells-from-another-person-1.21730?WT.ec_id=NEWS-20170330&spMailingID=53740049&sp
https://www.nature.com/articles/d41586-019-00656-2?utm_
source=Nature+Briefing&utm_campaign=fb45cec6f6-briefing-dy-20190225&utm_
medium=email&utm_term=0_c9dfd39373-fb45cec6f6-42544483

INFARCT: Cutoff of blood supply causing tissue death, resulting in a scarred area.
http://www.omicsonline.org/biomarkers-in-acute-myocardial-infarction-2155-9880.1000222.pdf

INFECTION: Invasion of foreign organisms, such as bacteria or viruses, into the body.
http://www.ph.ucla.edu/epi/faculty/detels/epi220/detels_agents.pdf

INFLAMMATION: The body's response to infection or injury, including redness, swelling, and heat. The specific responses are geared to killing the infectious agent and repairing the damaged tissue.
http://journal.frontiersin.org/article/10.3389/fimmu.2017.00017/full?utm_
source=newsletter&utm_medium=email&utm_campaign=Immunology-w4-2017

INFLAMMAGING: Increasing chronic, sterile, low grade inflammation seen as aging progresses. Increased numbers of peripheral immune molecules in older people, with relevance to cognition and age-related disease. https://www.frontiersin.org/articles/10.3389/fimmu.2020.02045/full?utm_source=F-AAE&utm_medium=EMLF&utm_campaign=MRK_1429095_35_Immuno_20200910_arts_A https://www.nature.com/articles/s41574-018-0059-4 https://pubmed.ncbi.nlm.nih.gov/25417146/

INFLUENZA: Contagious respiratory illness caused by influenza virus. http://journals.lww.com/epidem/Abstract/2015/11000/Review_Article___The_Fraction_of_Influenza_Virus.13.aspxhttps://www.nature.com/articles/s41574-018-0059-4
http://www.cdc.gov/mmwr/volumes/65/rr/rr6505a1.htm

INFORMATION TECHNOLOGY: IT. Computerized paperless data keeping, analysis, and transmission.
https://www.intel.com/content/www/us/en/healthcare-it/collaborative-care.html?cid=sem43700013297809532&intel_term=technology+for+healthcare&gclid=Cj0KEQjw6am-BRCTk4WZhLfd4-oBEiQA3ydA3lK6NZjCN51AIK72GMKucyGNX297Xgy6h66th96XBwcaAhYO8P8HAQ&gclsrc=aw.ds

INHIBINS: Peptides made in granulosa cells of ovarian follicles that inhibit secretion of follicle stimulating hormone (FSH).
http://www.medicinenet.com/script/main/art.asp?articlekey=22571
http://press.endocrine.org/doi/abs/10.1210/endo-124-1-552

INSOMNIA: Sleeplessness.

INSULIN: Polypeptide hormone, produced by the beta cells of the islets of Langerhans in the pancreas, that regulates blood glucose
http://onlinelibrary.wiley.com/doi/10.1002/bip.20734/full

INSULIN RESISTANCE: Lowered level of response to insulin.
http://emedicine.medscape.com/article/122501-overview

INTEGRIN: A receptor glycoprotein on a cell surface involved in the adhesion of the cell to other cells such as T-cells.
https://www.ncbi.nlm.nih.gov/books/NBK26867/

INTELLIGENCE: Ability to acquire and apply knowledge and skills.
https://www.lexico.com/en/definition/intelligence

INTERFERON: A protein that can inhibit virus replication.
https://www.drugs.com/drug-class/interferons.html
http://journal.frontiersin.org/article/10.3389/fimmu.2017.00062/full?utm_source=newsletter&utm_medium=email&utm_campaign=Immunology-w7-2017

INTERSTITIAL CYSTITIS: Painful Bladder Syndrome (BPS).
http://emedicine.medscape.com/article/2055505-overview

INTERSTITIAL SPACE: Small, narrow, fluid containing space between tissues
https://www.ncbi.nlm.nih.gov/pmc/articles/PMC3139075/
https://www.thefreedictionary.com/interstitial+space

INTERSTITIUM: Fluid filled interstitial space draining to lymph nodes, supported by a network of collagen bundles. Visualized by laser endomicroscopy in relation to the extrahepatic bile duct, and other tissues that are subject to intermittent compression, including the submucosa of the gastrointestinal tract, and the urinary bladder.
https://www.nature.com/articles/s41598-018-23062-6

INTRAUTERINE ENVIRONMENT: The environment in which the growing fetus lives.

INTRAUTERINE GROWTH RETARDATION: IUGR. Fetal growth restriction.
http://www.uptodate.com/contents/fetal-growth-restriction-evaluation-and-management

ISCHEMIA: Inadequate blood supply to an organ, resulting in inadequate oxygenation.

KAPOSI'S SARCOMA: Malignancy with cutaneous lesions caused by HHV8: human herpesvirus 8. Tends to occur in immunosuppressed individuals, notably those with AIDS (Autoimmune Deficiency Syndrome).
http://emedicine.medscape.com/article/279734-overview

KERATOPLASTY: Conductive keratoplasty. CK. Eye surgery utilizing radio frequency energy to change the shape of the cornea.

KILLER CELL: Natural killer (**NK**) cells are derived from hematopoietic stem cells in bone marrow. They kill cancer cells by secreting **perforins** (cytolytic proteins) and **granzymes** (proteases : enzymes that catalyze degradation of protein)

https://www.ncbi.nlm.nih.gov/pmc/articles/PMC4346487/

https://en.wikipedia.org/wiki/Granzyme

http://medical-dictionary.thefreedictionary.com/perforin

http://www.dictionary.com/browse/protease

http://journal.frontiersin.org/article/10.3389/fimmu.2016.00492/full

http://journal.frontiersin.org/article/10.3389/fimmu.2017.00293/full?utm_source=newsletter&utm_medium=email&utm_campaign=Immunology-w12-2017

http://journal.frontiersin.org/article/10.3389/fimmu.2017.00683/full?utm_source=F-AAE&utm_medium=EMLF&utm_campaign=MRK_307979_35_Immuno_20170622_arts_A

http://journal.frontiersin.org/article/10.3389/fimmu.2017.00760/full?utm_source=F-AAE&utm_medium=EMLF&utm_campaign=MRK_320984_35_Immuno_20170706_arts_A

http://journal.frontiersin.org/article/10.3389/fimmu.2017.00930/full?utm_source=F-AAE&utm_medium=EMLF&utm_campaign=MRK_352999_35_Immuno_20170808_arts_A

http://journal.frontiersin.org/article/10.3389/fimmu.2017.00774/full?utm_source=F-AAE&utm_medium=EMLF&utm_campaign=MRK_333189_35_Immuno_20170720_arts_A

http://journal.frontiersin.org/article/10.3389/fimmu.2017.01061/full?utm_source=F-AAE&utm_medium=EMLF&utm_campaign=MRK_398354_35_Immuno_20170921_arts_A

KINASE: Enzyme important in the carbohydrate metabolism and energy output of cells. **Protein-Tyrosine Kinases (PTK's)** regulate signaling in the cell. If PTK signaling is disrupted, malignant transformation of the cell can result.

http://www.ncbi.nlm.nih.gov/pubmed/10966463

http://www.sciencedirect.com/science/article/pii/S1043661813001771

https://www.empr.com/news/vitrakvi-larotrectinib-advanced-solid-tumors-ntrk-gene-fusion-approval/article/816725/?utm_source=newsletter&utm_medium=email&utm_campaign=mpr-dailydose-cp-20181129&cpn=obgyn_all%2cobgyn_md%2ccambia_august2018&hmS

LABOR: Period from the onset of regular uterine contractions with dilatation and effacement of the cervix and descent of the fetus through the birth canal culminating in delivery of the baby.

LACTIC ACIDOSIS: Increased plasma lactate. See: The Care of the Older Person: Critical Care of the Older Person: Astrid Pilgrim, Michael R. Pinsky; How To Diagnose And Treat Delirium: Haiban Yin. RMC Publishing, LLC www.careoftheolderperson.com
http://emedicine.medscape.com/article/167027-overview

LACTOSE INTOLERANCE: Inability to digest lactose, a disaccharide in milk made up of glucose and galactose.
http://emedicine.medscape.com/article/187249-overview

LAPAROSCOPY: a minimally invasive surgical technique in which a fiberoptic telescope (laparoscope) is introduced into the abdominal cavity through a small incision near the lower margin of the umbilicus.

LASER: **L**ight **A**mplification by **S**timulated **E**mission of **R**adiation. A narrow, often powerful, beam of light which does not spread and is monochromatic. This is a directed light beam, not nuclear radiation.
http://www.azooptics.com/Article.aspx?ArticleID=44
https://www.nature.com/articles/s41551-016-0008?WT.mc_id=
EMI_NBME_1701_LAUNCHISSUE_PORTFOLIO&spMailingID=
53217285&spUserID=MTc3MDI4ODk5NQS2&spJobID=
1083253126&spReportId=MTA4MzI1MzEyNgS2

LEPTIN: Hormone produced by adipocytes involved in fat storage regulation. Acts on hypothalamus to suppress appetite.
http://www.sciencedirect.com/science/article/pii/S0083672905710128

LEUKEMIA: Malignant form of white blood cells in the blood stream, commonly arising from the bone marrow.
http://www.ncbi.nlm.nih.gov/pmc/articles/PMC3396664/

LIBIDO: Sexual drive. See: The Care of the Older Person: After the Menopause: Ronald M. Caplan RMC Publishing, LLC
https://en.wikipedia.org/wiki/Flibanserin
http://www.medscape.com/viewarticle/871481?nlid=110609_2581&src=WNL_

mdplsnews_161111_mscpedit_

obgy&uac=66536PR&spon=16&impID=1232827&faf=1

https://www.fda.gov/news-events/press-announcements/fda-approves-new-treatment-hypoactive-sexual-desire-disorder-premenopausal-women

http://www.addyi.com

LIFE: The capacity to metabolize, grow, reproduce, function and change (adapt). The classic vital functions to assess continuing life are brain activity, respiration and cardiac activity. The **VITAL ORGANS** without which life cannot be sustained are the brain, heart, lungs, liver and kidneys.

https://www.google.com/search?rlz=1C1CHBF_enUS821US821&sxsrf=

ALeKk007mA8gEJfS83a8KXD_XDCjMxHuOg%3A1600519500079&ei=TP1lX_2y

BK-xytMPyqa7yAo&q=life+definition&oq=+life+definition&gs_lcp=CgZwc3ktYW

IQARgAMgwIABCxAxBDEEYQ-QEyBggAEAcQHjIGC

LIFE EXPECTANCY: The age to which a person or a selected population group might live. See: The Care of the Older Person: Introduction: Jose Morais. RMC Publishing, LLC

www.careoftheolderperson.com

https://www.zionmarketresearch.com/report/home-healthcare-market

http://science.sciencemag.org/content/360/6396/1459

http://onlinelibrary.wiley.com/doi/10.1002/sres.2420/full

http://www.cdc.gov/nchs/data/hus/2011/022.pdf

http://www.statcan.gc.ca/tables-tableaux/sum-som/l01/cst01/health26-eng.htm

http://www.cdc.gov/nchs/data/databriefs/db267.pdf

http://mdlinx.pdr.net/internal-medicine/news-article.cfm/6986115/?utm_source=in-house&utm_medium=message&utm_campaign=mh-im-dec16

http://journals.plos.org/plosbiology/article?id=10.1371/journal.pbio.2002458#pbio.2002458.ref039 http://science.sciencemag.org/content/360/6396/1459

https://www.cdc.gov/nchs/data/hus/2017/027.pdf

https://www.jwatch.org/fw114817/2018/11/30/us-life-expectancy-down-overdose-and-suicide-rates?query=pfwTOC&jwd=000012066693&jspc=OBG

LIPOFUSCIN: Brown-yellow lipid containing residues of lysosomal digestion. Considered to be a "wear and tear" pigment.

The Care of the Older Person: Critical Care of the Older Person:

Astrid F. Pilgrim, Michael R. Pinsky https://en.wikipedia.org/wiki/Lipofuscin#:~:text=Lipofuscin%20is%20the%20name%20given,nerve%20cells%2C%20and%20ganglion%20cells.

LIPOSUCTION: Surgical removal of fat by suction.

LIQUID BIOPSY: Blood testing for circulating tumor DNA (ctDNA). Identifies cancer mutations useful as biomarkers, many associated with targeted drug.
http://www.ncbi.nlm.nih.gov/pmc/articles/PMC4356857/
http://www.nature.com/nrclinonc/posters/liquidbiopsies/nrclinonc_liquidbiopsies_poster_web.pdf
http://www.nature.com/news/liquid-biopsies-success-highlights-power-of-combining-basic-and-clinical-research-1.21883?WT.ec_id=NATURE-20170427&spMailingID=53937339&
https://www.nature.com/articles/s41551-017-0065?WT.mc_id=EMI_NBME_1704_APRILISSUE_PORTFOLIO&spMailingID=53957850&spUserID=MTc3MDI4ODk5NQS

LOW DENSITY LIPOPROTEIN: LDL. Complex of lipids and proteins that transports cholesterol in the blood. Significant factor in the formation of arteriosclerotic plaques.
http://www.ncbi.nlm.nih.gov/pubmed/10073963

LUNG CANCER: Malignant tumor in the lung. Major cause of cancer deaths. Predominant type is Non- Small Cell Lung Cancer (**NSCLC**), strongly linked to tobacco smoking.
https://cancerstaging.org/references-tools/quickreferences/Documents/LungMedium.pdf
https://www.ncbi.nlm.nih.gov/pmc/articles/PMC3864624/
https://www.ncbi.nlm.nih.gov/pmc/articles/PMC4367711/
https://www.ncbi.nlm.nih.gov/pmc/articles/PMC5107578/
http://www.jtcvsonline.org/article/S0022-5223(17)31171-6/fulltext#sec1.6
https://www.frontiersin.org/articles/10.3389/fimmu.2020.01996/full?utm_source=F-AAE&utm_medium=EMLF&utm_campaign=MRK_1407965_35_Immuno_2020082

LUTEINIZING HORMONE: LH. Secreted by the anterior pituitary, surges prior to ovulation. Acts on the ovary.
http://emedicine.medscape.com/article/2089268-overview

LYME DISEASE: Tick-borne illness caused by Borrelia burgdorferi. Other tick-borne illnesses include babesiosis, anaplasmosis, ehrlichosis, and Rocky Mountain Spotted Fever.
http://www.ncbi.nlm.nih.gov/pmc/articles/PMC3542482/

LYMPH NODE: Small and bean shaped, lymph nodes are present throughout the body. They are composed of lymphoid tissue, and are connected by lymph channels. The lymphatic system is important in the immune response, in fighting infection. Cancerous cells can enter the lymphatic system and drain to lymph nodes, enlarging them. Cancer surgery often involves the removal of affected lymph nodes, or lymph nodes that are likely to be affected by a cancer.
https://www.boundless.com/physiology/textbooks/boundless-anatomy-and-physiology-textbook/lymphatic-system-20/lymph-cells-and-tissues-193/lymph-nodes-963-3100/

LYMPHOCYTE: A form of white blood cell. B cells and T cells are two main types.
http://www.ncbi.nlm.nih.gov/pubmedhealth/PMHT0022042/

LYMPHOMA: A solid malignant tumor often composed of cells that resemble lymphocytes. Can arise at various sites within the body and invade the bloodstream.
http://www.bloodjournal.org/content/125/1/22

LYNCH SYNDROME: Autosomal dominant inherited predisposition for colon and endometrial cancers.
https://www.ncbi.nlm.nih.gov/pmc/articles/PMC2933058/
https://www.sgo.org/wp-content/uploads/2016/10/2016-SGO-Genetics-Toolkit3.pdf

LYSOSOMES: Organelles in the cell containing enzymes that degrade biologic polymers including proteins, carbohydrates and lipids.
https://www.ncbi.nlm.nih.gov/books/NBK9953/

MACHINE LEARNING: How computers learn from data. Intersection of statistics and computing algorithms.
https://www.ncbi.nlm.nih.gov/pmc/articles/PMC5831252/
https://www.sciencedirect.com/science/article/pii/S093336571730009X
https://www.techemergence.com/machine-learning-in-pharma-medicine/

https://www.healthcareitnews.com/projects/ai-and-machinelearning?
mkt_tok=eyJpIjoiWVRJNE5qTmpPRE01WmpabSIsInQiOiJCckta
VzljSVRpVVpWQ3FYa2lEazc1WHlQSGc5bUV3YXlwTFVtbEdv
M2RjSVY

MACROPHAGE: A large phagocytic white blood cell.
http://www.cell.com/immunity/fulltext/S1074-7613(14)00235-0

MACULAR DEGENERATION: Deterioration of the macula, the area surrounding
the fovea near the center of the retina in the eye.
https://www.ncbi.nlm.nih.gov/pmc/articles/PMC3732788/
https://www.nature.com/articles/nbt.4114.epdf?referrer_access_
token=8BtrAvy5kx0RIQxVHmwBfNRgN0jAjWeI9jnR3ZoTv0PJSqIFs
8CVMGLKXeHOLTvVGIDHNZm

MALNUTRITION: Improper intake and processing of foodstuffs. See: The Care
of the Older Person: Could My Patient Be Malnourished? Jose A. Morais, RMC
Publishing, LLC 2018, 2019 www.careoftheolderperson.com
https://www.ncbi.nlm.nih.gov/pubmed/16782522

MAMMOGRAPHY: Xray breast imaging.
http://emedicine.medscape.com/article/346529-overview
http://www.jwatch.org/na42993/2016/12/13/when-stop-
surveillance-mammography-older-breast-cancer?query=etoc_
jwwomen&jwd=000012066693&jspc=OBG

MAO INHIBITORS: Monoamine oxidase inhibitors, sometimes still used in the
treatment of depression. Monoamine oxidase enzymes catalase oxidation and
inactivation of monoamine neurotransmitters, including dopamine, noradrenaline,
adrenaline and serotonin.
http://www.webmd.com/depression/symptoms-depressed-anxiety-12/
antidepressants

MEDIASTINUM: Space in the thorax between the pleural sacs, notably containing
the heart and its great vessels.
https://www.youtube.com/watch?v=2POIlBe2xR4

MEDULLA (OBLONGATA): Part of the brain in the brainstem that controls
involuntary activities necessary for life.

https://www.neuroscientificallychallenged.com/blog/know-your-brain-medulla-oblongata

MEIOSIS: Cell division resulting in cells (gametes) with a single set of chromosomes, half the number of chromosomes present in the parent cell. https://www.khanacademy.org/science/biology/cellular-molecular-biology/meiosis/a/phases-of-meiosis

MELANOMA: Tumor of melanin-forming cells. http://www.medicaljournals.se/acta/content/?doi=10.2340/00015555-2035&html=1 https://www.cell.com/cell/fulltext/S0092-8674(17)30952-2

MENOPAUSE: Cessation of menses. See: The Care of the Older Person: After the Menopause: Ronald M. Caplan RMC Publishing, LLC https://www.ncbi.nlm.nih.gov/pmc/articles/PMC3285482/

MENSTRUATION: Blood and shedding endometrium from the uterus beginning approximately fourteen days after ovulation in a non-pregnant cycle. https://www.ncbi.nlm.nih.gov/pubmed/16160098

MERS: Middle East Respiratory Syndrome-Related Corona Virus: First reported in Saudi Arabia in 2012 https://www.niaid.nih.gov/diseases-conditions/covid-19

METABOLIC ACIDOSIS: Increase in plasma acidity. Excess production of acid with inadequate buffer, bicarbonate, to neutralize it. Insufficient renal excretion of acid. http://www.nature.com/nrneph/journal/v6/n5/abs/nrneph.2010.33.html

METABOLIC SYNDROME: Central (abdominal)obesity, hypertension, and insulin resistance. High levels of triglycerides, low levels of HDL. http://www.ncbi.nlm.nih.gov/pmc/articles/PMC3966331/

METABOLISM: Molecular chemical reactions within living tissue. http://www.biology-pages.info/C/CellularRespiration.html

METAPLASIA: A benign cell change. In a common type, glandular epithelium is transformed into squamous epithelium. https://en.wikipedia.org/wiki/Squamous_metaplasia

METASTASIS: Cancer cells at a distance from the primary tumor.
https://www.nature.com/articles/d41586-018-05445-x?utm_source=briefing-dy&utm_medium=email&utm_campaign=briefing&utm_content=20180618
https://www.cancer.gov/publications/dictionaries/cancer-terms/def/metastasis

METFORMIN: Oral anti-hyperglycemic agent used in Type 2 Diabetes. Decreases hepatic glucose production. Implications in other disease states, weight loss and possibly lifespan
https://www.ncbi.nlm.nih.gov/pmc/articles/PMC3398862/

MICROBIOME: Bacteria that inhabit the gut.
http://jamanetwork.com/journals/jama/fullarticle/2594788

MICROGLIA: Immune, phagocytic, central nervous system (brain and spinal cord) cells implicated in Alzheimer's.
https://www.frontiersin.org/articles/10.3389/fimmu.2019.00790/full?utm_source=F-AAE&utm_medium=EMLF&utm_campaign=MRK_973135_35_Immuno_20190425_arts_A

MICROSURGERY: Surgery performed with visualization through a microscope, often involving anastomoses of small blood vessels.

MIGRAINE: Vascular headaches involving the blood vessels of the brain.
http://www.ncbi.nlm.nih.gov/pmc/articles/PMC3663475/
https://www.jwatch.org/fw113584/2017/11/30/migraine-prevention-two-calcitonin-gene-related-peptide?query=pfwTOC&jwd=000012066693&jspc=OBG
http://www.pdr.net/drug-summary/Imitrex-Tablets-sumatriptan-succinate-201
https://www.ncbi.nlm.nih.gov/pubmed/29800211
https://www.thelancet.com/journals/lancet/article/PIIS0140-6736(18)32534-0/fulltext
https://www.empr.com/ajovy/drug/34876/
https://www.ptcommunity.com/journal/article/full/2018/10/616/emerging-therapies-patients-difficult-treat-migraine?utm_source=PT_NL_2018-10-16_nsp_v9&utm_campaign=PT+NL+18-10-16&utm_medium=email https://www.empr.com/news/ajovy-migraine-prevention-fremanezumab-vfrm-preventative-migraine/article/796090/?utm_source=newsletter&utm_medium=email&utm_campaign=mpr-promo-20181105&chttps://jamanetwork.com/journals/jamaneurology/fullarticle/2681442

https://jamanetwork.com/journals/jamaneurology/fullarticle/2681442
https://onlinelibrary.wiley.com/doi/10.1111/head.13456

MIS-C: Multisystem Inflammatory Syndrome in Children: Coincident with COVID19 pandemic. Clinically similar to **Kawasaki disease,** Kawasaki disease shock syndrome and toxic shock syndrome. Can present with fever, hypotension, gastrointestinal symptoms, rash, and myocarditis.
https://www.uptodate.com/contents/coronavirus-disease-2019-covid-19-considerations-in-children

MITOCHONDRIA: Intracellular organelle in which respiration and energy production occur.
https://jamanetwork.com/journals/jamaneurology/fullarticle/2681442
http://citeseerx.ist.psu.edu/viewdoc/download?doi=10.1.1.572.8830&rep=rep1&type=pdf
http://www.cell.com/cell-metabolism/fulltext/S1550-4131(16)30502-2
http://mdlinx.pdr.net/neurology/news-article.cfm/6907659?utm_source=in-house&utm_medium=message&utm_campaign=medhead
https://link.springer.com/article/10.1007/s10815-017-1006-3/fulltext.html?wt_mc=alerts.TOCjournals
https://www.deepdyve.com/lp/springer-journal/quantitative-and-qualitative-changes-of-mitochondria-in-human-Gh20vR9aBa?key=bioportfolio

MITOSIS: Cell division resulting in daughter cells identical to the parent cell.
https://www.khanacademy.org/science/biology/cellular-molecular-biology/meiosis/a/phases-of-meiosis

MOBILITY: Ability to move freely and easily. See The Care of the Older Person: Why Does My Patient Have Gait and Balance Disorders?: Olivier Beauchet RMC Publishing, LLC
https://www.mayoclinic.org/diseases-conditions/movement-disorders/symptoms-causes/syc-20363893
https://en.oxforddictionaries.com/definition/mobility

MOHS SURGERY: Surgery in which thin layers of cancer containing skin are stepwise removed and examined microscopically, until only cancer free tissue remains.
http://emedicine.medscape.com/article/2212475-overview

MOLECULAR PROFILING (of cancer patients): The use of Next Generation Sequencing (NGS) gives rise to Personalized therapy with selective genome and immune-targeted drugs (see Precision Medicine, NGS)
https://www.nature.com/articles/s41591-019-0407-5

MONOCLONAL ANTIBODY: An antibody that will go to a specific receptor site. "Monoclonal" refers to the fact that the antibody protein is derived from one clone of cells, all of which are identical. A particular neutralizing IgG1 monoclonal antibody known as **Bamlanivimab,** directed against the spike protein of SARS-CoV-2 virus that causes COVID-19, received an Emergency Use Authorization in the USA from the FDA in 2020.
http://www.ncbi.nlm.nih.gov/pmc/articles/PMC4491443/ https://www.fda.gov/media/143603/download

MONTREAL COGNITIVE ASSESSMENT: MoCA: Test to detect mild cognitive impairment and Alzheimer's disease. The Care of the Older Person: Chapter: "Doctor, my wife is getting forgetful": Serge Gauthier RMC Publishing, LLC www.careoftheolderperson.com
http://dementia.ie/images/uploads/site-images/MoCA-Test-English_7_1.pdf
http://www.mocatest.org/
https://www.sciencedirect.com/topics/neuroscience/montreal-cognitive-assessment

MOTORIC COGNITIVE RISK SYNDROME (MCR): Predementia syndrome combining cognitive complaint and slow gait.
http://biomedgerontology.oxfordjournals.org/content/71/8/1081

MRI: **Magnetic Resonance Imaging**. An advanced imaging technique that uses a powerful magnet to alter polarity.
https://onlinelibrary.wiley.com/doi/full/10.1002/jmri.23642

MSG: Monosodium glutamate.
http://www.mayoclinic.org/healthy-lifestyle/nutrition-and-healthy-eating/expert-answers/monosodium-glutamate/faq-20058196

MULTIPLE MYELOMA: Plasma cell (a type of white blood cell derived from B cell) malignancy. Anemia and osteolytic (bone reabsorbing) skeletal lesions usually present. A monoclonal (M) protein can usually be detected in the blood serum and urine.
https://www.mdedge.com/oncologypractice/article/154492/multiple-

myeloma/crb-410-update-multiple-myeloma-response-rates?oc_
slh=1de3dcf7eb6395af6b796baf8538c

https://www.ncbi.nlm.nih.gov/pmc/articles/PMC5223450/

https://www.cancer.gov/publications/dictionaries/cancer-terms?
cdrid=46230

https://www.cancer.gov/publications/dictionaries/cancer-terms?
cdrid=45810

MUTATION: Abnormal recombinations of the chromosomes. Permanent alteration in DNA sequence. Alteration in a genome, that may or may not be harmful to the individual.
http://www.nature.com/scitable/definition/recombination-226
http://www.ncbi.nlm.nih.gov/pubmed/23266571
https://academic.oup.com/annonc/article/29/1/30/4616649

MYELIN: Insulating sheath around nerve fibers.
http://www.news-medical.net/health/Myelin-Function.aspx

MYELITIS: Inflammation of the spinal cord https://en.wikipedia.org/wiki/
Myelitis#:~:text=Myelitis%20is%20inflammation%20of%20the,as%20paralysis%20
and%20sensory%20loss.

MYELODYSPLASTIC SYNDROME (MDS): Bone marrow cancer with insufficient presence of normal blood cells, and presence of abnormal blood cells.
https://www.cancer.gov/publications/dictionaries/cancer-terms/def/
myelodysplastic-syndrome

MYELOPEROXIDASE: MPO. Enzyme in neutrophils linked to cardiovascular disease.
http://www.ncbi.nlm.nih.gov/gene/4353
http://www.ncbi.nlm.nih.gov/pubmed/26567811/

MYOCARDIAL INFARCTION: Irreversible injury to heart muscle.
http://www.clevelandclinicmeded.com/medicalpubs/diseasemanagement/
cardiology/acute-myocardial-infarction/
https://arxiv.org/abs/1708.09843

MYOCARDIUM: Heart muscle.
https://www.boundless.com/physiology/textbooks/boundless-anatomy-

and-physiology-textbook/cardiovascular-system-the-heart-18/the-heart-172/
myocardial-thickness-and-function-867-10251/

MYOCYTE: Heart muscle cell.
https://www.sciencedaily.com/releases/2016/04/160421145756.htm

MYOMECTOMY: Surgical removal of fibroids from the uterus.

NANOTECHNOLOGY: Engineering of tiny machines, often for the monitoring, prevention, and treatment of disease.
http://tedx.tumblr.com/post/35204848311/fight-cancer-with-nanotechnology-sylvain-martel
https://iopscience.iop.org/journal/0957-4484;jsessionid=3420F74BB331365A7161E71B24C8121C.c4.iopscience.cld.iop.org
https://www.frontiersin.org/articles/10.3389/fimmu.2017.00069/full?utm_source=newsletter&utm_medium=email&utm_campaign=Immunology-w6-2017
https://www.nature.com/articles/s41551-017-0029?WT.mc_id=LDN_NBME_1801_FIRSTANNIVERSARY_PORTFOLIO

NARRATIVE MEDICINE: Narrative competence: Listening to and understanding related stories , and appropriately responding.
http://www.ncbi.nlm.nih.gov/pmc/articles/PMC3034473/

NEPHROPATHY: Kidney disease or damage.
http://www.ncbi.nlm.nih.gov/pmc/articles/PMC3084647/
https://en.wikipedia.org/wiki/Kidney_disease

NEPHROSIS: Generally refers to degenerative disease of the renal (kidney) tubules
http://medical-dictionary.thefreedictionary.com/nephrosis

NEPHROTIC SYNDROME: Excretion of significant amounts of protein in the urine, along with decreased serum albumin (a protein), and edema (swelling due to fluid accumulation)
http://emedicine.medscape.com/article/244631-overview

NEURAL TUBE DEFECT: Birth defect of brain, spine, or spinal cord.
http://www.ncbi.nlm.nih.gov/pmc/articles/PMC4023229/

NEURODEGENERATION: Progressive loss of brain function associated with aging. https://www.ncbi.nlm.nih.gov/pubmed/30258237

NEURODEGENERATIVE DISEASES: Diseases which cause progressive loss of cognitive and/or motor function.

https://www.ncbi.nlm.nih.gov/pubmed/23305823

https://www.ncbi.nlm.nih.gov/pubmed/30258237

NEUROGENESIS: Formation of neurons

https://www.nature.com/articles/nature25975https://www.nature.com/articles/s41591-019-0375-9?utm_source=nm_etoc&utm_medium=email&utm_campaign=toc_41591_25_4&utm_content=20190405&WT.ec_id=NM-201904&sap-outbound-id=A2CA93DADBF79C1C13E7D04CDCA72468DD68FEE3

NEUROIMMUNE COMMUNICATION: Interaction between the nervous and immune systems, influencing each other.

http://www.nature.com/ni/journal/v18/n2/full/ni.3676.html

http://www.nature.com/neuro/journal/v20/n2/full/nn.4496.html

NEUROMORPHIC ENGINEERING: Designing hardware and physical models of neural and sensory systems.

https://www.frontiersin.org/journals/neuroscience/sections/neuromorphic-engineering

http://compneuro.uwaterloo.ca/research/nef/overview-of-the-nef.html

NEURON: Specialized nervous system cell that can be stimulated and conducts impulses.

http://www.ncbi.nlm.nih.gov/books/NBK21535/ https://www.nature.com/articles/s41593-018-0205-2.epdf?shared_access_token=60bklwIRkphHPPY3R_u069RgN0jAjWel9jnR3ZoTv0M_ZnMCyHI8KbNyV63mNxsudkNYBmXFIhQDgOHiquMVMmq6S_Ta_jrenQf

NEUTROPHIL: A white blood cell containing granules that are enzyme containing sacs.

http://jem.rupress.org/content/210/7/1283.full

NEXT GENERATION SEQUENCING (NGS): Rapid (high throughput) DNA sequencing. Used for molecular profiling of tumor samples in order to individualize treatment.

https://www.ncbi.nlm.nih.gov/pmc/articles/PMC5808190/

https://www.ncbi.nlm.nih.gov/pmc/articles/PMC4494749/

NICOTINAMIDE RIBOSIDE: NR: A form of Vitamin B3 (nicotinic acid, Niacin). Converts to **NAD**, Nicotinamide Adenine Dinucleotide, a coenzyme in cells that is involved in energy metabolism
http://www.ctl.cornell.edu/events/ctvf12/Sauve.pdf
http://jpet.aspetjournals.org/content/324/3/883.full

NITRITES: Ester or salt of nitrous acid. Vasodilator.
http://circ.ahajournals.org/content/117/16/2151

NNT: Number Needed to Treat. Epidemiological measure of the effectiveness of a medical intervention. The number of patients who need a specific treatment to prevent one additional bad outcome
The Care of the Older Person: Stroke Prevention in the Elderly: Liam Durcan: RMC Publishing, LLC 2021.
https://patient.info/doctor/numbers-needed-to-treat#:~:text=The%20number%20 needed%20to%20treat,the%20adverse%20outcome%20being%20prevented.

NUCLEAR POWER: Energy produced by atomic reaction.
http://www.nei.org/Knowledge-Center/How-Nuclear-Reactors-Work

NUCLEAR WASTE: Radioactive byproducts usually from operation of a nuclear reactor.
http://www.nrc.gov/reading-rm/doc-collections/fact-sheets/radwaste.html
http://www.nrc.gov/reading-rm/doc-collections/fact-sheets/radwaste.html

NUCLEASE: Enzyme that catalyzes the cleavage of phosphodiester bonds between nucleotides.
http://www.nature.com/onc/journal/v21/n58/full/1206135a.html?foxtrotcallback=true
https://www.ncbi.nlm.nih.gov/pubmed/24690881
https://www.ncbi.nlm.nih.gov/pubmed/24690881

NUCLEIC ACID: Substance found in the cytoplasm of cells, as well as in chromosomes, and in viruses. Four specific nucleic acids: **adenine** (A), **cytosine** (C), **guanine** (G), and **thymine** (T) are arranged in pairs on each rung of the ladder of DNA. They code the sequences of amino acids that make up proteins.
http://www.rsc.org/Education/Teachers/Resources/cfb/nucleicacids.htm

NUCLEOSOME: The basic structural unit of chromatin.
https://en.wikipedia.org/wiki/Chromatin
https://www.nature.com/scitable/topicpage/dna-packaging-nucleosomes-and-chromatin-310

NUCLEOSIDE: Compound found in DNA or RNA made up of a purine or pyrimidine (nitrogenous) base linked to a sugar. Lacks the phosphate group(s) of a nucleotide. Nucleosides used as antiviral and anticancer agents.
https://www.google.com/search?sxsrf=ALeKk01w3ybsI878-V5kuWH4SuYetqPY
rg:1593538669885&q=Dictionary&stick=H4sIAAAAAAAAONQesSoyi3w8sc9YS
mZ https://www.diffen.com/difference/Nucleoside_vs_Nucleotide

NUCLEOTIDE: Building block (subunit) of **nucleic acid**. Nitrogenous base plus ribose or deoxyribose plus one or more phosphate groups. Malfunction can lead to cancer.
https://en.wikipedia.org/wiki/Nucleotide

NUCLEUS: A central structure, surrounded by its own membrane, in the cell. The nucleus contains the chromosomes.
https://micro.magnet.fsu.edu/cells/nucleus/nucleus.html
https://micro.magnet.fsu.edu/cells/nucleus/nucleus.html

NURSING: Breastfeeding.

OBESITY: More than 20% above expected body weight, Body Mass Index (BMI) of 30 or more.
http://www.ncbi.nlm.nih.gov/pubmed/22171945
https://www.ncbi.nlm.nih.gov/pubmed/27386756
http://www.cell.com/cell/fulltext/S0092-8674(16)30213-6
https://www.frontiersin.org/articles/10.3389/fimmu.2017.01745/full?utm_
source=F-AAE&utm_medium=EMLF&utm_campaign=MRK_491010_35_I
https://jamanetwork.com/journals/jama/article-abstract/2685153?utm_
source=silverchair&utm_campaign=jama_network&utm_content=weekly_
highlights&cmp=1&utm_medium=email

ONCOLOGIST: Physician who specializes in the treatment of cancer.
http://www.oncologypractice.com/jcso/specialty-focus/lung/single-article-
page/genomic-oncology-moving-beyond-the-tip-of-the-iceberg/0a952f61278bdd07
e9d7db4e7c6d1fcb.html

OPHTHALMIC NERVE: Branch of the trigeminal nerve that gives sensory fibers to the ciliary muscle of the eye, lacrimal gland, eyelids, forehead, and mucous membrane of the nose.
http://www.ncbi.nlm.nih.gov/pubmed/11842844

OPIOID: Naturally occurring and synthetic potentially addictive substances that act on specific (opioid) receptors to produce effects including pain relief. Major cause of drug abuse, addiction, and death.
https://www.drugabuse.gov/drugs-abuse/opioids
https://www.drugabuse.gov/drugs-abuse/opioids/opioid-crisis
https://www.fda.gov/Drugs/DrugSafety/InformationbyDrugClass/ucm337066.htm

OSTEOBLAST: Cell that synthesizes bone.
www.nature.com/articles/boneres20169

OSTEOCLAST: Cell that reabsorbs bone. The Care of the Older Person: After the Menopause: Ronald M. Caplan RMC Publishing, LLC www.careoftheolderperson.com
http://www.ncbi.nlm.nih.gov/pubmed/1873485
https://www.nature.com/articles/s41413-018-0040-9

OSTEOPENIA: Reduced bone mass. Less severe than osteoporosis.
medicine.medscape.com/article/330598-overview

OSTEOPOROSIS: Reduced bone mass due to depletion of calcium and bone protein.
https://www.karger.com/Article/FullText/431091
http://www.thelancet.com/journals/lancet/article/PIIS0140-6736(17)31613-6/fulltext
https://mydigimag.rrd.com/publication/?i=470718&ver=html5&p=30&utm_source=PT+eTOC+2018-02+prospect+no+spons&utm_campaign=PT1802_Digital_Edition_Alert&utm_medium=email#{"page":"30"
https://www.medscape.com/viewarticle/914567?src=WNL_recnl_190722_MSCPEDIT_obgyn&uac=66536PR&impID=2036955&faf=1

OVARIAN CANCER: Cancer of the ovary.
https://www.ncbi.nlm.nih.gov/pmc/articles/PMC5365187/
https://www.uptodate.com/contents/screening-for-ovarian-cancer

OVARY: The primary female sex organ. Almond shaped, 3 centimeters long. Two ovaries, one on either side of the uterus in the pelvis.
http://emedicine.medscape.com/article/1949171-overview

http://www.fertstert.org/article/S0015-0282(17)31879-4/
fulltext?elsca1=etoc&elsca2=email&elsca3=
0015-0282_201710_108_4_&elsca4=Obstetrics%20and%20Gyn
https://www.fertstert.org/article/S0015-0282(18)31744-8/fulltext?dgcid=raven_
jbs_etoc_email
https://www.frontiersin.org/articles/10.3389/fimmu.2018.02009/full?utm_
source=F-AAE&utm_medium=EMLF&utm_campaign=MRK_779779_35_
Immuno_20180927_arts_A

OVULATION: During the menstrual cycle, several fluid filled follicles, each
containing an ovum, develop. One becomes the dominant follicle. The other
follicles regress. At midcycle, the dominant follicle ruptures, releasing the egg,
which is then picked up by the fimbria of the fallopian tube.
https://www.ncbi.nlm.nih.gov/books/NBK279054/

OVUM: Pleural: ova. The oocyte. The egg. A single cell present in the female ovary
that eventually can be fertilized by a single sperm cell from the male. The ovum
before fertilization has only twenty three chromosomes. These pair with the twenty
three chromosomes from the spermatozoon to create a genetically new individual
with forty six chromosomes.
http://www.theodora.com/anatomy/the_ovum.html

PALLIATIVE CARE: Team support system of enhanced physical, psychosocial, and
spiritual quality of life in the face of life-threatening illness. Prevention and relief of
suffering and pain. Affirmation of life, and regarding dying as a normal process.
http://www.who.int/cancer/palliative/definition/en/
https://www.surgical.theclinics.com/article/S0039-6109(19)30088-X/pdf
https://www.sciencedirect.com/science/article/pii/
S0039610919300891?dgcid=author

PAPANICOLAOU SMEAR: Cells in cervical mucus examined microscopically .
https://www.google.com/search?q=photographs+of+normal+and+
ascus+cells&rlz=1C1CHBF_enUS694US694&espv=2&biw=1745&bih=
883&tbm=isch&tbo=u&source=univ&sa=X&ved=
0ahUKEwittZaMp57PAhUELyYKHeGjBJcQsAQIGw

PARATHYROID HORMONE: PTH. Secreted by parathyroid glands. Regulates blood levels of calcium and phosphorus.
http://www.ncbi.nlm.nih.gov/pubmed/19395963

PARKINSONISM: Parkinson disease. Chronic progressive debilitating neurologic condition arising in the basal ganglia of the brain. Loss of dopaminergic cells. Decreased dopamine production in substantia nigra. The Care of the Older Person: Why Does My Patient Have Gait & Balance Disorders?: Olivier Beauchet. RMC Publishing, LLC www.careoftgheolderperson.com
http://www.neurobiologyofaging.org/article/S0197-4580(16)30060-4/abstract
https://www.nature.com/articles/s41531-017-0015-3?WT.mc_id_EMI_PARKD_1708_PMC&WT.ec_id=INTERNAL&
spMailingID=54985332&spUserID=MTc3MDI4ODk
https://www.frontiersin.org/articles/10.3389/fneur.2018.00809/full
https://jamanetwork.com/journals/jamanetworkopen/fullarticle/2723412?utm_source=silverchair&utm_medium=email&utm_campaign=article_alert-jamanetworkopen&utm_content=etoc&utm_term=030119

PARP: A group of enzymes important in DNA repair. Poly Adenosine diphosphate (ADP) Ribose Polymerase. https://www.sciencedirect.com/science/article/pii/S0923753419386478

PARP INHIBITORS: used in **BRCA** associated breast, ovarian and pancreatic cancer, prostate cancer.
https://www.nejm.org/doi/pdf/10.1056/NEJMoa1903387#:~:text=This%20article%20was%20published%20on,2019%2C%20at%20NEJM.org.&text=Patients%20with%20a%20germline%20BRCA1,antitumor%20activity%20in%20this%20population.
https://www.hematologyandoncology.net/archives/may-2015/parp-inhibitors-in-ovarian-and-other-cancers/
https://www.fda.gov/drugs/resources-information-approved-drugs/fda-approves-olaparib-germline-brca-mutated-metastatic-breast-cancer_
https://www.fda.gov/drugs/drug-approvals-and-databases/fda-approves-olaparib-hrr-gene-mutated-metastatic-castration-resistant-prostate-cancer

PATHOLOGIST: Physician specializing in the diagnosis of disease by inspecting organs and tumors, both by direct vision and microscopically.

PATIENT-GENERATED HEALH DATA: PGHD: Wearable monitoring devices.
https://pages.mobihealthnews.com/WP-Fitbit-Mediashark-2018-10_LP-Multiplying-the-Value-of-Wearables-and-Patient-Generated-Health-Data2.
html?topic=analytics%2C%20mobile%2C%20patientengagement&utm_source=epush&utm_medium=email&utm_campa

PCI: Percutaneous coronary intervention. Coronary angioplasty. Stent introduced by catheter and placed in coronary artery.
http://emedicine.medscape.com/article/161446-overview
http://emedicine.medscape.com/article/161446-technique

PEPTIDE: Two or more amino acids linked together.
https://www2.chemistry.msu.edu/faculty/reusch/virttxtjml/protein2.htm

PERIMENOPAUSE: The time shortly before menopause.

PERIPHERAL ARTERY OCCLUSIVE DISEASE: Narrowing and blockage of smaller arteries. **CLAUDICATION:** Thigh pain with exercise is a symptom.
http://emedicine.medscape.com/article/460178-overview

PERSONALITY TYPE: Psychologic classification of individuals.
http://mbtitoday.org/carl-jung-psychological-type/

PESSARY: Device placed in the vagina for support.

PET SCAN: Positron Emission Tomography. The person being imaged is given sugar, which is tagged by radioactive isotope. Malignant cells tend to metabolize sugar at a higher rate, because they are actively growing and dividing. The increased radioactive uptake measured at a given site in the body infers that there may be a malignant tumor at that site.
https://journals.lww.com/thoracicimaging/Fulltext/2013/01000/Overview_of_Positron_Emission_Tomography,_Hybrid.4.aspx

PHAGOCYTOSIS: The engulfing of a cell fragment or foreign body by a cell.
http://www.dictionary.com/browse/phagocytosis

PHENOTYPE: The observable properties, characteristics and traits of an organism produced by the interaction of the genotype and the environment.
https://en.wikipedia.org/wiki/Phenotype

PHEROMONE: Chemical substance released by an individual that stimulates the behavior of other individuals.
http://www.scientificamerican.com/article/are-human-pheromones-real/

PHLEBITIS: Inflammation of the walls of a vein.
http://emedicine.medscape.com/article/463256-overview

PHYTOESTROGENS: Naturally occurring estrogen like compounds in plants.
http://www.ncbi.nlm.nih.gov/pmc/articles/PMC3074428/

PITUITARY GLAND: Endocrine gland attached to the base of the brain that secretes hormones that act on other endocrine glands.
http://teachmeanatomy.info/neuro/structures/pituitary-gland/

PLACENTA: Disc-shaped organ that forms in pregnancy, nourishes and supports the developing fetus, and secretes hormones. The surface that is in contact with the mother's uterine wall is composed of many tiny villi. The fetal blood circulates within these villi, which are bathed on their outside by maternal blood from arteries in the uterine wall. Exchange between mother and fetus of nutrients, waste products of metabolism, oxygen and carbon dioxide continuously occurs through the external lining of each villus. After the baby is delivered, the placenta detaches from the wall of the uterus, and is itself delivered.
https://www.nichd.nih.gov/about/meetings/2014/Documents/BurtonWashington2014.pdf

PLASMA (BLOOD): Fluid part of the blood that carries the blood cells
https://www.ncbi.nlm.nih.gov/pubmedhealth/PMHT0022021/

PLASMID: Circular molecule of DNA found in bacteria.
https://www.nature.com/scitable/definition/plasmid-plasmids-28

PLATELET: Cell fragment in blood involved in blood clotting.
https://www.ouhsc.edu/platelets/platelets/platelets%20intro.html

PMDD: Premenstrual dysphoric disorder. Premenstrual mood and behavioral changes.

PMS: Premenstrual syndrome. Various symptoms just prior to, or with the onset of, a period. May include depression, anxiety, bloating, constipation, diarrhea, breast tenderness, weight gain, and headache.

PNEUMONIA: Lung inflammation with congestion.

https://www.ncbi.nlm.nih.gov/pmc/articles/PMC4072047/

https://www.ncbi.nlm.nih.gov/pmc/articles/PMC4072047/

https://www.ncbi.nlm.nih.gov/pmc/articles/PMC4072047/

POLAR BODY: Small cells resulting from two meiotic divisions of the oocyte. Contain the same DNA as the oocyte.

http://www.ncbi.nlm.nih.gov/pmc/articles/PMC3164815/

POLIOMYELITIS: Infectious disease caused by the poliovirus that can result in paresthesias, meningitis and paralysis. Widespread use of effective vaccines has largely eliminated this disease from many societies.

https://www.cdc.gov/polio/what-is-polio/index.htm#:~:text=Related%20 Pages,move%20parts%20of%20the%20body). https://www.ncbi.nlm.nih.gov/ pmc/articles/PMC4212416/

POLLUTION: Presence in, or introduction into, the environment of harmful substances.

POLYGENIC RISK SCORE: (Genetic Risk Score) Estimating the risk conferred by a number of DNA variants in genes to result in a disease onset or other outcome.

https://jamanetwork.com/journals/jama/fullarticle/2730627?guestAccess Key=6579bb87-9479-4cfd-a93c-d39102a0fb5f&utm_source=silverchair&utm_ medium=email&utm_campaign=article_alert-jama&utm_

POLYP: Benign growth arising from a stalk. Polyps occur in the interior of the uterus and may protrude out the cervical os. Polyps in the large intestine may be malignant. Polyps can grow on the vocal cords, and other areas.

POLYPHARMACY: Simultaneous use of multiple drugs, more than are medically necessary. See: The Care of the Older Person: Polypharmacy and Deprescribing in the Elderly: Louise Mallet RMC Publishing LLC www.careoftheolderperson.com

https://www.ncbi.nlm.nih.gov/pmc/articles/PMC3864987/

https://jamanetwork.com/journals/jama/fullarticle/2714515?guestAccess Key=06cab41f-eab9-4441-85a3-53b6c4725e5e&utm_source=silverchair&utm_ medium=email&utm_campaign=article_alert-jama&utm

POSTMENOPAUSAL BLEEDING: Vaginal bleeding occurring after the menopause.

https://www.ncbi.nlm.nih.gov/pmc/articles/PMC3951032/

PRECISION MEDICINE: Studying how the genomic variation in an individual or their disease (tumor sample) influences drug response. Identification of the specific mutations in a tumor, so that targeted therapy can be brought to bear. See Next Generation Sequencing (NGS)
http://stm.sciencemag.org/content/7/300/300ps17.full
https://academic.oup.com/annonc/article/29/1/30/4616649

PREIMPLANTATION GENETIC DIAGNOSIS: PGD. Chromosomal analysis of the polar body (See: Polar body), or of a single embryonic cell.
http://emedicine.medscape.com/article/273415-overview

PRETERM INFANT: Formerly called prematurity. A baby born before thirty eight weeks of intrauterine life.
http://www.adelaide.edu.au/news/news88982.html

PROBIOTICS: Microorganisms, usually bacteria, with health benefits.
http://www.medicinenet.com/script/main/art.asp?articlekey=11901

PROGENITOR CELL: Activated in tissue repair; differentiate to replace damaged tissue. If signal to differentiate not processed, progenitor cells can keep on reproducing, leading to mutations
http://stemcell.childrenshospital.org/about-stem-cells/adult-somatic-stem-cells-101/what-are-progenitor-cells/

PROGESTERONE: A female sex hormone, made in the ovary, prominent in the second half of the menstrual cycle.
https://en.wikipedia.org/wiki/Progesterone

2002. Shyamala, G., Y.-C. Chou, S. G. Louie, R. C. Guzman, G. H. Smith, and S. Nandi. 2002. Cellular expression of estrogen and progesterone receptors in mammary glands: Regulation by hormones, development and aging. J. Steroid Biochem. Mol. Biol. 80:137–148.

PROGESTIN: A progesterone-like substance.

PROGRAMMED CELL DEATH: See Apoptosis for references

PROKARYOTE: Single celled organism without a distinct nucleus and no specialized organelles (except ribosomes). Includes Bacteria.
http://www.dictionary.com/browse/prokaryote

PROLACTIN: Hormone secreted by the anterior pituitary that stimulates lactation.
http://www.ncbi.nlm.nih.gov/pubmed/11015620

PROLAPSE: Downward displacement of an organ.
http://emedicine.medscape.com/article/276259-overview

PROSTAGLANDINS: Group of fatty acids that stimulate contractility of uterine and other smooth muscle.
http://www.ncbi.nlm.nih.gov/pmc/articles/PMC3081099/

PROSTATE: Gland located below the bladder and surrounding the urethra in males. Prostatic fluid is secreted via ducts that open into the urethra.
http://www.ncbi.nlm.nih.gov/pubmedhealth/PMH0072475/
http://www.ncbi.nlm.nih.gov/pmc/articles/PMC4633657/
http://jamanetwork.com/journals/jama/fullarticle/2618352?utm_medium=alert&utm_source=JAMAPublishAheadofPrint&utm_campaign=11-04-2017

PROSTATE CANCER: Cancer of the prostate gland.
https://www.ncbi.nlm.nih.gov/pubmed/28655021
http://www.nejm.org/doi/full/10.1056/NEJMoa1715546?query=main_nav_lg

PROTEIN: A specific sequence of amino acids. Specific proteins are elaborated by specific genes. Proteins have vital functions within the body. They make up the structure of various organs and are involved in their function. They make up the hormones, and the enzymes which facilitate chemical reactions in the body. They are involved in immune response. A specific protein, the **mTOR protein** seems to have a role in aging. **Rapamycin** is one drug that is an mTOR inhibitor. **Metformin** inhibits the mTOR protein indirectly.
https://en.wikipedia.org/wiki/Proteome https://www.ncbi.nlm.nih.gov/pmc/articles/PMC3398862/ https://www.ncbi.nlm.nih.gov/pmc/articles/PMC3972801/#:~:text=Rapamycin%20forms%20a%20gain%2Dof,)%20complex%201%20(mTORC1).&text=Only%20mTORC1%20is%20acutely%20sensitive%20to%20inhibition%20by%20rapamycin.

PROTEOMICS: The study of all the proteins in the body, how they function and interact.
http://proteomics.cancer.gov/whatisproteomics

PROTEOSTASIS: Dysfunction in protein homeostasis that can be seen in aging people. https://www.nature.com/articles/s41580-019-0101-y

PROTON PUMP INHIBITORS: Drugs that inhibit acid secretion by gastric parietal cells. Used in gastroesophageal reflux disease (**GERD**). https://www.ncbi.nlm.nih.gov/pmc/articles/PMC5221858/

PTK: Protein-tyrosine kinase. Regulates signaling in the cell. http://www.ncbi.nlm.nih.gov/pubmed/9393984

PULMONARY EMBOLUS: PE. Blood clot in the lung. http://emedicine.medscape.com/article/300901-overview

RADIATION: Emission of energy as electromagnetic waves or as moving subatomic particles, especially high energy particles that cause ionization. Ionizing radiation has enough energy to remove electrons from the orbit of an atom, causing the atom to be charged (ionized). http://www.who.int/ionizing_radiation/about/what_is_ir/en/

RECEPTOR SITE: Distinctively shaped area on a cell surface, designed to receive a specific substance. http://www.merckmanuals.com/professional/clinical-pharmacology/pharmacodynamics/drug%E2%80%93receptor-interactions https://www.empr.com/news/vitrakvi-larotrectinib-advanced-solid-tumors-ntrk-gene-fusion-approval/article/816725/?utm_source=newsletter&utm_medium=email&utm_campaign=mpr-dailydose-cp-20181129&cpn=obgyn_all,obgyn_md,cambia_august2018&hmS

RECOMBINANT DNA TECHNOLOGY: Rearranging DNA molecules, manufacturing recombinant DNA. Recombinant DNA molecule constructed from segments obtained from different DNA molecules. https://en.wikipedia.org/wiki/Recombinant_DNA

RECOMBINATION: Genetic recombination. Interchange of chromosomal parts or genes. Breaking and rejoining DNA strands, forming new DNA molecules. https://en.wikipedia.org/wiki/Genetic_recombination https://www.nature.com/scitable/topicpage/dna-is-constantly-changing-through-the-process-6524876

RECTOCELE: Bulging of the anterior wall of the rectum into the posterior wall of the vagina.
https://www.ncbi.nlm.nih.gov/pmc/articles/PMC2967328/

REGENERATIVE MEDICINE: Creation of new organs, tissues, and body parts from stem cells, which are placed on a dissolvable matrix: tissue engineering, along with self-healing by the body's systems.
http://www.nature.com/articles/npjregenmed20167
https://www.nature.com/articles/s41536-017-0008-1?WT.mc_id=EMI_
RegMed_1704&spMailingID=53890539&spUserID=
MTc3MDI4ODk5NQS2&spJobID=114328
https://www.nature.com/articles/npjregenmed20167?WT.mc_id=
EMI_RegMed_1706&spMailingID=54243481&spUserID=
MTc3MDI4ODk5NQS2&spJobID=1181517

REJECTION: HOST VS GRAFT: Immunologic response by organ recipient to allograft, damaging it. Immune cells in the transplanted organ can also attack the host: Graft vs. host response.
http://emedicine.medscape.com/article/430449-overview#a4

RENIN: Proteolytic enzyme elaborated by juxtaglomerular cells of the kidneys that acts on angiotensin.
https://www.britannica.com/science/renin-angiotensin-system

RENIN-ANGIOTENSIN SYSTEM: RAS. A mechanism of acute renal hypertension. Renal artery compression or occlusion causing ischemia of the renal cortex results in renal juxtaglomerular cells converting prorenin into renin. Renin acts on angiotensinogen in the bloodstream from the liver, converting it to angiotensin I, which is converted to angiotensin II by angiotensin-converting enzyme. Angiotensin II acts on aldosterone producing cells in the adrenal cortex, causing aldosterone production, leading to sodium retention and increased plasma volume. This leads to an increase in blood pressure, and increased blood flow, including to the kidneys, resulting in stretching of renal afferent arterioles, giving negative feedback so that renin secretion tends to return towards normal. Renin-angiotensin systems are present in various other tissues, in addition to the kidneys.
http://www.ncbi.nlm.nih.gov/pubmed/17878513

REPROGRAMMING: (Cellular Reprogramming): Using the expression of four genes (**Yamanaka Factors**) to convert any cell into **induced pluripotent stem cells (iPSCs)**

https://www.salk.edu/news-release/turning-back-time-salk-scientists-reverse-signs-aging/

http://www.cell.com/cell/fulltext/S0092-8674(16)31664-6

RESVERATROL: Polyphenolic compound in red wine that may be partly responsible for the beneficial cardiovascular effects that have been attributed to red wine.

http://lpi.oregonstate.edu/mic/dietary-factors/phytochemicals/resveratrol

RETICULOENDOTHELIAL SYSTEM, also called: **MONONUCLEAR PHAGOCYTE SYSTEM (MPS):** Widespread system in reticular (thin banding fibers) connective tissue that forms antibodies to counteract foreign antigens.

https://en.wikipedia.org/wiki/Mononuclear_phagocyte_system

RETINOPATHY: Disease of the retina

http://www.ncbi.nlm.nih.gov/pmc/articles/PMC3874488/

RH ISOIMMUNIZATION: Immune response of Rh Negative mother to her Rh positive fetus. First Rh positive child usually not affected.

http://emedicine.medscape.com/article/797150-overview

RIBOSOME: The protein manufacturing machine. Complex molecular machine one millionth of an inch in diameter. Tiny organ (organelle) in the cytoplasm of the cell. Made up of proteins and ribosomal RNA (rRNA)- the active component in protein synthesis. At the ribosome, the genetic code is read and translated into proteins. Amino acids are carried to the ribosome by transfer RNA (tRNA) . The genetic code instructions for making a protein are carried to the ribosome by messenger RNA (mRNA) from the DNA in the cell nucleus. At the ribosome, the tRNA recognizes the sequence of the genetic code on the mRNA and lines up the amino acids in the proper order. The ribosome catalyzes the formation of bonds between the amino acids.

https://micro.magnet.fsu.edu/cells/ribosomes/ribosomes.html

RNA: Ribonucleic acid. **Messenger RNA** (mRNA) is essentially a copy of a piece of one strand of DNA. Proteins are not made from the DNA of the gene. A template of RNA is made from the gene DNA. The RNA is then processed. The processing involves splicing of RNA. This spliced RNA, the template upon which the protein is made (protein synthesis), is called **messenger RNA** (mRNA). mRNA goes to the ribosome in the cell cytoplasm, where it meets the **transfer RNA** (tRNA) carrying the amino acids. Under the influence of **ribosomal RNA** (rRNA), the amino acids are bound together to form the protein (see **Ribosome**).

http://www.nature.com/scitable/definition/ribonucleic-acid-rna-45
https://jamanetwork.com/journals/jama/fullarticle/2712406?guestAccess
Key=22414c3e-162a-4ff0-8b50-5477ff58735b&utm_source=silverchair&utm_
campaign=jama_network&utm_content=weekly_highlights&cmp=1&utm_
medium=email https://www.nature.com/collections/hibdgeeijf?utm_
source=nature&utm_medium=tpe&utm_campaign=exrna-outlook&sap-outbound-
id=F54F4C2E18504F080DE

RNA EDITING: Making discrete changes to nucleotide sequences. (See **Nucleotide**) Can change proteins without making permanent changes to DNA.
https://www.google.com/search?q=rna+editing+definition&rlz=1C1CHBF_en
US821US821&sxsrf=ALeKk00BTRIVfqmQj4UbehB8M429Om-0aA:160459741631
7&tbm=isch&source=iu&ictx=1&fir=e1WL4n9BGtSUIM%252CCUK3YbinpbKiN
M%252C%252Fm%252F0855vy&vet=1&usg=   https://translational-medicine.
biomedcentral.com/articles/10.1186/s12967-019-2071-4 **https://www.nature.com/
articles/d41586-020-00272-5**

RNA INTERFERENCE: RNAi : Pathway that regulates gene expression
https://jamanetwork.com/journals/jama/fullarticle/2712406?guestAccessKey=2
2414c3e-162a-4ff0-8b50-5477ff58735b&utm_source=silverchair&utm_campaign=-
jama_network&utm_content=weekly_highlights&cmp=1&utm_medium=email
https://www.ncbi.nlm.nih.gov/probe/docs/techrnai/
https://www.nature.com/nrg/multimedia/rnai/animation/index.html
https://www.ncbi.nlm.nih.gov/pmc/articles/PMC5542916/
https://www.nature.com/articles/d41586-018-05867-7?WT.ec_id=NATURE-
20180816&utm_source=nature_etoc&utm_medium=email&utm_campaign=
20180816&spMailingID=57190125&spUserID=MjA1NjIyNjc4OAS2&spJobID=
1462154550&spReportId=MTQ2MjE1

ROBOTICS: A robot is a machine capable of automatically carrying out complex actions, programmable by computer.
https://jamanetwork.com/journals/jama/fullarticle/2712406?guestAccess

Key=22414c3e-162a-4ff0-8b50-5477ff58735b&utm_source=silverchair&utm_
campaign=jama_network&utm_content=weekly_highlights&cmp=1&utm_
medium=emailt

Robotic surgery is carried out via robotic telemanipulation. The surgeon's movements at a console are translated to surgical instruments previously placed into the patient by minimally invasive technique.
http://allaboutroboticsurgery.com/surgicalrobots.html

SARCOMA: A virulent form of malignant, solid tumor.
http://sarcomahelp.org/reviews/who-classification-sarcomas.html

SARS: **S**evere **a**cute **r**espiratory **s**yndrome. SARS-CoV caused by a corona virus. First traced to Asia 2002.
http://www.cdc.gov/sars/about/fs-sars.html
https://www.niaid.nih.gov/diseases-conditions/covid-19
https://www.frontiersin.org/articles/10.3389/fimmu.2020.01880/full?utm_source=
F-AAE&utm_medium=EMLF&utm_campaign=MRK_1417202_35_Immuno_202009

SCAR: Cicatrix. Connective tissue in which fibroblasts form granulation tissue. Older scars are composed of dense collagenous tissue.

SCURVY: Disease caused by lack of Vitamin C (ascorbic acid).
http://www.medicalnewstoday.com/articles/155758.php

SELF-DESTRUCT GENES: Genes that cause cell death (apoptosis).
http://www.nature.com/mt/journal/v23/n9/full/mt2015139a.html

SENOLYTICS: Drugs that kill **senescent**, non-dividing cells that accumulate in aging organs.
https://www.nature.com/news/to-stay-young-kill-zombie-cells-1.22872?WT.ec_
id=NEWS-20171026&spMailingID=55224149&spUserID=MTc2NjY4OTM5NgS2&s
http://www.cell.com/cell/fulltext/S0092-8674(17)30246-5
https://www.ncbi.nlm.nih.gov/pubmed/22048312
https://www.ncbi.nlm.nih.gov/labs/journals/j-am-geriatr-soc/new/2017-09-05/
http://onlinelibrary.wiley.com/wol1/doi/10.1111/jgs.14969/full

SENSITIVITY: (In medical testing) Probability that a test result will be positive when the disease is present.
https://www.medcalc.org/calc/diagnostic_test.php

SEPSIS: Systemic inflammatory response to infection.
http://www.ncbi.nlm.nih.gov/pmc/articles/PMC3684427/

Consensus Definitions for Sepsis and Septic Shock | Critical Care Medicine | JAMA | The JAMA Network

SERM: Specific estrogen receptor modulator. A class of drugs used during the menopause to prevent osteoporosis. Some drugs in this class are protective against the formation of breast cancer.
http://www.ncbi.nlm.nih.gov/pmc/articles/PMC3624793/

SEROTONIN: 5HT. 5-hydroxytryptamine. A monoamine neurotransmitter derived from tryptophan.
https://en.wikipedia.org/wiki/Serotonin

SEROTONIN/NOREPINEPHRINE REUPTAKE INHIBITORS: SNRI'S. Medications used in depression. See: The Care of the Older Person: An Overview of Late-Life Depression: Artin Mahdanian, Silvia Monti De Flores. RMC Publishing, LLC
www.careoftheolderperson.com
http://pharmacologycorner.com/serotonin-5ht-receptors-agonists-antagonist/ #serotonin%20agonists

SHBG: Sex hormone binding globulin. Protein elaborated in the liver that binds and transports testosterone, dihydrotestosterone (DHT), and estradiol as inactive forms in blood.
https://en.wikipedia.org/wiki/Sex_hormone-binding_globulin

SHINGLES: Delayed cutaneous manifestation by **Herpes Zoster** (Varicella: chicken pox) virus. Preventive vaccine available.
http://annals.org/aim/fullarticle/2671913/recommended-immunization-schedule-adults-aged-19-years-older-united-states
http://bmjopen.bmj.com/content/4/6/e004833

SIALOMUCIN: Mucopolysaccharide containing sialic acid. Component of lung airway secretion.
http://www.ncbi.nlm.nih.gov/gene/8763

SICKNESS (ILLNESS): Inability of individuals to pursue their goals and purposes because of impairments in function considered to be in the domain of medicine
Boudreau, JD, Cassell, EJ, Fuks, A: Physicianship and the Rebirth of Medical Education. Oxford University Press 2018

SIGNAL TRANSDUCTION (CELL SIGNALING): Transmission of molecular signals from cell surface receptors to the cell interior.
https://www.tocris.com/pharmacologicalBrowser.php?ItemId=187888#.V8hjh7ZTFwE

SINGLE CELL BIOLOGY: The study of the individual cell.
https://genomebiology.biomedcentral.com/articles/10.1186/s13059-016-0941-0
http://www.nature.com/news/single-cell-biology-1.22241
https://www.frontiersin.org/articles/10.3389/fimmu.2018.02425/full?utm_source=F-AAE&utm_medium=EMLF&utm_campaign=MRK_812127_35_Immuno_20181030_arts_A

SIRTUIN GENES: Genes that exert anti-aging effect in yeast. Increased sirtuin activity may be related to the mechanism by which caloric restriction extends life span.
https://www.ncbi.nlm.nih.gov/pubmed/18419308

SOMATIC CELL NUCLEAR TRANSFER: Therapeutic cloning. Nucleus is taken from an adult cell and placed into an ovum whose own nucleus has been removed. These embryonic stem cells are induced to form specialized cells needed by the adult from whom the adult cell nucleus was taken.
http://www.hhmi.org/biointeractive/somatic-cell-nuclear-transfer-animation

SPECIFICITY:(In medical testing) Probability that a test result will be negative when the disease is not present.
https://www.medcalc.org/calc/diagnostic_test.php

SPERMATOZOON: The male germ (sex) cell, derived from the testicle. It has a head, body and tail, and is motile. The spermatozoon swims up the female reproductive tract, eventually fertilizing (fusing with) the egg (ovum) in the

fallopian tube.
https://www.boundless.com/physiology/textbooks/boundless-anatomy-and-physiology-textbook/the-reproductive-system-27/physiology-of-the-male-reproductive-system-253/spermatogenesis-1234-9350/

SPINDLE NUCLEAR TRANSFER: Removal of the nuclear spindle from a maternal oocyte and transferring that spindle to a donor oocyte from which the spindle has been removed, in order to obviate a mitochondrial mutation. The donor oocyte containing the maternal nuclear spindle is then fertilized.
https://www.ncbi.nlm.nih.gov/pmc/articles/PMC4005382/
https://www.sciencenews.org/blog/science-ticker/first-%E2%80%98three-parent-baby%E2%80%99-born-nuclear-transfer

SPLICING: The reattaching of the two ends of a stringlike material, after a piece has been removed. In **GENE SPLICING,** DNA is cut and a gene inserted.
http://www.premierbiosoft.com/tech_notes/gene-splicing.html

SSRI: **S**elective **S**erotonin **R**euptake Inhibitor: Medications used in depression. Inhibit reuptake of serotonin, so increase serotonin activity. See: The Care of the Older Person: An Overview of Late-Life Depression; Artin Mahdanian, Silvia Monti De Flores. RMC Publishing, LLC www.careoftheolderperson.com
http://www.rxlist.com/the_comprehensive_list_of_antidepressants-page2/drugs-condition.htm#ssris https://www.ncbi.nlm.nih.gov/books/NBK554406/#:~:text=Mechanism%20of%20Action&text=As%20the%20name%20suggests%2C%20SSRIs,such%20as%20dopamine%20or%20norepinephrine.

STATINS: Drugs that reduce circulating LDL (low density lipoprotein) by encouraging the LDL receptor to increase uptake. Decreased production of LDL-C (low density lipoprotein cholesterol) results.
https://www.drugs.com/drug-class/hmg-coa-reductase-inhibitors.html

STEM CELL: An undifferentiated cell that has the potential to become a specialized cell with a specific function, such as a blood cell or a muscle cell.
http://stemcells.nih.gov/info/basics/1.htm
http://fhs.mcmaster.ca/main/news/news_2016/life_saving_blood_stem_cells.html

STEM CELL TRANSPLANT: Injection of stem cells into the body to replace damaged or diseased tissue, blood.

http://www.cancer.gov/about-cancer/treatment/types/stem-cell-transplant
http://journal.frontiersin.org/article/10.3389/fimmu.2016.00470/full

STENT: Self expanding tube placed in a blood vessel to keep that vessel patent. May be drug-eluting.
https://www.sciencedaily.com/releases/2015/03/150316135610.htm

STEREOTACTIC RADIOSURGERY: SRS. Precisely focused radiation to scar and close the blood vessels of an arteriovenous malformation (AVM) in the brain.
http://www.irsa.org/radiosurgery.html

STEREOTAXIS: Method in neurosurgery for locating points within the brain using an external three dimensional frame.

STRESS: Response to physical, mental or emotional pressure https://www.cancer.gov/publications/dictionaries/cancer-terms/def/stress

STROKE: Cerebrovascular accident. Damage to the brain by a blood clot in a vessel supplying the brain, or by hemorrhage into the brain.
http://www.neurology.org/content/early/2016/09/16/WNL.0000000000003238.abstract
http://www.empr.com/news/repatha-heart-attack-stroke-prevention-pcsk9-inhibitor/article/711332/?DCMP=EMC-MPR_DailyDose_cp_20171204&cpn=obgyn_all&hmSubId=&hmEmail=hIe6FnTBLUDNqAesd8d7sd9Sz-y1cfMN0&NID=1538223656&c_id=&dl=0&spMailingID=18599771&spUserID=MTgxMDk3OTQyMDM0S0&spJobID=1160335565&spReportId=MTE2MDMzNTU2NQS2
http://www.acc.org/latest-in-cardiology/ten-points-to-remember/2018/01/29/12/45/2018-guidelines-for-the-early-management-of-stroke hs://www.nature.com/articles/s41746-017-0015-z?utm_source=Springer_Nature_website&utm_medium=Website_links&utm_content=AngWan-SN-OD-Neuroscience-Global&utm_campaign=SNOR_USG_SFN18ttp

SUBUNIT: Ribosomal nucleic acid (rRNA) molecules (see "Ribosome")
http://www.microbe.net/simple-guides/fact-sheet-ribosomal-rna-rrna-the-details/

SUDDEN INFANT DEATH SYNDROME: SIDS, Unexplained death during sleep of a seemingly healthy baby.
http://emedicine.medscape.com/article/804412-overview

SUICIDE: Intentional, voluntary taking of own life. Contributory factor influencing average lifespan.
http://healthjournalism.org/blog/2014/04/exploring-risk-factors-rates-of-suicide-in-seniors/

SUPERAGER: Person 80 years or older with episodic memory ability at least as good as average middle-age adult. Significantly thicker brain cortex than same-age peers.
http://jamanetwork.com/journals/jama/article-abstract/2614177

T-LYMPHOCYTE: **T-Cell**. White blood cell that is immunologically competent. Responsible for cell-mediated immunity. Can attack surface antigens on malignant cells, if activated by prior presentation of the antigen.
https://en.wikipedia.org/wiki/T_cell
https://www.frontiersin.org/articles/10.3389/fimmu.2018.00233/full?utm_source=F-AAE&utm_medium=EMLF&utm_campaign=MRK_554072_35_Immuno_20180227_arts_A

TALENS: Transcription **A**ctivator-**L**ike **E**ffector **N**ucleases. Utilized to alter genes. See **Transcription, Nuclease.**
https://www.ncbi.nlm.nih.gov/pmc/articles/PMC3547402/

TARGETED AREA CORRECTION SEQUENCING: Detection of mutations and rearrangements indicative of cancer in cell-free plasma DNA.
https://www.ncbi.nlm.nih.gov/pmc/articles/PMC4755822/
http://journals.plos.org/plosgenetics/article?id=10.1371/journal.pgen.1005816
http://journals.plos.org/plosone/article?id=10.1371/journal.pone.0064271
http://journals.plos.org/plosgenetics/article?id=10.1371/journal.pgen.1005816

TARGETED THERAPY: Drug designed to reverse the effects of a specific mutation
http://www.ncbi.nlm.nih.gov/pubmed/23470539

TELOMERASE: Enzyme that maintains and repairs the telomere.
http://study.com/academy/lesson/what-is-telomerase-definition-function-structure.html

TELOMERE: The end of a chromosome. It is made up of DNA. The telomere gives stability to the end of the chromosome, preventing abnormal recombinations (mutations). The Care of the Older Person: Introduction: Jose Morais. RMC Publishing, LLC

www.careoftheolderperson.com
https://en.wikipedia.org/wiki/Telomere
https://link.springer.com/article/10.1007/s10815-017-0967-6/fulltext.html?wt_mc=alerts.TOCjournals

TEMPLATE: The pattern from which copies are made.
https://engineering.ucsb.edu/~shell/che170/DNA-notes.pdf

TESTIS: The male gonad.
http://emedicine.medscape.com/article/1949259-overview

TESTOSTERONE: The prominent androgen in the male. Male sex hormone. Present in lesser amounts in women.
http://www.livescience.com/38963-testosterone.html

THALLIUM STRESS TEST: Radioisotope uptake monitoring and myocardial perfusion assessment while patient is on a treadmill.
http://pubs.rsna.org/doi/full/10.1148/rg.317115090

THROMBOPHLEBITIS: Inflammation of the wall of a vein in conjunction with thrombosis.

THROMBOSIS: Blood clotting in a blood vessel.

THYMUS GLAND: Lymphoid gland of the immune system located in the neck that produces T-Cells.
http://biology.about.com/od/anatomy/ss/thymus.htm

TIA: Transient ischemic arteriospasm. Constriction of blood vessels in the brain with no permanent damage.

TISSUE ENGINEERING: Combining cells, scaffolds, and biologically active molecules to create new tissue.
https://www.nibib.nih.gov/science-education/science-topics/tissue-engineering-and-regenerative-medicine

TISSUE TYPING: Tissue antigens of prospective organ donor and recipient compared for histocompatibility. HLA (human leukocyte antigen) typing.
http://www.encyclopedia.com/topic/Tissue_Typing.aspx

TOTIPOTENTIALITY: Capability of a cell to differentiate into unlimited number of cell types.
http://medical-dictionary.thefreedictionary.com/totipotential+cell

TOXEMIA: The hypertensive disorders of pregnancy.

TPA: Tissue plasminogen activator. Protein involved in the breakdown of blood clots.
http://pharmacologycorner.com/thrombolytic-agents-mechanism-of-action-indications-contraindications-and-side-effects/
http://atvb.ahajournals.org/content/29/8/1151.full

TRABECULA: Supporting structures of connective tissue.

TRANSCRIPTION: Transfer of genetic code information between nucleic acids. The process by which the genetic code on the DNA gets into the mRNA template (see DNA, RNA).
http://www.vcbio.science.ru.nl/en/virtuallessons/cellcycle/trans/

TRANSCRIPTOME: Gene readouts (transcripts) of all the DNA in a cell by RNA
https://www.genome.gov/13014330/transcriptome-fact-sheet/

TRANSFORMATION ZONE: The outer cervix is lined by squamous cells, much like the vaginal lining. The inner canal of the cervix is lined by tall cylindrical cells. Where these two layers meet, there is an area of microscopic activity where the cylindrical columnar cells are being transformed, or over-ridden, by squamous cells. This is a benign process called **squamous metaplasia**. This area is called the transformation zone. It is in this area of cell activity that cancer of the cervix most commonly arises.

TRANSLATION: The process by which the genetic code of mRNA becomes proteins.
https://bioweb.uwlax.edu/GenWeb/Molecular/Theory/Translation/translation.htm

TRANSLATIONAL MEDICINE: Mechanisms by which new drugs and tests get from the laboratory into the hands of physicians for administration to patients, and the mechanisms for ensuring that patients get necessary services.
https://www.ncbi.nlm.nih.gov/pmc/articles/PMC2829707/
http://www.medscape.com/viewarticle/871305nlid=110427_2581&src=WNL_

mdplsnews_161104_mscpedit_
obgy&uac=66536PR&spon=16&impID=1228473&faf=1

TRANSPLANTATION: Transfer of organ or tissue from one individual to another.
http://www.ajog.org/article/0002-9378(70)90382-0/abstract?cc=y=
http://www.who.int/transplantation/organ/en/

TRIGEMINAL NERVE: The fifth cranial nerve.
http://emedicine.medscape.com/article/1873373-overview

TRIGLYCERIDE: Ester formed from glycerol and three molecules of fatty acids.
https://en.wikipedia.org/wiki/Triglyceride https://www.ncbi.nlm.nih.gov/
pmc/articles/PMC6376873/

TRIPTANS: Serotonin (5HT) receptor agonists. Medications that constrict blood
vessels in the brain and are used in the treatment of migraine.
http://archneur.jamanetwork.com/article.aspx?articleid=782346

TROPHOBLAST: Outer ring of cells around the blastocyst cavity that becomes the
placenta.
http://discovery.lifemapsc.com/in-vivo-development/trophoblast/trophoblast

TROPONINS: Proteins released when heart muscle is damaged. Can be detected
in blood circulation and be used to predict cardiovascular disease (CVD) risk.
https://www.ahajournals.org/doi/pdf/10.1161/CIRCULATIONAHA.118.038772

TUBERCULOSIS: Infectious disease especially affecting the lungs caused by
mycobacterium tuberculosis.
http://www.thelancet.com/journals/lanres/article/PIIS2213-
2600(15)00063-6/abstract

TUMOR: Abnormal growth. May be benign or malignant.

TUMOR GRADE: Appearance, abnormality of malignant tumor cells.
https://www.cancer.gov/about-cancer/diagnosis-staging/prognosis/tumor-
grade-fact-sheet

TUMOR INFILTRATING LYMPHOCYTE (TIL): Immune cell from a patient's
blood that has moved into a tumor to attack it. TIL's can be removed from the
tumor, activated, then given back to the patient.

https://www.cancer.gov/publications/dictionaries/cancer-terms/def/tumor-infiltrating-lymphocyte

TUMOR SPECIFIC ANTIGEN (TSA): Protein or other molecule produced in tumor cells that sets off an immune response in the host. Used as tumor markers to identify tumor cells in the body. Used in the immunologic treatment of cancer. Also, **Tumor Associated Antigens (TAA)** that are significantly more abundant in cancer cells than in other tissue. CEA Antigen, Prostate-Specific Antigen, CA125, CA19-9

https://www.researchgate.net/publication/9314460_Demonstration_of_Tumor-Specific_Antigens_in_Human_Colonic_Carcinomata_by_Immunological_Tolerance_and_Absorption_Techniques

https://www.researchgate.net/publication/12453745_Self_recognition_in_the_Ig_superfamily_Identification_of_precise_subdomains_in_carcinoembryonic_antigen_required_for_intercellular_adhesion

TUMOR STAGE: Extent of the malignant tumor: its size and spread.

https://www.cancer.gov/about-cancer/diagnosis-staging/staging

TUMOR SUPPRESSOR GENE (Antioncogene): Genes, such as the TP59 gene, that elaborate tumor suppressor proteins that control cell growth. Mutations (DNA changes) in these genes are associated with cancer. Tumor Protein 53 (TP53) that also has a role in germ cell survival, is another example.

https://www.cancer.gov/publications/dictionaries/cancer-terms?cdrid=46657

https://www.nature.com/articles/d41586-017-07291-9?WT.ec_id=NEWSDAILY-20171123&utm_source=briefing&utm_medium=email&utm_campaig

http://www.fertstert.org/article/S0015-0282(17)32096-4/fulltext?elsca1=etoc&elsca2=email&elsca3=0015-0282_201801_109_1_&elsca4=Obstetrics%20and%20Gyn

TURBINATES: Shelves of bone covered by thick mucous membrane that project into the nasal passages.

http://emedicine.medscape.com/article/874771-overview

UBIQUITIN-PROTEASOME SYSTEM : A protein clearance mechanism with implications in aging and age-related diseases

https://link.springer.com/article/10.1007/s10815-016-0842-x?wt_mc=alerts.TOCjournals

http://www.nature.com/ncomms/2014/141208/ncomms6659/fig_tab/ncomms6659_F1.html

ULTRASONOGRAPHY: Imaging by reflecting high energy "sound" waves off objects. The waves have higher frequency than sound that can be heard by humans. Four dimensional sonography refers to images being seen in real time.
https://www.ncbi.nlm.nih.gov/pubmed/20541656
http://medical-dictionary.thefreedictionary.com/ultrasonography

ULTRAVIOLET RAYS: UV. Short wavelength solar rays that are invisible to the human eye.
http://medical-dictionary.thefreedictionary.com/ultraviolet+rays

UMBILICAL CORD: The cord that connects the developing fetus to the placenta. Blood circulates in the cord via two arteries and one vein: the umbilical vein carrying nutrients and oxygen from the placenta to the fetus, and the umbilical arteries carrying waste products of metabolism and carbon dioxide away from the fetus, back to the placenta.
https://www.ncbi.nlm.nih.gov/books/NBK53254/

UMBILICAL CORD BLOOD: Fetal blood that circulates via the umbilical cord.
http://www.webmd.com/parenting/baby/features/banking-your-babys-cord-blood#1
http://journal.frontiersin.org/article/10.3389/fimmu.2017.00087/full?utm_source=newsletter&utm_medium=email&utm_campaign=Immunology-w6-2017
https://www.nature.com/nature/journal/vaop/ncurrent/full/nature22067.html

URETHRA: The passage from the urinary bladder to the vulva in the female, and to the penile meatus in the male.

URETHROCELE: Bulging of the urethra into the anterior vaginal wall.

URINARY INCONTINENCE: Involuntary loss of urine. Stress incontinence, urgency incontinence and neurogenic incontinence are types. See: The Care of the Older Person: Incontinence In Older Adults: Samer Shamout, Lysanne Campeau. RMC Publishing, LLC www.careoftheolderperson.com
http://jamanetwork.com/journals/jama/article-abstract/2595508

UTERUS: The womb. Its endometrial lining undergoes decidual change to receive the implanting fertilized egg (zygote). During labor, muscular rhythmic contractions of the uterine wall gradually send the fetus through the birth canal.

VACCINE: A killed or attenuated (variant) virus given by mouth or injection to activate the body's immune system against the actual dangerous virus. In the case of COVID-19, mRNA vaccines are being used. If a vaccinated person comes in contact with the actual virus, the person's activated immune system kills the virus before it can cause harm. Anticancer vaccines that target malignant cells are now being developed and are in use. The Care of the Older Person: Are the Immunizations of my patient up to date? Dominique Tessier. RMC Publishing, LLC www.careoftheolderperson.com
https://www.jci.org/articles/view/80009
http://journal.frontiersin.org/article/10.3389/fimmu.2017.00800/full?utm_source=F-AAE&utm_medium=EMLF&utm_campaign=MRK_333189_35_Immuno_20170720_arts_A tps://jamanetwork.com/journals/jama/fullarticle/2714651?guestAccessKey=1f4ca6ea-c69b-48ab-909f-713499b43cf8&utm_source=silverchair&utm_medium=email&utm_campaign=article_alert-jama&utm_content=etoc&utm_term=120518
https://jamanetwork.com/journals/jama/fullarticle/2714651?guestAccessKey=1f4ca6ea-c69b-48ab-909f-713499b43cf8&utm_source=silverchair&utm_medium=email&utm_campaign=article_alert-jama&utm_content=etoc&utm_term=1205181
https://jamanetwork.com/journals/jama/fullarticle/2770485?guestAccessKey=c95ea2e7-ea01-40d0-90fbe95cd2a1ba7e&utm_source=silverchair&utm_medium=email&utm_campaign=article_alert-jama&utm_content=olf&utm_term=090320
https://www.nap.edu/catalog/25917/framework-for-equitable-allocation-of-covid-19-vaccine https://www.nature.com/articles/d41586-020-02856-7?utm_source=Nature+Briefing&utm_campaign=7f2b123fc5-briefing-dy-20201014&utm_medium=email&utm_term=0_c9dfd39373-7f2b123fc5-42544483 https://www.ncbi.nlm.nih.gov/pmc/articles/PMC7218962/
https://www.cdc.gov/vaccines/covid-19/hcp/mrna-vaccine-basics.html#:~:text=mRNA%20vaccines%20take%20advantage%20of,virus%20that%20causes%20COVID%2D19.

VAGINA: The female genital tract extending inwards from the vulva. Closed at rest with the anterior wall resting on the posterior wall. Its muscular, elastic wall is lined by a mucous membrane that has a normal secretion. The cervix protrudes into the inner end, the vaginal vault.

VALUE-BASED MEDICAL CARE: Quality of care relative to its cost. Quality is assessed in the areas of outcomes, safety and service. Outcomes includes measurement of mortality rates, complications, and resultant functional status of patients. Safety includes attention to infection rates, accidental falls, and medication errors. Service assesses patient satisfaction, wait times, access to treatment and procedures, and affordability.
https://wire.ama-assn.org/education/value-based-care-elusive-concept-enters-curriculum?&utm_source=BHClistID&utm_medium=BulletinHealthCare&utm_term=120616&utm_content=MorningRounds&utm_campaign=BHCMessageID
http://jamanetwork.com/journals/jama/fullarticle/2594716

VARICOSE VEINS: Veins that bulge out due to damage to their valves.
http://emedicine.medscape.com/article/462579-treatment

VASOPRESSIN: Antidiuretic hormone (**ADH**). Formed in the hypothalamus and released from the posterior pituitary. Acts on renal collecting system, increasing water permeability and decreasing urine formation. Acts on vascular smooth muscle, causing vasoconstriction.
http://www.cvphysiology.com/Blood%20Pressure/BP016

VEGETATIVE SYMPTOMS: Disturbances of functions necessary to maintain life: See: The Care of the Older Person: An Overview of Late-Life Depression: Artin Mahdanian, Silvia Monti De Flores. RMC Publishing, LLC www.careoftheolderperson.com
https://en.wikipedia.org/wiki/Vegetative_symptoms

VEGF: Vascular Endothelial Growth Factor. Angiogenic factor that promotes growth in vascular endothelial cells. Has a role in tumor angiogenesis.
http://www.nature.com/nrc/journal/v8/n8/full/nrc2403.html
http://perspectivesinmedicine.cshlp.org/content/2/10/a006577.full

VEIN: A blood vessel that carries blood from the body towards the heart, usually transporting carbon dioxide and waste products of metabolism. Exceptions include the pulmonary vein, which carries oxygenated blood from the lungs to the heart for redistribution throughout the body, and the umbilical vein in the fetus, which carries oxygenated blood from the placenta to the fetal heart for redistribution throughout the fetal body.

VILLUS: A tiny projection from a surface.

VIRUS: An infecting agent so small that it cannot be seen under a light microscope. Viruses are made up of DNA or RNA. They can only replicate (divide) by invading into a host cell and causing that cell to manufacture more virus. http://www.ncbi.nlm.nih.gov/books/NBK21523/

VITAL ORGAN: Organ necessary for life, including the heart, lungs, brain, kidneys and liver.

VITAMIN: A substance that in small amounts is essential to metabolism, that naturally occurs in food. The Care of the Older Person: Could My Patient Be Malnourished?: Jose Morais. RMC Publishing, LLC www.careoftheolderperson.com http://annals.org/article.aspx?articleid=1767855

VULVA: The female external genitalia. Includes: labia majora, labia minora, clitoris, vestibule, urethral orifice, mons pubis.

WEST NILE VIRUS: A mosquito borne flavivirus that can cause encephalitis and meningitis.
http://www.cdc.gov/westnile/symptoms/

XENOBOT: Tiny robot constructed from living (frog} cells with the aid of Artificial Intelligence (AI)
https://www.smithsonianmag.com/innovation/scientists-assemble-frog-stem-cells-first-living-machines-180973947/

YAMANAKA FACTORS: Four genes that are important in cellular reprogramming to pluripotent stem cells.
https://www.ncbi.nlm.nih.gov/pubmed/19030024

ZIKA VIRUS: Mosquito borne. The fetuses of infected pregnant women have an increased incidence of microcephaly. There is an increased incidence of Guillain-Barre Syndrome with flaccid paralysis. Ref: Yale School of Medicine News, 08/26/2016
http://www.bloomberg.com/news/articles/2016-08-19/zika-may-cause-brain-damage-in-adults-too

http://www.contagionlive.com/news/zika-research-reveals-virus-may-
negatively-impact-adult-neural-stem-cells?utm_source=Informz&utm_medium=
Contagion+Live&utm_campaign=Contagion_Live_Trending_News_9-5-16
http://jamanetwork.com/journals/jama/fullarticle/2593701
https://www.mdlinx.com/obstetrics-gynecology/top-medical-news/
article/2017/01/02/3?utm_source=in-house&utm_medium=message&utm_
campaign=in-the-news-jan17

ZONA PELLUCIDA: The glycoprotein outer envelope of the ovum.
http://www.ncbi.nlm.nih.gov/pubmed/10497324

ZYGOTE: Fertilization (fusion of ovum and spermatozoon) results in a new
cell: the zygote, which has forty six chromosomes including either an X or Y
chromosome from the spermatozoon, and an X chromosome from the ovum.
The zygote is therefore either XX (female) or XY (male). The zygote develops to
a blastocyst stage with an inner cell mass that becomes the embryo, a fluid filled
blastocyst cavity, and an outer ring of cells around the blastocyst cavity called the
trophoblast, which becomes the placenta.
http://www.biology-online.org/dictionary/Zygote

BIBLIOGRAPHY & SUPPLEMENTAL BIBLIOGRAPHY

End of Each Chapter
The links under entries in the Glossary
And see **www.rcaplanmd.com**

www.ingramcontent.com/pod-product-compliance
Lightning Source LLC
Chambersburg PA
CBHW080042280326
41935CB00014B/1759